Bucci (Ed)

Glaucoma: Decision Making in Therapy

Springer
Berlin
Heidelberg
New York
Barcelona
Budapest
Hong Kong
London
Milano
Paris
Santa Clara
Singapore
Tokyo

M. G. Bucci (Ed)

Glaucoma: Decision Making in Therapy

Springer

Editor

Massimo G. Bucci
Eye Clinic
University of Rome "Tor Vergata"
C.I. Columbus
Via della Pineta Sacchetti, 506
00136 Rome

ISBN-13: 978-3-540-75021-5 e-ISBN-13: 978-88-470-2196-9
DOI: 10.1007/978-88-470-2196-9

Library of Congress Cataloging-in-Publication Data. Glaucoma: decision making in therapy (edited by) Massimo G. Bucci. p. cm. Based on the International Congress on Glaucoma held in Rome on 2-4 February 1996. Includes bibliographical references and index. ISBN 3-540-75021-5 1. Glaucoma-Treatment-Decision making-Congresses. I. Bucci, M. (Massimo) II. International Congress on Glaucoma (1996: Rome, Italy) [DNLM: 1. Glaucoma-diagnosis-congresses. 2. Glaucoma-therapy-congresses. WW 290 G550143 1997] RE871.G5454 1997 617.7'41-dc20 DNLM/DLC for Library of Congress 96-25619

Softcover reprint of the hardcover 1st edition 1996

Typesetting: Graphostudio, Milan

Preface

The volume reports lectures and discussions presented at the International Congress on Glaucoma, held in Rome on 2-4 February, 1996.

The Congress has been designed to clarify and possibly to define the fundamental steps for managing glaucoma patients.

"Decision making in therapy" does not mean that the conference sessions have been devoted to therapeutic problems only, even if semeiologic and diagnostic problems are pertinent when aimed at successful therapy.

Actually, it is necessary to distinguish the onset of glaucoma from ocular hypertension, to decide if and how to start treatment and the methods to assess its effectiveness, to understand if the failure of medical therapy justifies surgery and, above all, if intraocular pressure is, in any case, the most important risk factor to treat.

Particular relevance has been given to normal-pressure glaucoma, whose physiopathological and clinical characteristics are still highly controversial. Two round tables were devoted to the recent advances in the treatment of glaucoma, which aims at lowering intraocular pressure, directly improving the eye trophism and regenerating the areas damaged by the disease.

All ophthalmologists, particularly the younger ones, have had the opportunity to capitalize on the experience and knowledge of distinguished experts from different parts of the world.

This has been an invaluable and perhaps unique opportunity for all of us to express our doubts and to enhance our scientific background.

Glaucoma still represents one of the most frequent causes of blindness in the western countries. Therefore, it is imperative to allow all ophthalmologists to be continuously informed about the most recent advances on this severe disease.

Massimo G. Bucci

Preface

Contents

MEDICAL THERAPY

UP-DATING ON HYPOTENSIVE AND NON HYPOTENSIVE GLAUCOMA THERAPY

NORMAL TENSION GLAUCOMA

SURGICAL TREATMENT

UP-DATING ON HYPOTENSIVE AND NON HYPOTENSIVE GLAUCOMA THERAPY

Contributors

PHYSIOPATHOLOGY

Anatomic-Functional Aspects of Aqueous Humor Inflow

L. Scullica

Eye Clinic, Catholic University, Largo A. Gemelli 8, 00168 Roma, Italy

The production and outflow of the aqueous humor (AH) represents an important and certainly one of the most interesting aspects of ophthalmic physiology. The AH has, in fact, several functions including:

1. A hydrostatic function, as it determines the ocular pressure, which in turn affects optical function.
2. An optical function, as the AH maintains both the cornea's curvature and the refractive index of the corneal stroma. The AH has an index of refraction very close to that of the cornea and, since it is cell-free and has a low protein content it does not reflect or refract light.
3. A nutritional function for the cornea and the crystalline lens whose metabolic final products it draws off.
4. An immunological defense function, as a carrier of antibodies and drugs [1].

The quantity of AH which is in the eye varies between 250 and 300 μl, 50 of which are in the anterior chamber and 200-250 of which are in the posterior chamber. The AH's components are derived from the blood and therefore the AH is affected by the blood's chemical composition, with changes occurring based on nourishment, drugs, stress and time of day [2]. The AH even changes considerably according to the integrity of the hemato-ophthalmic barrier, which is related to the diameter of the intraocular vessels, to the pressure existing in these vessels and to the composition of the blood.

The composition of the AH and the relation amongst its different components are considerably different than those of the plasma from which the AH is derived, since in the normal AH the concentration of several substances is less than or exceeds the plasma concentration. The concentration of chlorides, lactates, sodium, uric acid, and above all ascorbates, whose concentration is almost 70 times greater than in the plasma, is greater in the AH. By contrast, iron, glucose, cholesterol, creatinine, calcium, bilirubin, triglycerides, and particularly total proteins (plasma concentration 6.2 g/dl) are lacking in the AH.

The difference in the concentration of substances in the AH vs the plasma made us abandon our original concept that the AH was a simple blood filtrate. Instead, it has been proposed a mechanism of AH secretion that operates together with a simple diffusion mechanism. This alternative concept was made possible due to our ability to analyze the AH of the posterior chamber.

We have seen that ascorbates and bicarbonates are present in the AH of the posterior chamber in a quantity greater than that found in the plasma. Thus, for these substances there had to be a mechanism of active transport of a secretory type.

The presence of certain enzymatic systems supports this hypotesis, for instance, carbonic anhydrase. This enzyme is responsible for the transport of bicarbonates into the AH. Inhibition of carbonic anhydrase reduces by 50% the formation of AH [3].

Several transport systems with pump functions have been located but are still poorly understood. Some of these systems transport substances into the AH while others remove noxidous substances. Substances concentrated in large quantities in the AH include ascorbates and different aminoacids which are also found in the lens where they are needed.

Similar to what occurs in the pigmented epithelium of the retina, the passage of water and metabolites into and out of the AH is probably mediated by the activity of ciliary and pigmented epithelium. This active system of transport predominates over ultrafiltration during normal conditions.

Replenishment of the AH takes place by continuous downflow through the corneoscleral trabeculate. The consequence is constant circulation from the site of production to the area of downflow and from the posterior to the anterior chamber through the pupillary foramen.

It has been known for more than 200 years that the ciliary body is the site of AH production. This finding was based on the presence of an iris bombé pupil seclusion and on the regular production of AH found in congenital aniridia, in spite of the absence of the iris.

The anterior area of the ciliary body can be divided into two parts: (1) the posterior, flat ciliary ring or pars plana ciliaris, and (2) the anterior pars plicata ciliaris, made out of approximately 70 radial plicae, the ciliary processes. These play a very important role in the production of AH.

Ciliary processes are made of vascular bundles surrounded by a stroma of loose connective tissue and covered by the ciliary epithelium, with the interposition of a basal thin layer, an anterior continuation of Bruch's membrane that divides the chorio capillary layer from the pigmented epithelium in the posterior part of the uvea. This basal thin layer, similar to Bruch's choroidal membrane, is divided into three strata: an elastic one outside, a cuticular one inside, and an intermediate one made out of loose connective tissue.

The angioarchitecture of the ciliary processes is very important to the production of AH and its regulation.

Vascularization of ciliary processes was first studied by Maggiore [4] and Kiss [5]. More recently, we have studied the ciliary processes in the rabbit's eye [6-9].

The vascular bundles come from ciliary arteries that originate from a large arterial circle of the iris which is formed by the long posterior ciliary arteries once they have pierced the ciliary muscle.

These vessels fray out in a system of capillaries whose caliber is much bigger than that of the capillaries of the iris. Indeed, ciliary capillaries look more like venules and are fenestrated as well.

The special connections found between the endothelia cells of the ciliary process capillaries are identical to the ones observed in the vessels of the choriocapillary layer and liver sinusoids and are typical of those segments of the vascular tree where there is a diffusion of substances.

Proteins and macromolecules which create a high osmotic pressure in the interstice, pass through these permeable vessels. The ciliary epithelium works actively in order to selectively bring ions and water to the posterior chamber and so it opposes this pressure.

Ciliary capillaries are drained by a vein, the marginal vein of the ciliary process, which, according to the circumstances, can either fray out in a second capillary system on the level of the orbiculus ciliaris, acting as a portal-type venous vessel, or meet directly in the system of vorticose veins [6, 8].

The two strata of cells that cover the basal thin layer from the inside are the homologues of the two original layers of the optic cup. The outside layer nearer to the capillaries is made up of pigmented cells, homologous to the cells of the pigmented epithelium of retina. The inner layer, which looks more superficial than the axial plane of the ciliary process, represents the continuation of the retina.

The pigmented cells are connected to the overhanging cells which form the ciliary epithelium by adhesion plates (desmosomes) and by very small finger-like expansions towards the basal part of the ciliary epithelium [10, 11]. In the anterior part of the ciliary process, cells are directly connected with the capillary wall and with the stromal cells, sending out a syncytium of extensions while in the posterior portion epithelium has a smooth surface [12, 13].

Ciliary epithelium is formed by cylindric cells which are taller in the posterior part of the ciliary body but flatten anteriorly. The association amongst these cells is not very tight and there are vesicular spaces and fissures. The intimate structure of the ciliary epithelial cells has been particularly studied in order to determine whether these cells exhibit a secretory activity. In fact, granules with specifically staining mitochondria, endoplasmic reticulum, and Golgi complex have been found using histological methods [14].

By electron microscopy, interdigitations of cellular membranes characteristic of a secretory activity have been shown in the cellular corpus and between cells [10, 15-19]. These invaginations and interdigitations of cellular membrane are also found where there is active fluid transport, e.g., in kidney tubules [20] and in ependymall cells of the corium plexus [21]. They are the site of an intense phosphatase alkaline activity, demonstrating significant metabolic activity connected with fluid transport [22].

After paracentesis of the anterior chamber, or after the disruption of the hemato-ophtalmic barrier, vacuoles were found in the cells of the ciliary epithelium. These vacuoles have been interpreted as the expression of an active transport mechanism [10, 13, 23].

Regarding the ciliary processes of the rabbit [24, 25] there is both an architectural aspect and an histochemical aspect to be considered.

At the anterior part, or head of the ciliary process, the zonular fibers do not insert and can thus be defined as the free part of the ciliary process. The posterior part includes the corpus of the ciliary process and zonular part.

Histochemically, the ciliary epithelium of the free part is generally formed by flat cells and normally does not react to Gomori's stain for the alkaline phosphatase, while the cells of the zonular part react in a characteristic way. Moreover, the wide capillaries which form the capillary system of the anterior part of ciliary process are always reactive to Gomori's stain, in contrast to what occurs in the zonular part [25, 26].

The innervation of the ciliary corpus is extremely rich and depends on the posterior long and short ciliary nerves that accompany the arteries. The nerves form a plexus in the ciliary muscle and around the vessels of the ciliary processes. The nerve plexus is especially rich between the two strata of the epithelium [27, 28]. Many sensitive nerve fibers, with club-shaped terminations, have been observed.

Under normal conditions, the participation of the iris in producing AH is very little, certainly less than 10% [29].

Unlike the capillaries of the ciliary processes, those of the iris have wider epithelial walls, a smaller diameter and are impermeable to circulating proteins and macromolecules.

The vessels of these processes are sensitive to histamine and respond by becoming permeable to circulating macromolecules. This response is found after paracentesis in dogs, cats, and rabbits but not in monkeys.

The pigmented epithelium has a specific myoepithelial function and forms the dilatator muscle of the iris, while the inner stratum, a continuation of the ciliary epithelium of the retina, is intensely pigmented.

Some experiments using peroxidases have shown that when this substance is injected into the vessels it spreads to the cells of the anterior stratum but is stopped by the cells of the posterior stratum, which are equipped with zonulae occludents similar to the corresponding ciliary cells. However, we still know very little about the participation of these elements in the formation of AH.

The anterior surface of the iris is limited by cells similar to those of the stroma, which are probably fibroblasts, since they lack a basal membrane or characteristics of endothelial cells. The anterior stromal sheet is crossed by fascicles of connective tissue fibers. Since these fibers are not continuous, free substances found in the stroma can diffuse into the anterior chamber without any obstacles.

AH production can be measured by means of fluorophotometry [30]. Using this method it was found that the production of AH is not constant. During the day, AH production in humans is approximately 3.8 μl/min while at night it is reduced to less than 1.5 μl min [31]. By contrast in the rabbit eye, the opposite is found, i.e., AH production is greater at night [33].

This rhythmical pattern of AH production is also maintained under conditions of constant darkness [34], as are other biorhythms. It must thus be considered as a true circadian rhythm ruled by the nervous system, truly autonomic through adrenergic control [35]. In fact, cervical ganglionectomy or decentralisation of cervical sympathetic ganglia reduces the increased nocturnal flux in rabbits. The same occurs after topical administration of timolol [36]. This adrenergic control seems to have an effect mainly on the β-receptors of ciliary epithelial cells but other receptors are probably also involved.

Epinephrine, administered intravenously or by topical instillation, causes an increase in AH flux in humans, especially during sleep, probably because epinephrine partly stimulates β adrenergic receptors. If these receptors are inhibited by timolol the systemic effect prevails [38].

According to Gharagozloo and Brubaker [39], at least two types of adrenergic receptors (ß and α) can be located in the cells of the ciliary epithelium: ß-receptors have a stimulating effect on adenylcyclase while α2 receptors have an inhibiting effect.

The activation of adenylcyclase causes an increase in the production of cyclic AMP and, as a consequence, protein phosphorylation and increased production of AH. The α2 receptors act in the opposite way. While ß receptors can be blocked by the action of timolol, reduced cyclic AMP production can also be caused by activation of α2 receptors, as happens after instillation of apraclonidine, an α2 receptor agonist.

Apraclonidine, however, has no additional effect if it is administered at the same time as timolol, while it causes a further reduction in AH production in eyes already treated with timolol and during sleep. This might be due to the existance of adrenergic receptors at sites other than the ciliary epithelium. Funk and Rohen [40] have demonstrated that the afferent arterioles of the ciliary corpus are specifically sensitive to adrenergic α1 agents.

Farenbach and colleagues [41] have also demonstrated that apraclonidine causes an intense vasoconstriction of the radial arterioles, which travel from the arterial ring of the iris to the ciliary processes. This adrenergic influence on the circulation of the ciliary processes was also emphasized in previous studies on the circulation of the rabbit ciliary body, where it was possible to demonstrate an angioarchitectonic disposition of the ciliary processes remarkably different from that found in response to vasokinetic drugs.

The above described mechanisms underlying AH production are physiological and follow a circardian rhythm determined by the adrenergic system. Under these conditions, AH is as clear as water as it has a low protein concentration. Its chemical composition, however, varies while passing from the ciliary body to the trabeculate, due to the continuous addition of components coming from the adjoining structures. In response to various extrinsic factors, all of the structures that block the indiscriminate passage or simple diffusion of plasma substances through the so-called hemato-ophthalmic barrier may be altered. Thus, proteins and cells can flow into the AH and modify its composition.

The hemato-ophthalmic barrier has two components: the first is epithelial and is located at the level of the nonpigmented cells of the ciliary processes and of the homologous cells of the iris, where the occluding zonules connecting the top of these cells oppose the passage of circulating macromolecules which diffuse, by a more or less controlled mechanism, from the open capillaries of the ciliary processes to the AH.

The second is located in the iris at the level of the endothelial cells of capillaries.

The lack of a barrier at anterior surface of the iris could also allow, in some circumstances, that some substances carried in the blood, pass the stroma of the ciliary processes or of the choroid and diffuse into the iris through its root, thereby moving into the AH of the anterior chamber [42].

Moreover, the regular flow of AH through the trabeculate is supported by a general pressure existing in the eye. When the ocular pressure is artificially lowered, the direction of the flux of the ocular fluids is reversed and a large quantity of plasma proteins enter the anterior chamber of the canal of Schlemm, which then fills with blood [42].

Not only an intact hemato-ophthalmic barrier, but also unidirectional flux of AH is necessary to maintain the contents of the anterior chamber clear. When the barrier is altered, for reasons decribed below, the circulating macromolecules which are normally blocked by the barrier, pass into the AH, whose composition becomes close to that of plasma.

This AH is also called plasmoid aqueous.

Following rupture of the hemato-ophthalmic barrier, substances diffuse more easily into the AH and in inverse proportion to their molecular weight, their solubility in lipids, their dimension and their degree of dissociation. Rupture of the blood-aqueous barrier may be due to the following reasons: (1) traumatic; (2) nervous; (3) immunogenetic; (4) endogenous; (5) exogenous; (6) radiant.

Traumas are the most frequent cause of the rupture and include paracentesis of the anterior chamber, accidents, surgical trauma to the iris or the lens, and contusion.

A nervous rupture can occur because of the stimulation of the trigeminal nerve, while rupture of the barrier for immunogenetic reasons occurs in uveitis or following experimental administration of bovine serum albumin.

Amongst the endogenous reasons for the hemato-ophthalmic barrier rupture we remember histamine, bradykinin, prostaglandins and arachidonic acid, serotonin, and acetylcholine. Exogenous agents that induce rupture include chemical, acid, or basic burns, formaldehyde, and azotized mustard. Finally, ionic radiation, infrared radiation, ultraviolet radiation, and microwaves can all damage the blood-aqueous barrier.

Nonetheless, mechanism by which rupture occurs and the site where it takes place are not al-ways the same, as we have demonstrated [43, 44].

In rabbits, paracentesis of the anterior chamber leads to stagnation at the level of the head of the ciliary processes, with a subsequent drop in the venous pressure of the choroid and consequently of the vorticose vein to which the dorsal veins, that drain blood into the ciliary processes, are directly or indirectly connected.

The same thing does not happen following stimulation of trigeminal nerve [44].

In animals stimulated mechanically in the first branch of the trigeminal, we obtain initially a myosis with congestion of the iris and hypertonia.

An angiographic study in these conditions, using a solution of ink or neoprene latex, shows edema and stagnation at the base of the ciliary corpus and in the iris, associated with areas of cilioiridial nonperfusion.

The instillation of 2% formaldehyde in the conjunctival sac causes a similar condition, with edema and evidence of poor circulation in the lower part of the ciliary corpus and in the iris.

The prior administration of aspirin does not modify the circulatory effects produced by formaldehyde but does modify the circulatory effects of paracentesis, reducing stagnation at the head of the ciliary processes and causing ischemia mainly of the iris.

As aspirin interferes with prostaglandins, starting from arachidonic acid, it was thought that rupture of the hemato-ophthalmic barrier by formaldehyde does not involve release of prostaglandins, because the circulatory effects remain the same.

Instead, regarding paracentesis, the hemodynamic situation is modified probably because the administration of aspirin disturbs the balance between prostaglandins and catecholamines, with the latter prevailing and thereby enhancing vasoconstriction of the vessels of the iris [44, 45].

The changing of the proteic composition of the aqueous humor is in any case not dependent on the modifications of flux of A.H. [46].

References

1. Scullica L (1986)La dinamica dell'acqueo, concetti attuali sulla produzione e il deflusso dell'umore acqueo. Boll D'Oculist 65 Suppl 2:47-64
2. Moses RA (1970) Adler's Physiology of the eye; clinical applications. The CV Moses Co, Saint Louis
3. Becker B (1959) Basic carbonic anhidrase and the formation of aqueous humor. Amer J Ophthalmol 47:342
4. Maggiore L (1924) Su alcune particolarità del comportamento dei vasi sanguigni del segmento anteriore dell'uvea con particolare ri-guardo alla vascolarizzazione del muscolo ci-liare ed ai rapporti tra la circolazione endo ed extra-bulbare. Tipografia delle Scienze, Roma
5. Kiss F (1949) A szem vérkeringese. Szemeszt 1:1
6. Scullica L (1957) Studi sulla angiotettonica della "tunica vasculosa bulbi" (Ricerche Lepus Cuniculus). Biologica Latina, 10 Suppl VI
7. Scullica L (1958) Modificazioni morfologiche della rete vascolare dei processi ciliari dell'orbicolo ciliare consecutive al trattamento con farmaci vasocostrittori e vasodilatatori. Gior It di Oftalmologia 11:252
8. Scullica L (1962) Observation of uveal blood flow pattern in excised arterially perfused rabbit eyes. Amer J Ophthalm 54:1057
9. Scullica L (1979) The uveal vascular system: its importance and involvement with anterior chamber opening. Docum Ophthal Proc Series, Dr Junk bv Publishers, The Hague, Boston-London 21:311
10. Pappas GD, Smelser GK (1958) Studies on the ciliary epithelium and the zonule. I Electronic microscope observations on changes induced by alteration of normal aqueous humor formation in the rabbit. Amer J Ophthalm 46 II: 299
11. Bairati A Jr, Orzalesi N (1966) The ultrastructure of the epithelium of the ciliary body study of the function complexes and of changes

associated with the production of plasmoid aqueous humor. Zeitschr f Zellf 69:635-658
12. Rohen vJ (1957) Ueber zwei morphologische und funktionelle verschiedene Abschnitte des Zillarkorpers. Ophthalmologica 133:103
13. Santoro A, Scullica L (1960) Appunti sull'ultrastruttura del segmento anteriore dei processi ciliari del coniglio albino. Boll Soc It Biol Sper 36:396
14. Duke-Elder S (1961) System of Ophthalmology Vol.II Henry Kimpton, London
15. Holmberg A (1957) Ultrastructural changes in the ciliary epithelium following inhibition secretion of aqueous. Thesis. Stockolm
16. Holmberg A (1959) Some characteristic components of the ciliary epithelium. Amer J Ophthalm. 48:426
17. Pease D (1956) Infolded basal plasma membrane found in epithelia noted for their water transport. J Biophys Biochem Cytol Suppl 2: 203
18. Pappas GD, Smelser GK, Brandt PW (1959) Studies on the ciliary epithelium and the zonule. Arch Ophthalm 62:959
19. Brini M, Porte L (1959) Bull Soc Franç Ophtal 72:56
20. Rhodin J (1954) Correlation of ultrastructural organization and function in normal and experimentally changed proximal convoluted tubule cells of the mouse kidney. Stockholm
21. Maxwell DS, Pease DC (1956) The electron microscopy of the choroid plexus. Biophys and Biochem Cytol 2:467
22. Fumagalli Z, Scullica L (1959) A proposito di particolari rapporti tra le cellule dell'epitelio ciliare. Biologica Latina 12:865
23. Carlini V (1910) Die veranderungen des iris - und ciliarepithels nach punktion der vorderkammer. Graefe's Arch Ophthal 77:96
24. Scullica L (1959) Osservazioni sulla minuta struttura dei processi ciliari del coniglio. Mon Zool It 67, Suppl
25. Scullica L (1959) Ricerche istochimiche sulla attivita fosfomonoesterasica alcalina dei processi ciliari del coniglio. Boll d'Ocul 1959 38: 889
26. Scullica L (1960) Ricerche istochimiche sul comportamento della attivita fosfatasica alcalina dei processi ciliari del coniglio albino in diverse condizioni sperimentali. Ann di Oftalmologia e Clinica Ocul 86:341
27. Yamada E (1988) Intraepithelial nerve fibers in the rabbit ocular ciliary epithelium. Arch Histol Cytol 51:43
28. Yamada E (1989) Further observations on the intraepithelial nerve fibers of rabbit ciliar epithelium. Arch Histol Cytol 52:1991
29. Bill A (1977) Basic physiology of the drainage of aqueous humor. Exp Eye Res Suppl 25:291,
30. McLaren JW, Brubaker RFA (1988) Scanning ocular fluotophotometer. Invest Ophthalm and Vis Sci 1988 29:1285-1293
31. Sheridan PT, Brubaker RF, Larsson LI, Retting ES, Young F Jr (1994) The effect of oral dexamethasone on the circadian rhythm of aqueous humor flow in humans. Invest Ophthal-mol Vis Sci 35:1150-1156
32. Anjou Cin (1961) Influence of light on the 24-hour variation in aqueous flare density and intraocular pressure in normal rabbits' eyes. Acta Ophthalmol (Copenh.) 39:852
33. Smith SD, Gregory DSA (1992) Circadian rhythm of aqueous flow underlies the circadian rhythm of IOP in NZW rabbit. Invest Ophthal-mol Vis Sci 30:339
34. Gregory DS, Aviado DG, Sears ML (1985) Cervical ganglionectomy alters the circadian rhythm of intraocular in New Zeland white rabbits. Curr Eye Res 4:1273
35. Ericson LA (1958) Twenty-four hourly variations of the aqueous flow. Arch Ophthalmol 36:1-95 (Suppl 50)
36. Yoshitomi T, Gregory DS (1991) Ocular adrenergic nerves contribute to control of the circadian rhythm of aqueous flow in rabbits. Invest Ophthalmol Vis Sci 32:52-528
37. Kacere RD, Dolan JW, Brubaker RF (1992) Intravenous epinephrine stimulates aqueous formation in the human eye. Invest Ophthalmol Vis Sci 33:2861-2865
38. Retting ES, Larsson LI, Brubaker RF (1994) The effect of topical timolol on epinephrine stimulated aqueous humor flow in sleeping humans. Invest Ophthalmol Vis Sci 35:554-559
39. Gharagozloo NZ, Brubaker RF (1991) Effect of apraclonidine in long-term timolol users. Opthalmology 98:1543-1546
40. Funk, Rohen JW (1990) ARVO. Quoted by [39]
41. Farenbach (1990) ARVO. Quoted by [39]
42. Raviola G (1977) The structural basis of the blood-aqueous barriers. Exp Eye Res Suppl 25:27-63
43. Scullica L, Romeo G, Candela E (1975) Effetti sul corpo ciliare della paracentesi della camera anteriore. Atti LVI Congr Soc Oftalm It, Roma; p 210
44. Scullica L, Bisantis C, Romeo G, Candela E (1976) Circolazione del corpo ciliare e rottura della barriera ematoftalmica. Atti LVII Congr Soc Oftalm Ital, Firenze, p 305
45. Scullica L, Bisantis C, Romeo G, Candela E (1978) The circulation in the ciliary processes and effect of rupturing of ophthalmic barrier. 5th Congress European Society Opthalmology, Hamburg 1976. Ferdinand Enke Verlag, Stuttgart
46. Murray DL, Bartels S (1993) The relationship between aqueous humor flow and anterior chamber protein concentration in rabbits. Invest Ophthalmol Vis Sci 34:370-376

Intraocular Pressure as a Risk Factor in Glaucoma

B. Boles Carenini and B. Brogliatti

Eye Clinic of the University of Turin, Via Juvarra 19, 10122 Turin, Italy

Over the years, there have been several definitions of glaucoma in the literature. These include:

"Glaucoma is an eye disease in which the complete clinical picture is characterized by ***increased intraocular pressure***, excavation and degeneration of the optic disc, and typical nerve fibre bundle damage, producing defects in the field of vision" [1].

"The glaucomas are now best defined as a related group of clinical syndromes characterized by damage to the optic nerve and loss of visual function obeying a characterized pattern usually ***associated with a statistically defined elevated intraocular pressure***" [2].

"Glaucoma means a condition in which the optic nerve is damaged by ***intraocular pressure higher*** than the eye can tolerate" [3].

And yet, again, a more complex definition describes glaucoma as "a quite composite ocular condition whose essentialities are aqueous circulation disorders which are ***translated into intraocular pressure values usually higher than normal*** and which, of their own accord, or facilitated by other factors, induce around the optic disc nerve fibre degenerative phenomena causing mainly perimetric sensory deficits" [4].

Every one of these definitions points to hypertension as the primary cause in the genesis of the functional damage. Opinions differ as to what mechanism hypertension uses to induce the injury and death of the sensory elements.

There is a school of thought which considers the characteristic glaucomatous damage a direct consequence of ocular hypertension (***mechanical hypothesis***). This theory states that the ocular hypertension induced by diminished aqueous humour outflow causes direct damage to the papillary nerve fibres and the pathogenetic mechanism is a progressive, initially reversible, modification of the lamina cribrosa (a structural modification with changes of pore size and collagen characteristics) which later impedes both orthograde and retrograde axoplasmatic flow with resulting damage to the implicated ganglion cell body.

Other investigators say that the mechanism of damage is duplex (***mechano-vascular hypothesis***). The ocular hypertension causes compression of the small vessels of the laminar and prelaminar portion of the optic nerve head and of the choroidal small vessels from which they originate. Because of an insufficient self-regulatory mechanism, blood flow decreases, with a resulting level of ischaemia that produces injury and final destruction of the nervous tissue.

Whatever the pathogenetic mechanism is that causes the damage (direct action on the fibres or through prior action on the vessels), the "first cause" in both hypotheses is aqueous dynamic decompensation leading to intraocular hypertension.

And for some forms of glaucoma, including malformative glaucomas, closed-angle glaucomas, many secondary glaucomas, some iatrogenic glaucomas, and experimental glaucomas, there seems to be no reasonable doubt about the fundamental cause-and-effect relationship between ocular hypertension and functional anatomic damage.

In particular, models of experimentally induced glaucoma in monkey [5], by laser damage to the trabecular meshwork with resulting outflow facility reduction and a parallel increase in intraocular pressure, clearly show that glaucomatous damage, like the natural disease in humans, can be caused entirely by the mechanical compression due to ocular hypertension through either orthograde or retrograde axonal flow blockage.

Similar results were produced by Quigley and Addicks [6], who caused intraocular pressure (IOP) elevation in primate eyes by anterior chamber injections of autologous fixed red blood cells. Transport of axonal material was blocked at the scleral lamina cribrosa by IOP elevations up to 50 mm Hg. In those eyes with an elevated IOP for longer than 1 week, the loss of anterior disk nerve fibres combined with posterior and lateral movements of the lamina cribrosa led to an increase in optic disk cupping.

All the same, studies in humans also have shown that provoked transitory increases of IOP produce posterior optic disk cupping, which regresses when the pressure returns to normal. The electronic microscope has also been used to demonstrate that early damage of the nerve fibres in human glaucomatous eyes is in the laminar region of the nerve, where clear signs of axoplasmatic blockage can be seen. That the damage is of mechanical origin is indicated by the fact that no selective capillary loss has been observed there [7, 8].

Other recent studies have shown that occlusion of a large part of the choroidal ducts (observed histologically in glaucomatous eye choroids) induces a pressure gradient increase in the remaining pervious ducts, which become dilated and thus increase choroid thickness. Since the choroid is situated inside a semirigid structure, the sclero-corneal tunic, its volume increase causes a secondary IOP increase [9]. This theory might be called ***vasculo-mechanical***, since its pathogenetic "first cause" is vascular, which is then translated into a hypertension, the chief factor in the subsequent damage.

Nonetheless, clinical observations have demostrated special situations such as:

1. Some subjects seem to support pressure levels above the statistical norm for a long time with no sign of damage.
2. Some subjects develop serious glaucomatous damage with only modest hypertension.
3. Some subjects present damage of a frankly glaucomatous type without altered pressure values (normal pressure or low critical pressure glaucoma).

These observations have led other authors to propound a ***purely vascular*** theory according to which open-angle glaucoma would be a disease independent of ocular pressure and the glaucomatous damage would be caused by an earlier ischaemic compression of the optic nerve, due to presumed microvascular alterations of the optic disc. After this, there would be a release of unknown stimuli capable of producing ocular hypertension. This would, therefore, be a symptom, and not the cause of the glaucomatous damage [10].

If we take each of the clinical observations set out above point by point, certain considerations emerge.

First, some subjects live with pressure levels above the statistical mean without showing signs of damage. This is, as far as we can find in the literature, a possibility unattested by follow-ups long enough to sufficiently confirm it [11-14].

In fact, it is well-known that the glaucomatous disease has such a slow course that, so it has been calculated, 7 to 10 years are required for the first signs of damage to be ophthalmoscopically apparent.

Furthermore, the time of disease appearance is certainly influenced by factors such as the subject's age, refraction, and state of health; that is, by all the commonly denominated risk factors [15-20].

Observation of a 40-50 year-old patient with altered IOP values but no evident signs of anatomo-functional damage cannot permit us to assert that this subject is not affected by glaucoma, because our methods of evaluation might not be sensitive enough to detect very early damage. We must remember that, until recently, glaucoma diagnosis was closely linked to demonstration of perimetric and ophthalmoscopic damage, while today diagnosis is possible much earlier by means of accurate study of the retinal nerve fibre aspect [21, 22] and electrophysiological demonstration of ganglion cell damage [23-26].

Second, as to the possibility that some subjects develop serious glaucomatous damage in the presence of moderate hypertension, it is first necessary to standardize what is meant by "normal intraocular pressure" or "moderate hypertension".

In the normal population the mean IOP is 15.4 mm Hg (s.d. 2.5) when measured in the sitting position and 16.5 mm Hg (s.d. 2.8) when measured in the lying position.

These results agree with those obtained at our clinic: in a study carried out on 250 eyes of undoubtedly non-glaucomatous subjects, IOP was measured with the no-contact Keeler tonometer, with which measurements can be made in both positions. We found a mean IOP of 14.1 mm Hg (s.d. 1.8) in the sitting position and 15.3 mm Hg (s.d. 1.8) in the lying position.

However, IOP varies with age and, therefore, a pressure value found in an elderly subject means something different than when the same value is found in a young subject, especially if myopia is present.

Moreover, it is certain that IOP, like other physiological parameters, is subject to circadian variation, with the result that an IOP value measured only once in 24 h is not sufficiently probative [27-32].

The literature data suggest that a normal eye's mean circadian variation is 6.5 mm Hg (s.d. 1.4), while that of a simple hypertensive eye is 8.1 mm Hg (s.d. 2.5). Still more irregular, and dependent also on the basal pressure value, is the circadian variation of a pharmacologically untreated glaucomatous eye, i.e., between 5.8 and 18.4 mm Hg [33]. Table 1 lists the mean values of circadian variations in untreated glaucomatous eyes, as found by various authors. These variations would be more pronounced in eyes with accelerated anatomo-functional damage [41, 42].

Tonographic studies by Stepanik [43] and Boles Carenini [34] have confirmed the importance of outflow resistance, the variations of which can be correlated with the typical daily IOP fluctuations. This provides further evidence of parallelism between IOP circadian rhythm and systemic venous pressure (SVP) circadian variations. In open-angle glaucoma, the SVP is higher in the morning hours, when pressure spikes are more frequent, as compared with normal subjects' values. Indispensable, therefore, are accurate tonometric curves including at least four readings within 24 h to expose the presence and amount of fluctuations. In fact, an eye with an IOP of 18 mm Hg at 10 a.m. can, on the basis of circadian mean variation and according to the data cited above, if normal, achieve a pressure of 24.5 mm Hg; if "simple ocular hypertensive," of 26.0 mm Hg; and, if untreated glaucomatous, of 36.0 mm Hg. It seems difficult, confronted with these figures, to be able to assert that one is dealing with a moderate hypertension.

Table 1. Mean range of circadian intraocular pressure variations in glaucomatous eyes not receiving therapy

Author	Number of eyes	Mean ±SD(mmHg)	Reference
Boles Carenini[34] (1955)	38	7.2±4.5	[34]
Drance[29] (1960)	138	11.0±5.7	[29]
Katavisto[35] (1964)	329	11.3±4.2	[35]
Kitazawa[33] (1975)	27	5.8±8.8	[33]
Worthen[30] (1975)	14	18.4 ±8.4	[30]
Greenidge[36] (1983)	32	10.2±4.7	[36]
Dannheim[37] (1976)	10	10.6±6.3	[37]
Merrit[[38](1979)	20	8.6±3.7	[38]
Smith[39] (1985)	800	5.8 ±3.0	[39]
Yamagami[40] (1993)	228	4.8±1.8	[40]

Studies reported in the literature indicate a difference in the circadian tonometric curves of open-angle and angle-closure glaucoma: in the former, the spikes are diurnal and, for the most part, matutinal [34, 44-46], while in the latter, they are nocturnal [44].

Nonetheless, based on these data we cannot limit our investigations to only the mornings, since, according to Zeimer [32], the probability of finding the daily maximum spike in the morning is no greater than 40% to 50%, because there does not exist a "type curve" for the glaucomatous subject.

Circadian IOP curves can be classified into two major groups: [1] ***regular***, with pressure spikes occurring always in the same time intervals; [2] ***irregular***, with pressure spikes occurring randomly throughout the day on different study days.

Regular curves, in turn, can be subdivided into five categories [35]: (1) morning type (17%); (2) day type (50%); (3) night type (11%); (4) flat type (9%); and (5) varying type (12%).

The first two types figure the most in terms of percentage.

Bito [47] claims there are at least three types of IOP elevation, sometimes even coexisting in the same patient. These are:

1. Maintained ocular hypertension, in which IOP is sufficiently high around the clock to cause optic nerve damage, at least when blood pressure declines.
2. Episodic ocular hypertension, which involves an exaggerated circadian hypertensive

phase, or IOP elevated above the circadian baseline for a few minutes or a few hours, possibly in association with an activity, a physiological state, or a behaviour pattern.
3. IOP spiking, in which sharp IOP increases, lasting for a few seconds or minutes, are even more likely than episodic ocular hypertension to be behaviour-related.

Some patients may, of course, exhibit more than one of these patterns, such as IOP spikes superimposed on episodic ocular hypertension.

Everything said so far can be used to challenge those who hold that there are subjects with serious glaucomatous damage without altered pressure values. It seems to us indisputable to maintain that, before being able to label someone with certainty as "ocular hypertensive" and another as having "low critical pressure" glaucoma, a serious, accurate and protracted study of their ocular pressure behaviours is necessary, avail being taken of opportune provocative tests.

It is evident, therefore, that measuring and interpreting tonometric data remain problematic, and that the solution will come when technology provides us with the means to constantly monitor each patient's IOP. It is our firm belief that the number of ocular hypertensives and of patients affected by glaucoma without hypertension will then plummet.

As far as ocular hypertensives are concerned, the number of cases will probably be reduced to the few that fall to the right of 21 mm Hg on the gaussian pressure curve and the percentage prevalence of ocular hypertension (6%-8%) with respect to primary open-angle glaucoma POAG (0.5%-2%), as indicated by some [48], will change considerably in favour of a POAG increase.

Also, regarding subjects with low critical pressure glaucoma, their number will be reduced, since it will be shown in many of them that the IOP normality is only apparent. Instead, it will be possible to show that, in the course of the day, these individuals have pressure spikes, misconstrued, but responsible for the anatomo-functional damage. We should like to describe a recent case. In this patient, the tension curve values never exceeded 13-15 mm Hg, but a cupped disc and typical perimetric deficits were noted. In different provocation tests, the IOP reached values around 36.0 mm Hg only after the water-drinking plus dark test was applied.

Another problem is that of how vulnerable each eye is. The same tensional values can act as pathogenic "noxae" differently in eyes which are structurally different as regards their sensitivity to pressure stress. Even tensional values within the statistical norm can be injurious when clinical sensitivity is greater than normal. It would, therefore, be immensely useful, particularly for therapeutic purposes, to have a method capable of indicating each person's critical IOP value, above which there is anatomo-functional damage. However, even if we were able to know the critical IOP value for each individual eye (and even if this value were below the statistical mean), IOP would still play a fundamental role in the pathogenesis of glaucoma. The relationship between elevated IOP and optic nerve damage in POAG fulfillis Koch's postulates, which state that: (1) the causative agent is always present when the disease is present; (2) administration of the causative agent can bring on the disease; and (3) elimination of the causative agent eliminates the disease.

To conclude, we would like to emphasize that the term glaucoma should be used to describe a condition due to a tensional imbalance caused by an alteration in the aqueous dynamics. In particular, in chronic simple glaucoma, the course is: (1) Trabecular meshwork modification, due perhaps to structural differences of the trabecular collagen (Grehn, personal comm.) [49-52], forms an obstacle to aqueous outflow from which hypertension arises. (2) The increased IOP acts at the point of least resistance of the bulbar wall, i.e., on the lamina cribrosa of the optic disc, which by measuring collagen VI has been shown to be appreciably different from that of the non-glaucomatous eye. (3) The caving-in of the lamina cribrosa, through the action on the optic nerve fibres and because of the action on the vessels which leave the optic nerve head, leads to glaucomatous damage.

Thus, IOP ought not to be considered as a risk factor, but as the true and proper cause of glaucoma, whose initiation may be facilitated by various risk factors, even those of a vascular nature (general vascular condition, altered hamorrheology, lack of autoregulation, etc.) which, by themselves, without hypertension, cannot give rise to glaucoma. Hence, we affirm, along with Duke-Elder [53] that: "Changes within the nerve head without a raised ocular tension and without a reduced coefficient of aqueous outflow, should not be considered as due to glaucoma but to ischaemic vascular disease."

References

1. Kolker AE, Hetherington J Jr (1970) In: Becker-Shaffer's diagnosis and therapy of the glaucomas. Mosby, St. Louis, p 206
2. Hart WM Jr. (1989) In: Ritch R, Shields MB, Krupin T (eds): The glaucomas. Mosby, St. Louis, p 789
3. Spaeth GL (1993) Development of glaucomatous changes of the optic nerve. In: Varma R, Spaeth GL, Parker KW (eds) The optic nerve in glaucoma. JB Lippincott, Philadelphia, p 63
4. Miglior M, Bagolini B, Boles Carenini B, Orzalesi N, Scullica L, Zingiriam M, Monduzzi M (ed) (1989) Oftalmologia clinica. Monduzzi, Bologna, p 408
5. Gaasterland DE, Kupfer C (1974) Experimental glaucoma in the rhesus monkey. Invest Ophthalmol Vis Sci 13: 455-457
6. Quigley HA, Addicks LM (1980) Chronic experimental glaucoma in the primates II. Effects of the extended intraocular pressure elevation on optic nerve head and axonal transport. Invest Ophthalmol Vis Sci 19:137-152
7. Quigley HA, Addicks EM, Green WR, Maumenee QE (1981) Optic nerve damage in human glaucoma. Arch Ophthalmol 99:635-649
8. Quigley HA, Hohman RM, Addicks EM, Green WR (1984) Blood vessels of the glaucomatous optic disk in experimental primate and human eyes. Invest Ophthalmol Vis Sci 25:918-931
9. Cristini G, Cennamo G (1991) Presumibile azione vasogenica dell'ipertensione oculare nel glaucoma primario. Min Oftalmol 33:201-203
10. Krakau CET (1981) Intraocular pressure elevation – cause or effect in chronic glaucoma? Ophthalmologica 182, 141-147
11. Bonomi L (1991) Possibili fattori di vulnerabilità del nervo ottico nel glaucoma. Min Oftalmol 33:183-190
12. Kitazawa Y, Harie T, Aoki S, et al. (1977) Untreated ocular hypertension. Arch Ophthalmol 95:-1180-1184
13. Bengtsson B (1981) Aspects of the epidemiology of chronic glaucoma. Acta Ophth [suppl] 146:1-64
14. Jampol LM, Board RJ, Maumenee AE (1978) Systemic hypotension and glaucomatous changes. Am J Ophthalmol 85:154-159
15. Bankes JL, Perkins ES, Tsolakis S, Wright JE (1968) Bedford glaucoma survey. Br Med J 1:791-796
16. Hollows FC, Graham PA (1966) Intraocular pressure, glaucoma, and glaucoma suspects in a defined population. Br J Ophthalmol 50:570-586
17. Leibowitz HM, Krueger DE, Maunder LR, et al. (1980) The Framingham Eye Study monograph: an ophthalmological and epidemiological study of cataract, glaucoma, diabetic retinopathy, macular degeneration, and visual acuity in a general population of 2631 adults, 1973-1975. Surv Ophthalmol (suppl) 24:335-610
18. Armaly MF (1966) On the distribution of applanation pressure and arcuate scotoma. In: Paterson G, Miller SJH, Paterson G (eds) Drug mechanisms in glaucoma. Little, Brown, Boston, pp 167-189
19. Leske MC (1983) The epidemiology of open-angle glaucoma: a review. Am J Epidemiol 118:166-191
20. Tielsch JM, Sommer A, Katz J, Royall RM, Quigley HA, Javitt J (1991) Racial variations in the prevalence of primary open angle glaucoma. The Baltimore Eye Survey. JAMA 266:369-374
21. Airaksinen PJ, Drance SM, Douglas GR, Schulzer M, Wijsman K (1985) Visual field and retinal nerve fiber layer comparison in glaucoma. Arch Ophthalmol 103:205-207
22. Sommer A, Katz J, Quingley HA, Miller NR, Robin AL, et al. (1991) Clinically detectable nerve fiber atrophy precedes the onset of glaucomatous field loss. Arch Ophthalmol 109:77-83
23. Korth M, Horn F, Jonas J (1993) Utility of the color pattern-electroretinogram (PERG) in glaucoma. Graefe's Arch Clin Ophthalmol 231:84-89
24. Mehaffey L, Holopigian K, Seiple W (1993) Electro-oculogram changes in patients with ocular hypertension and primary open angle glaucoma. Doc Ophthalmologica 83:103-110
25. Porciatti V, Falsini B, Brunori S, Colotto A, Moreti G (1987) Pattern electroretinogram as a function of spatial frequency in ocular hypertension and early glaucoma. Doc Ophthalmologica 65:349-355
26. Carli M, Steindler P, Ravagni M (1989) Perimetria computerizzata e potenziali visivi evocati in pazienti con glaucoma iniziale. Confronto tra due metodiche. Boll Ocul 68, [suppl] 6:107-111
27. Duke-Elder S (1952) The phasic variations in the ocular tension in primary glaucoma. Am J Ophthalmol 35:1-21
28. Ericson LA (1958) Twenty-four hourly variation of aqueous flow: examination with perilimbar suction cup. Acta Ophthalmol [suppl] 50:1-95
29. Drance SM (1960) The significance of the diurnal tension variations in normal and glaucomatous eyes. Arch Ophthalmol 64:494-501
30. Worthen D (1978) Intra-ocular pressure and its diurnal variation. In: Heilman K, Richardson KT (eds) Glaucoma–conceptions of disease. Thieme, Stuttgart, 54:66-72

31. Ferrario VF, Bianchi R, Giunta G, Roveda L (1982) Circadian rhythm in human intraocular pressure. Chronobiologia 9:33-69
32. Zeimer RC (1989) Circadian variations in intraocular pressure. In: Ritch R, Shields MB, Krupin T (eds) The glaucomas. Mosby, St. Louis, pp 319-335
33. Kitazawa Y, Horie T (1975) Diurnal variation of intraocular pressure in primary open-angle glaucoma. Am J Ophthalmol 79:557-566
34. Boles Carenini B (1955) Diurnal variations of systemic venous pressure compared with variations of tonographic readings and biomicroscopic aspect of aqueous veins. Am J Ophthalmol 39:793-808
35. Katavisto M (1964) The diurnal variations of ocular tension in glaucoma. Acta Ophthalmol Suppl 78:1-130
36. Greenidge KC, Spaeth GL, Fiol-Silva Z (1983) Effect of argon laser trabeculoplasty on the glaucomatous diurnal curve. Ophthalmology 90:800-803
37. Dannheim R (1976) Die Diagnose und Differentialdiagnose des Glaucoma chronicum simplex und des Glaucoma chronicum congestivum. Buch Augenarzt 69:171-174
38. Merritt JC, Reid LA, Smith R, Harris DF (1979) Diurnal intraocular pressure in juvenile open-angle glaucoma. Ann Ophthalmol 11:253-260
39. Smith J (1985) Diurnal intraocular pressure: correlation to automated perimetry. Ophthalmology 92:858-861
40. Yamagami J, Araie M, Aihara M, Yamamoto S (1993) Diurnal variation in intraocular pressure of normal-tension glaucoma eyes. Ophthalmology 100:643-650
41. Langley D, Swanljung H (1951) Ocular tension in glaucoma simplex. Brit J Ophthalmol 35:445-458
42. Phelps CD, Woodson RF, Kolker AE (1974) Diurnal variation in intraocular pressure. Am J Ophthalmol 77:367-377
43. Stepanik J (1954) Diurnal variations and their relation to visible aqueous outflow. Am J Ophthalmol 38:629-645
44. Kimura R (1966) Clinical studies on glaucoma Report 1. Acta Soc Ophthalmol Jpn, 70:1326-1330
45. Wilensky JT et coll (1982) Self-tonometry to manage glaucoma patients with apparently controlled intraocular pressure. Inv Ophthalmol Vis Sci 23:640-645
46. David R, Zangwill L, Briscoe D, Dagan M, Yagev R, Yassur Y (1992) Diurnal intraocular pressure variations: an analysis of 690 diurnal curves. Brit J Ophthalmol 76:280-283
47. Bito LZ (1994) Basic sciences in clinical glaucoma: a physiologic perspective with darwinian overtones. J Glaucoma 1: 193-205
48. Krupin T (1993) Manual of glaucoma: diagnosis and management. Churchill Livingstone, Edinburgh
49. Grierson J (1987) What is open angle glaucoma? Eye 1:15-28
50. Rohen JW (1983) Why is intraocular pressure elevated in chronic simple glaucoma? Ophthalmology 90:758-765
51. Segawa K (1979) Electron microscopic changes in the trabecular tissue in primary open angle glaucoma. Ann Ophthalmol 11:49-54
52. Lutjen-Drecoll E, Shimizu T, Rohrbach M, Rohen JW (1986) Quantitative analysis of "plaque material" in the inner and outer wall of Schlemm's canal in normal and glaucomatous eyes. Exp Eye Res 42:443-455
53. Duke-Elder S (1969) System of ophthalmology. Kimpton H, London, vol 9 pp 392-561

Early Optic Disc Glaucomatous Damage

H.A. Quigley

The Wilmer Ophthalmological Institute, The Johns Hopkins Hospital, 600 N. Wolfe Street, Baltimore, MD 21287-9205, USA

Thank you so much for inviting me to come. I'd like to talk now about what happens after the injury to the ganglion cells occurs. Dr. Boles Carenini has been talking about what some of these injuries might be but our attention has not been focused so acutely on how the ganglion cell dies. Here I will discuss some of the events that occur during the death of the ganglion cell and in this case in experimental glaucoma. We proposed that glaucoma is a disease in which the ganglion cell kills itself and that cell death might be something that we could stop through new forms of therapy. Based on information that is available in the world literature, it can be calculated that glaucoma affects 67 million people worldwide and is the second largest cause of blindness in the world. Thus, glaucoma is an extremely important area of study. I would define glaucoma as a condition that has two features: (1) retinal ganglion cell death (as far as we know, no other cells in the retina die in primary open angle glaucoma); (2) excavation of the optic disc, a term that best describes what occurs in the optic nerve head, which we can recognize clinically. It is becoming more common to define glaucoma without reference to a specific intraocular pressure (IOP) level. The features of disc excavation are well-known and include: collapse of the rim of the optic nerve as well as backward and outward rotation of the lamina cribrosa's connective tissue. Damage that excavation causes to the connective tissues of the nerve head is probably highly related to the fact that the site of injury, i.e., the place where the ganglion cells die, is the lamina cribrosa of the optic nerve head.

Axonal transport blockage has been studied by Anderson and Hendrickson and later by me in Doug Anderson's laboratory. Retrograde axonal transport can be shown to occur in axons normally. In other words, material can be seen moving in each nerve fiber in both directions, from the eye to the brain and from the brain back to the eye. The obstruction of transport is highly localized to areas right at the level of the optic nerve head and probably leads to the ganglion cell death. But how does it lead to the ganglion cells death? And, in fact, why do the cells die? Why don't they simply grow a new fiber? If axonal injury had occurred in the peripheral nervous system, the cell body would simply have grown a new axon. It has been said that central nervous system axons are not capable of growing a new fiber and yet every ganglion cell grew a fiber during embryological life. Thus, the genetic program for growing that axon is still present in the cell but is either turned off or the conditions for new axonal growth using this genetic program are not present. It is interesting to consider that at the embryological stage each of us has 3 million ganglion cells in our eye; yet we have only 1.5 million ganglion cells by the time the eye becomes mature. This means that half of the cells die by a process which is programmed in the cell. That program is referred to as apoptosis when it is a pathologically engendered state. Here, however, it is a message that the cell sends to itself. This situation occurs in our lymphatic system, our immunological system and interestingly it is used in our nervous system to eliminate nerve cells which are developed but do not properly link up or join to the appropriate cells. In the absence of such a process, our visual system would wind up with ganglion cells that were not topographically oriented in our visual system and would thus not work properly.

The apoptotic mechanism is rather interesting in that it involves the very quiet death of the cell by the switching on of an internal program by which the cell digests itself with enzymes; its DNA in the nucleus is digested and the cell is engulfed or phagocytosed by surrounding cells without disturbing the immediate environment. This is a very important aspect because, if there was a lot of disturbance and disruption of the surrounding cells, particularly in the retina, the normal delicate structure of the retina would be seriously disorganized.

Apoptosis can be contrasted with other mechanisms by which cells can die, e.g., necrosis, in which the cell literally bursts open and spills its contents into the surrounding space, engendering inflammation. While this is a grossly simplified comparison of the two processes, it is nonetheless important to consider the differences. I have a hypothesis for which there is some support and that is: ganglion cell death in glaucoma occurs because axonal movement of some critical material stops in the axons at the optic nerve head. Thus, material which is moving from the target cell in the brain back to the ganglion cell body in the retina is no longer transported. The level of this material in the ganglion cell body falls to a low level, starting programmed cell death in the ganglion cell body and the ganglion cell effectively commits suicide. In essence this might be similar to what occurs in the ganglion cell during embryological life, when the cell has not properly targeted and connected to a cell in the lateral geniculate body. Pathology recapitulates ontogeny. This fits with what we know about glaucoma clinically: that there is a quite rapid onset of cell death. Very few cells in a glaucomatous eye are in a reversible stage of dysfunction; if they were, then lowering the eye pressure or producing some other therapeutic event should dramatically improve the visual field. While central vision cannot be restored in a glaucoma patient, it can be in other conditions that affect the optic nerve.

Damage to the optic nerve caused by a tumor can be compared with damage due to glaucoma, as the two represent two different things affecting essentially the same cells but in slightly different ways and clinically they look very different. When a tumor affects an optic nerve, there's a selective loss of small ganglion cells, despite a general loss of vision and visual acuity. In glaucoma, by contrast, while there is some selectivity of loss of large ganglion cells, the general loss of vision and acuity is less than with tumor; however, glaucoma damage is largely irreversible. It may be that the tumor affects the transmission of nerve impulse more than it does axonal transport, at least for many of the ganglion cell axons. Of course, most tumors affect the optic nerve where it is myelinated. In a myelinated nerve, there is saltatory conduction. If the tumor is large and affects a segment of the optic nerve then it is probably affecting an area where conduction is going on in a myelinated segment. In this situation axonal transport is probably not affected very much and so axons do not die quite as quickly. In the case of glaucoma, damage is in a very localized area of the optic nerve which is not myelinated. It is possible then that the impulse is able to jump over the transport blockade. Of course the jump is passing along the membrane of the axon but it is able actually to get through, even though axonal transport is blocked and may still be quite functional, in terms of passage of the impulse. Only when the damage is such that the axon has finally reached the critical stage of programmed death does the impulse stop moving. This difference, between tumor and glaucoma, deserves considerably more study. If the above model is correct then function is affected by a tumor but axonal transport is not. The cell body and axon can recover because if you remove the tumor you still have a live axon. In glaucoma, once the cell death program starts, the process is basically irreversible.

Evidence exists for the process of apoptosis in human eye disease. It has already been demonstrated that apoptosis occurs in retinal degeneration following light toxicity damage to photoreceptors and when the retina is detached the photoreceptors die by apoptosis. In each case growth factor or small protein molecules can mediate the process, so we studied an experimental model of glaucoma by raising the pressure in the eyes of monkeys and found by light and electron microscopy, using a special stain for the process of apoptosis, that programmed cell death was indeed occurring. A special stain which looks for the DNA damage that is caused by apoptosis was utilized in a flat mounted group of ganglion cells of the retina. These are the capillaries running through the area near each ganglion cell body by microscopy. What happens if we damage the DNA in literally every ganglion cell is the cells' nuclei turn a bright orange. We examined individual ganglion cells in a rabbit who had its optic nerve transected; the ganglion cells of course died soon after. The cells were also studied in an experimental monkey that had elevated eye pressure, leading to apoptosis. In the ganglion cell bodies themselves, there were dramatic changes in the nucleus of glaucoma-affected cells. The nucleus becomes quite enlarged and looks very much like a fried egg. After the nucleus begins this process it breaks up into a number of small bodies referred to as apotoptic bodies. The chromatin forms tight little balls and ultimately the cells themselves become very small and are engulfed or phagocytosed by adjoining cells in the area. So the hypothesis is that the axon is injured, stopping the movement of material from the target cell of the brain back to the ganglion cell body such that the ganglion cell body initiates apoptosis. This "decision" can be affected by the delivery of certain growth factors, proteins that influence whether or not apoptosis is turned on, i.e., whether or not the enzymes that produce the effect of killing the cells are actually activated. Several of these growth factors are known to be present in retinal ganglion cells. Thus, it is quite possible that the life of a ganglion cell could be prolonged by stopping its suicide program. In the future a second approach to the treatment of glaucoma, besides lowering pressure may be administration of growth factors. Furthermore the cell itself is turning on or utilizing its genetic program to produce the method that kills itself. It is at least theoretically possible that genes that are known to inhibit the cell death program could be introduced into retinal ganglion cells. There have been publications in the last 12 months showing that various genes can be introduced into the retina and into ganglion cells with expression of the genes. It may be only a matter of time before someone attempts to slow down cell death program using such an approach. However, this process may only be temporary, as at present viral expression vectors are difficult to use and some of the introduced genes only function for a limited period of time before they stop working. A final feature of the cell death program may be that when a ganglion cell dies it releases its contents into the extracellular space. The cellular contents include the neurotransmitter glutamate, which is toxic to ganglion cells or any other neurons at high concentrations. There is now active research going on to look at whether glutamate-induced toxicity of retinal ganglion cells is a contributing feature in glaucoma.

Discussion

Question: M. Miglior

To Dr. Quigley. If we admit that apoptosis involves cells or compartment of cells in our body, for instance the cells of the optic nerve, we could also suppose to find out apoptosis along the trabecular cells. If so, we could possibly prevent the apoptotic damages at the trabecular level. What do you think of my opinion?

Answer: Quigley

Actually, you have asked me a question about the trabecular meshwork cells. Sitting near to me here is Dr. Alvarado and you may, I am sure, be familiar with the work in which Dr. Alvarado demonstrated that eyes with glaucoma have in general fewer trabecular meshwork endothelial cells than do eyes that are of the same age from persons without glaucoma. So, in addition to the fine structural details of the work that Dr. Alvarado has shown here, it's quite possible that there are simply fewer trabecular meshwork cells present in the eyes of someone with glaucoma.
I think we would love to know whether or not a glaucoma eye has differences in the intracellular pathways, and perhaps we should ask Dr. Alvarado if he likes to speculate or does he have evidence that the paracellular or transcellular pathway is different in glaucomatous eyes in comparison with eyes that are normal.
I don't know if you have any such information, but may be it is more relevant than my answer.

Answer: Alvarado

I am smiling because of my great respect for the skills of Dr. Quigley: his feet are faster than mine and he really docked the question which was directed at him. Thank you Harry. Actually, two things I have worked on, apoptosis turnout and eye with corneal endothelial syndrome where the endothelial cell changes that occur suggested that the process of apoptosis was going on. So I don't like the word suicide. Every morning I go across the Golden Gate bridge as I go to work and come back home. I always admire the beauty of the area and suicide is a horrendous act, something that you do against your will and despite your will to live. When we call it suicide we are bringing our own thought and philosophy into a process which is far no more normal. In fact, apoptosis is the best thing that cells can do to get out of the way for the sake of the organism. Suicide is something you do to destroy the organism. I don't like the word apoptosis, but getting back to the cells and the trabecular meshwork and linking optic neuropathy with trabeculopathy I actually think that there are many things we are already doing to protect the cells despite the fact that we didn't know we were doing such things. There are two factors that are extremely important to protect the cells.

One of them is the use of growth factors. The other one is the use of macrofages, and it turns out that trabeculoplasty is one of the best ways we can do both, recruiting macrofages to restore the vitality, health, population, and number of cells to the trabecular meshwork. What happens in glaucoma is a bit of a parcel, because the cells that die are distal internal to the justacanalicular where everyone believes the problem of glaucoma takes place. I have not found an explanation yet to link the death of cells in the corneal-sclera and uveal-sclera meshwork with what is going on in the justacanalicular tissue involving the trabecular cells and the cells in the Schlemm's canal, but I think it's a matter of future study before we understand well what's going on. Thank you Harry, I appreciate the opportunity you gave me.

Question:

My question is to Dr. Quigley. It is known that nitric oxide is involved in neuronal damage. Now my question is whether you have tried to prevent the apoptosis with nitric oxide inhibitors or by some other way. Now we have succeeded in preventing retinal ischemic damage with nitrous oxide.

Answer: Quigley

The question is if there has been any work in experimental glaucoma or human glaucoma that relates to nitric oxide inhibition. I am not aware that anyone has approached the subject in that way. There are fairly recent publications that have looked at the nitrous oxide system more to the front of the eye in the entire uvea and it may well be that such system is very directly involved in how fluid moves perhaps through the extracellular space at the ciliary body. And that may be involved in the unconventional routes of outflow. I don't know whether that would mean that there is a difference in the damage in the retina or not. I think that some of the experiments reported in retinal ischemia usually raise the eye pressure causing a damage to the retina; that's a very typical paradox because it is the easiest way to close off blood flow. But that's very different from primary open angle glaucoma. At present I am afraid we don't know. It's an exciting area as nitric oxide is something that arose due to the interest of people. Actually, Dr. Salomon Schneider and his crew were very actively involved and we set a sort of personal role in being interested in nitric oxide.

Question: Carella

To Prof. Boles. We should definitely establish whether these transient or persistent intraocular hypertensive peaks belong to glaucoma "sine ipertensione" or they are not detectable manifestations of the hypertensive glaucoma.
The ideal solution is to monitor the 24 hours intraocular pressure. Are you aware of any of such systems?

Answer: Boles Carenini

When a "method" will be available to monitor the intraocular pressure along 24 hours, then we will probably realize a reduction in the number of ocular hypertensive patients or glaucoma patients without ocular hypertensive value.
Such a monitoring system is still in experimental evaluation.

Question: Rama

To Prof. Alvarado. You clearly showed the importance of endothelial cells and the drug effects on these cells. I am wondering what is the effect on these cells with aging, what is their embriogenesis, and do these cells have the ability to regenerate ?

Answer: Alvarado

I want to repeat the question. It is in two parts I believe; the first one is what happens to the cells with aging, and then can these cells regenerate themselves? What happens to the cells with aging is that there is a gradual and progressive loss of cells as a function of age, and of time. That grade of loss is identical to the loss of cells in the corneal endothelium. It means that by the time you get to be one hundred years old you have lost 50% of the cells you had at birth as a normal individual.
By the time you are 55/60 years old and you have glaucoma you have lost the same number of cells that an individual 115/120 years old would have lost, so there is an accelerated but steady loss of cells in glaucomatous individuals. The second question has to do with regeneration. There are two processes both of which are bad. The first one occurs when the trabecular meshwork is injured as a function of age and not as a consequence of wounding. What happens is that the regeneration takes place in two ways. The cells in the innermost layer, the ones that are facing the anterior chamber, the ones that are holding the corneal endothelium from moving onto the trabecular meshwork, speaking in terms that make what happens clear, those cells will preserve a lining, so that although you have fewer cells the lining persists. Therefore that means, since the surface area hasn't decreased, that the cells must have increased in size. In doing that they cannot preserve the porosity of the innermost lining; therefore, the innermost lining looses its normal porosity, and the cells external to the innermost portion of the meshwork that are lost are not noticed as having been lost. The neighbouring cell doesn't respond in anyway. It does ignore that its neighbour has gone; the consequence of that is also deleterious, because those lining cells keep the aqueous channel lined with a nonthrombogenic endothelium, whose function is to permit the aqueous channel to collapse and even worse to come in contact.
You may begin to loose cells and the cells do not get replaced. This sticking of the aqueous channel becomes progressive, therefore the porosity of the corneal sclera meshwork also decreases.

Question: Bagolini

I was impressed by Dr. Quigley's presentation. According to literature data, in glaucoma the magnocellular system is more affected than the parvocellular one. Is there a reason for that?

Answer: Quigley

The question is perfectly clear, you are asking whether or not the larger ganglion cells die first because they are most susceptible to apoptosis or to some other mechanism.
From the literature it appears that the magnocellular system is more interested than the parvocellular system. My laboratory and two others have supported this idea, but unfortunately we don't have any reason to believe that we know why the big cells die more selectively faster or why ganglion cells die in glaucoma. The bigger cells appear to be dying somehow faster, if you look at the available data, but we don't to know yet why that is the case.

Question: Traverso

You have nicely shown that steroids decrease the paracellular flow. Are your data coming from normal human eyes, glaucomatous human eyes or steroids responders?

Answer: Alvarado

Normal eyes. The implication of your question is that glaucoma steroids inducement is created in susceptible individuals and that this is a generalized effect. We believe that the question of susceptibility depends on the time length of application as well as on dosage. So in vitro you could get the effect in all cell types, whether they are from normal or glaucomatous individuals.

Question: Bisantis

Dr. Alvarado said that a few substances allow the passage of aqueous not through the cells but among the cellular spaces and that they also induce a collapse of endothelial cells. I would like to ask if this mechanism may result in the functional loss of the endothelial cells by degeneration, apoptosis, necrosis or by other processes.

Answer: Alvarado

Again the question is whether the collapse of the trabecular structure, the 3-dimensional structure I talked about, causes an induced secondary change of two natures, two types; in one type of changing the extra-cellular matrix doesn't alter the cells and the other is simply a structural change where the fluid outflow is rerouted through a very small portion of cells so that those cells that are now selected to handle the amount of fluid flow will have an impact in fluid flow that will be greater than normal although the cells are normal.

Question: Carella

To Prof. Scullica. I would like to hear something more about the ciliary body circulation, especially regarding its derivations.

Answer: Scullica

Circulation in the ciliary bodies was extensively studied by Maggiore and by the Hungarian researchers. We also looked at these studies from the '50s to the '70s using the rabbit as an experimental model. The rabbit is a suitable model to study and to dissect vessels. By injecting neopren latex and Indian ink into the vessels we found that ciliary bodies circulation is not always the same, but it changes according to the general circulatory condition. Moreover, not all the ciliary bodies work at the same time. The circulation may be directed toward the vortex vein or through the capillary network. The functional reason for this network is not clear.

Question: Ravalico

To Dr. Alvarado. You mentioned the possible regeneration of endothelial cells by laser trabeculoplasty. We also found this possibility a few years ago. There is also the possibility to induce experimental glaucoma in Primates by increasing the extracellular matrix. Do you think it depends on the amount of laser treatment or is it related to other reasons ?

Answer: Alvarado

Actually, I should also mention that Dr. Van Burskirk and his group have very well documented the cellular proliferation and I should give credit to that group. The question you asked is actually one that involves the healing process that I mentioned earlier. The problem with laser trabeculoplasty is that it does induce some beneficial responses, but if you exceed the treated area you are going to invoke a response that will result in a loss of porosity. This is why one has to be very cautious in treating and retreating his patients. Thank you.

Microvasculature of the Optic Disc and Glaucoma

E. M. Van Buskirk and G.A. Cioffi

Devers Eye Institute, 1040 NW 22nd Avenue, Suite 200, Portland, OR 97210, USA

Introduction

Over the past several decades, increasing evidence has mounted to suggest that impairment of blood flow within the optic nerve head may contribute to the optic neuropathy of glaucoma in some subjects [1].

Diseases such as systemic hypertension, diabetes mellitus, Raynaud's syndrome, and migraine, associated with vascular and microvascular abnormalities, commonly are also associated with glaucoma [2].

Although the majority of glaucoma patients in Europe and North America appear to exhibit abnormally high levels of intraocular pressure, this is not true in Japan, compelling investigators to look elsewhere for causal factors at least in those patients [3].

Technology for clinical measurement of optic nerve blood flow is now burgeoning, with a variety of reports of abnormalities in some forms of glaucoma; but, to date, poor resolution of individual microvascular regions within the anterior optic nerve compromises interpretation of the data.

Good laboratory models of pressure induced glaucomatous optic neuropathy have been well and extensively studied [4].

Until recently, no models of optic nerve ischemia had been developed to permit comparison to the pressure model.

We have sought to understand as completely as possible the microvascular anatomy of the anterior optic nerve in primate and subprimate species [5] and then to model optic nerve ischemia by inducing controlled measurable vasoconstriction within the tissue.

Blood Supply to the Anterior Optic Nerve

The blood supply to the eye derives primarily from the ophthalmic artery, the first branch of the internal carotid artery. The ocular branches of the ophthalmic artery are the central retinal artery and one to five posterior ciliary arterial trunks that branch into the main posterior ciliary arteries. Most individuals have two to three posterior ciliary trunks which supply the medial and lateral posterior ciliary arteries. Each main posterior ciliary artery divides further into several short posterior ciliary arteries, just before or after entering the sclera.

The anterior portion of the optic nerve may be divided into four lamellar regions: the superficial nerve fiber layer, the prelaminar region, the laminar region, and the retrolaminar region, each with its own unique microvascular features. The superficial nerve fiber layer is supplied principally from the arterioles in the adjacent retina. Most of these vessels are capillaries originating in the peripapillary nerve fiber layer. These vessels, as with all capillary beds within the optic nerve, are not fenestrated and the tight junctions between their endothelial cells constitute the blood-ocular barrier. The temporal nerve fiber layer may have an additional arterial contribution from a cilioretinal artery when present. No direct choroidal contribution is observed in the superficial nerve fiber layer region.

The prelaminar region receives its arterial supply via direct branches of the short posterior ciliary arteries and via vessels originating from the arterial circle of Zinn and Haller

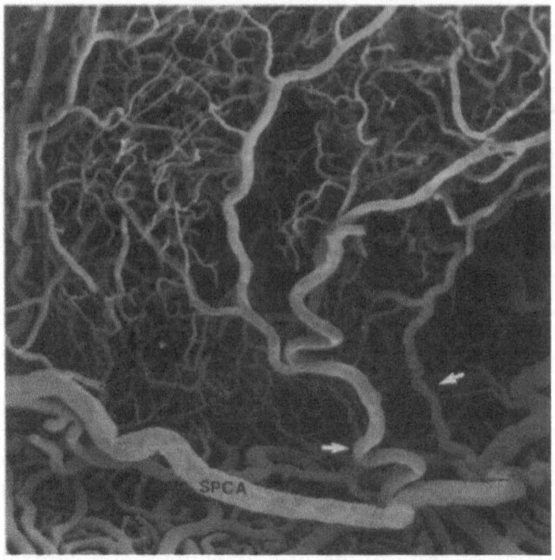

Fig. 1. Methacrylate corrosion casting of anterior optic nerve vasculature, lateral posterior view, showing the short posterior ciliary arterial supply (SPCA) in the rhesus monkey. Arterioles to the anterior optic nerve are indicated with *arrows*

(Figs. 1, 2). The posterior ciliary arterial system provides input to both the choroidal vessels and the arterial circle of Zinn and Haller. Our investigations have delineated only minimal anatomic vascular connections between the peripapillary choroid and anterior optic nerve. Branches from the short posterior ciliary arteries sometimes course through the choroid and supply the prelaminar region, but these vessels do not actually arise from the choroid.

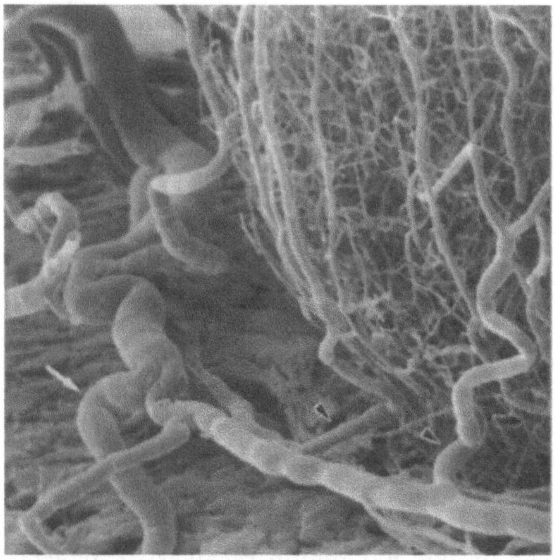

Fig. 2. Methacrylate corrosion casting of anterior optic nerve vasculature, lateral posterior view, showing the short posterior ciliary arterial supply in the human (eyebank) eye. Short posterior ciliary artery is shown branching to supply both the peripapillary choroid (*arrow*) and the anterior optic nerve (*arrowhead*)

The short posterior ciliary arteries, either directly or via the arterial circle of Zinn and Haller, also provide the principal arterial input to the laminar region of the optic nerve. As in the prelaminar region, the peripapillary choroid may contribute occasional, small arterioles to the lamina cribrosa region.

The precapillary vessels perforate the outer aspect of the lamina cribrosa before branching into an intraseptal capillary network (Fig. 3). Most of the blood supply to the retrolaminar portion of the optic nerve occurs through numerous perforating arterioles from the pia mater.

The central retinal artery does not branch to either the prelaminar or laminar region but does occasionally contribute small branches within the retrolaminar optic nerve.

The rich capillary beds of the peripapillary retina, the anterior optic nerve, and the retrolaminar region are anatomically confluent and form a continuous fine vascular network along the anterior optic nerve.

There is a subtle transition in the organization

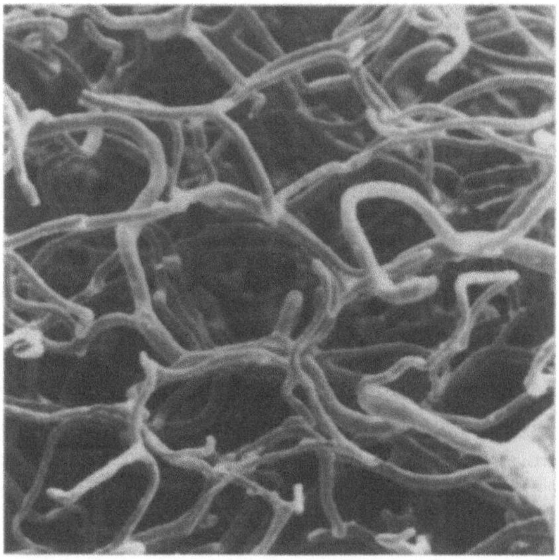

Fig. 3. Methacrylate corrosion casting of microvasculature within the septae of the lamina cribrosa of the optic nerve, enface view

of the capillaries from the complex and random arrangement of the prelaminar region to the horizontal network of laminar capillaries conforming to the pattern of the laminar connective tissue septae (Fig. 3). Although the longitudinal anastomoses of capillaries throughout the anterior optic nerve might be viewed as a protective mechanism against regional ischemia, flow resistance in these fine capillaries may be so high as to limit collateral flow.

The venous drainage of the anterior optic nerve is almost exclusively via the central retinal vein (Fig. 4). In the nerve fiber layer, blood is drained by small veins that converge and empty, ultimately, into the central retinal vein. In the prelaminar, laminar and retrolaminar regions, venous drainage also occurs via the central retinal vein or centripetal tributaries to the central retinal vein. Occasional small venules also connect the optic nerve and the peripapillary choroid, mainly within the prelaminar region. In the peripheral aspects of the laminar and retrolaminar regions, some optic nerve venous drainage may also be via pial veins, but these pial veins also drain into the central retinal vein as it exits the optic nerve.

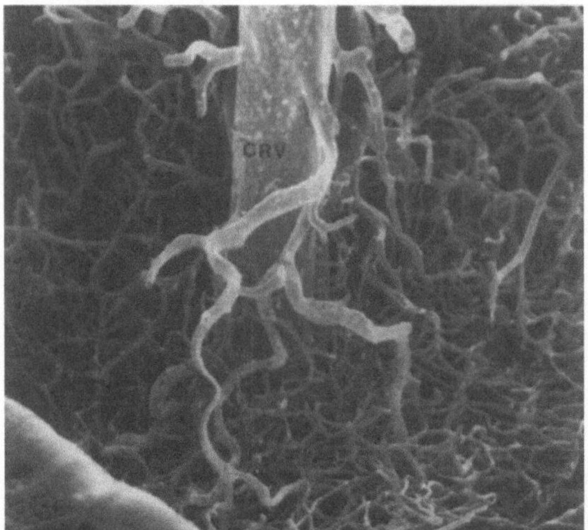

Fig. 4. Methacrylate corrosion casting of anterior optic nerve vasculature, lateral posterior view, showing the short posterior ciliary arterial supply (SPCA) in the rhesus monkey. Near half of the vessels posterior to the lamina have been dissected away to reveal the central retinal vein (CRV) draining the capillaries of the anterior optic nerve

A Laboratory Model of Chronic Optic Nerve Ischemia

Recently, we have developed an in vivo laboratory model of chronic vasoconstriction and vascular insufficiency of the anterior optic nerve [1, 6, 7]. In this model, dose-dependent vasoconstriction of the anterior optic nerve microvasculature of the rabbit has followed chronic, local delivery of endothelin-1 to the perineural region of the anterior optic nerve via osmotically driven minipumps.

Optic nerve blood flow has been determined by means of the colored microspheres technique [8]. The morphologic optic nerve changes over time have been monitored with a confocal scanning laser ophthalmoscope.

Long-term administration of endothelin-1 to the anterior optic nerve region induced a significant decrease in local blood flow of approximately 38%, compared to the contralateral eye. Control animals receiving only balanced salt solution from the minipump had no diminution in flow compared to the contralateral untreated eyes [7]. In the endothelin treated ischemic eyes, after 8 weeks of local administration of endothelin-1, multivariate analysis disclosed a small, but statistically significant, change in optic nerve morphology, as measured with a confocal scanning laser ophthalmoscope, compared to the control eyes. These changes were consistent with an increase in optic nerve cup volume and a decrease in optic neural rim area [7]. Blood flow and morphologic changes were independent of changes in intraocular pressure.

Endothelin-1 was chosen to induce chronic optic nerve ischemia not only because it is the most potent vasoconstrictor known, but it may also play a role in some regional ischemic processes throughout the body. In healthy young humans, the circulating levels of endothelin are very low [9]. In pathological conditions, such as an ischemic cerebrovascular insult, the plasma level of endothelin-1 has been reported to be elevated [10]. Experimentally, endothelin-1 has been shown to produce, in vivo, localized cerebral vasoconstriction, resulting in regional ischemic damage of the cerebral nervous tissues [11]. Endothelin-1 is a strong vasoconstrictive agent of the ocular circulation as well, and the vasomodulation potency of endothelial mediators increases with decreasing diameters of the blood vessel [12-15]. Recently, Moriya et al. [16] found a statistically significant increase in the levels of plasma endothelin-1 in patients with low tension glaucoma as compared to normal controls. This compound has been demonstrated to cause, in vivo, a dose-dependent vasoconstriction of the anterior optic nerve microvasculature in the rabbit [1-6]. The role of endothelin-1 in optic nerve pathology deserves further investigation.

The morphologic changes observed with scanning laser ophthalmoscopy suggest an optic nerve cupping with atrophy of the perineural rim resulting from chronic optic nerve ischemia. Such morphologic changes would be expected to occur in a glaucomatous optic neuropathy. However, anatomical differences between the optic nerve in humans and rabbits preclude a definitive comparison of the present results with human glaucomatous optic neuropathy. Most probably, an anterior ischemic optic neuropathy would cause similar morphologic changes in the rabbit optic nerve. The potential role of vascular insufficiency in glaucoma has been debated for over a century and remains controversial [17]. It has been difficult to settle these controversies with current experimental techniques. Experimental optic nerve atrophy similar to that seen in glaucoma patients can also be induced by an increased intraocular pressure [4, 18]. However, an increased intraocular pressure cannot account for the changes observed in the current study.

Possible Implications of Microvascular Anatomy for the Development of Glaucomatous Optic Neuropathy

Blood Flow and Watershed Zones

The primary arterial supply to the anterior optic nerve, in both human and nonhuman primates, derives from the short posterior ciliary arteries [19-21]. These vessels penetrate the optic nerve from its periphery. In contrast, the venous drainage for the anterior optic nerve occurs entirely through the central portion of the nerve by way of the central retinal vein. Therefore, the direction of the optic nerve blood flow is centripetal, from the peripheral arterial supply toward the central venous drainage. This is in contrast to virtually all other nonprimate mammals, which exhibit multiple, peripheral veins for drainage of the optic nerve [22-24]. The peripapillary choroid also derives its blood supply from branches of these same short posterior ciliary arteries, at the margin of the optic nerve. The venous drainage of the peripapillary choroidal region is via the vortex system, which is located more anteriorly in the eye. Therefore, the peripapillary blood flow is directed away from the optic disk margin toward the peripheral choroid. At the prelaminar and laminar levels of the optic nerve, the only vessels between the optic nerve and the peripapillary choroid are the small arterial and venous connections. There is a conspicuous absence of capillary beds in this area. Since arteriolar blood flow is directed away from the peripapillary region, either toward the choroid or the central optic nerve, and the peripapillary region is likely a low pressure system as compared to the rest of the choroid [25, 26], the area between the optic nerve and the peripapillary choroid may act as a "watershed zone." This region may be susceptible to localized ischemia during periods of decreased arterial perfusion. This "peripapillary watershed zone" between the optic nerve and the peripapillary choroid is somewhat different than the concept described by Hayreh [26]. However, if this concept of a peripapillary watershed region is combined with the vertically oriented watershed zones, the peripapillary region certainly becomes a potential site for ischemic damage, especially at the superior and inferior temporal regions. During periods of decreased systemic blood pressure or increased intraocular pressure, localized hypoperfusion may occur in these regions. The association between nocturnal hypotension and low tension glaucoma, further underscores the possibility that a peripapillary watershed zone could contribute to the nerve damage seen with glaucoma [27].

Choroid and Optic Nerve Perfusion

Because the choroidal vasculature and the anterior optic nerve vasculature are largely separated from each other, enhanced blood flow to the choroid may have no relation to increased optic nerve head perfusion, or could actually be detrimental.

The peripapillary choroid and the anterior optic nerve share a common arterial supply at the level of the posterior ciliary arteries. If blood flow is decreased at the posterior ciliary artery level, perfusion to both the peripapillary choroid and anterior optic nerve would be expected to decrease simultaneously. However, regional control is more likely at the smaller arterial and precapillary levels [22]. Therefore, increases or decreases in choroidal blood flow may not directly correlate with the blood flow of the anterior optic nerve. In fact, enhanced flow to the choroid could potentially redirect blood flow away from the optic nerve.

Venous Outflow

Finally, the presence of a single central venous outflow pathway is unique to primates [19, 20, 22, 28, 29]. This peculiarity of the venous outflow may partially underlie the susceptibility of the human optic nerve to ischemic disorders and may be related to the association of central retinal vein occlusion and open angle glaucoma. Since vascular perfusion is dependent not only on the arterial pressure but also on the venous outflow resistance, impaired venous outflow could also play an important role in the development of ischemic optic nerve disorders [22]. Compromise of outflow through this single vessel either by external pressure (i.e., intraocular pressure) or an anatomic anomaly may alter anterior optic nerve perfusion. The venous system has been largely ignored and considered non-contributory to the perfusion of this region. In light of this unique solitary outflow system, future investigation into the anatomy, the variations and vasomotor activity of the venous system may be warranted.

References

1. Cioffi GA, Orgul S, Onda E, Bacon DR, Van Buskirk EM (1995) An in vivo model of chronic optic nerve ischemia: the dose-dependent effects of endothelin-1 on the optic nerve microvasculature. Curr Eye Res. 14:1147-1153
2. Flammer J et al. (1992) The probable involvement of factors other than intraocular pressure in the pathogenesis of glaucoma. In: Drance SM, Van Buskirk EM, Neufeld AH (eds) Farmacology of Glaucoma, Williams and Wilkins, Baltimore, pp 273-283
3. Shiose Y (1990) Intraocular pressure. New perspectives. Surv Ophthalmol. 34:413-435
4. Quigley HA, Hohman RM, Addicks EM (1980) Chronic experimental glaucoma in primates. II. Effect of extended intraocular pressure elevation on optic nerve head and axonal transport. Invest Ophthalmol Vis Sci 19:137-52
5. Cioffi GA, Van Buskirk EM (1994) Vasculature of the anterior optic nerve and peripapillary choroid. In: Ritch R, Shields MB, Krupin (eds) The glaucomas, 2nd edn. CV Mosby, St. Louis pp 177-178
6. Cioffi GA, Van Buskirk EM (1994) Microvasculature of the anterior optic nerve. Surv Ophthalmol 38 (Suppl):S107-S117
7. Orgul S, Cioffi GA, Wilson DJ, Bacon DR, Van Buskirk EM (1996) An endothelin-1 induced model of chronic optic nerve ischemia in the rabbit. Invest Ophthalmol Vis Sci (in press)
8. Orgul S, Cioffi GA, Bacon DR, Van Buskirk EM (1996) Measurement of optic nerve blood flow with nonradioactive colored microspheres in rabbits. Microvas Res 51:175-186
9. Hartter E, Woloszczuk W (1989) Radioimmunoassay of endothelin. Lancet 1:909
10. Ziv I, Fleminger G, Djaldetti R, Achiron A, Meland E, Sokolovsky M (1992) Increased plasma endothelin-1 in acute ischemic stroke. Stroke 23:1014-1016
11. Sharkey J, Ritchie IM, Kelly PAT (1993) Perivascular microapplication of endothelin-1: a new model of focal cerebral ischemia in the rat. J Cardiovasc Pharmacol 13:865-871
12. Yao K, Tschudi M, Flammer J, Luscher TF (1993) Endothelium-dependent regulation of vascular tone of the porcine ophthalmic artery. Invest Ophthalmol Vis Sci 32:1792 1798
13. Haefliger IO, Flammer J, Luscher TF (1992) Nitric oxide and endothelin-1 are important regulators of human ophthalmic artery. Invest Ophthalmol Vis Sci 33:2340-2343
14. Haefliger IO, Flammer J, Luscher TF (1993) Heterogeneity of endothelium-dependent regulation in ophthalmic and ciliary arteries. Invest Ophthalmol Vis Sci 34:1722-1730
15. Meyer P, Flammer J, Luscher TF (1993) Endothelium-dependent regulation of the ophthalmic microcirculation in the perfused porcine eye; role of nitric oxide and endothelins. Invest Ophthalmol Vis Sci 34:3614-3621
16. Moriya S, Sugiyama Y, Shimizu K, Hamada J, Tokuoka S, Azuma I (1992) Low tension glau-

coma and endothelin (ET-1) Folia Ophthalmol Jpn 43:554-559
17. Van Buskirk EM, Cioffi GA (1992) Glaucomatous optic neuropathy. Am J Ophthalmol 113:447-452
18. Gaasterland DE, Tanishima T, Kuwabara T (1978) Axoplasmic flow during chronic experimental glaucoma. I Light and electron microscopic studies of the monkey optic nerve head during development of glaucomatous cupping. Invest Ophthalmol Vis Sci 17:838-846
19. Hayreh SS (1978) Structure and blood supply of the optic nerve. In: Heilmann K, Richardson KT (eds) Glaucoma: conceptions of a disease pathogenesis, diagnosis, therapy. Thieme, Stuttgart, pp 78-96
20. Lieberman MF, Maumenee AE, Green WR (1976) Histologic studies of the vasculature of the anterior optic nerve. Am J Ophthalmol 82:405-423
21. Olver JM, Spalton DJ, McCartney ACE (1990) Microvascular study of the retrolaminar optic nerve in man: the possible significance in anterior ischemic optic neuropathy. Eye 4:7
22. Cioffi GA, Van Buskirk EM (1994) Anatomy of the ocular microvasculature. Surv Ophthalmol 38 (Suppl):5107
23. Sugiyama K, Bacon DR, Cioffi GA et al. (1992) The effects of phenylephrine on the ciliary body and optic nerve head vasculature. J Glaucoma 1:156-164
24. Sugiyama K, Bacon DR, Cioffi GA et al. (1992) Optic nerve head microvasculature of the rabbit eye. Invest Ophthalmol Vis Sci 33:2251-2261
25. Geijssen HC (1991) Studies on normal-pressure glaucoma. Kugler, New York
26. Hayreh SS (1989) Blood supply of the optic nerve head in health and disease. In: Lambrou GN, Greve EL (eds) Ocular blood flow in glaucoma: means, methods, and measurements, Kugler & Ghedini, Amsterdam, pp 3-48
27. Hayreh SS (1976) The pathogenesis of optic nerve lesions in glaucoma. Trans Am Acad Ophthalmol Otolaryngol 81:197-213
28. Anderson DR, Hoyt WF (1969) Ultrastructure of the intraorbital portion of human and monkey optic nerve Arch Ophthalmol 82:506
29. Ernest JT, Potts AM (1968) Pathophysiology of the distal portion of the optic nerve. II. Vascular relationships. Am J Ophthalmol 66:380

The Vascular Factors in Glaucoma

S. M. Drance

Department of Ophthalmology, University of British Columbia, 2211 Wesbrook Mall, Vancouver, BC V6T 2B5, Canada

Introduction

All glaucoma population studies have confirmed that all levels of intraocular pressure (IOP) are risk factors for the disease and are both causative and dose related. Many patients however seem to develop the disease with normal and occasionally even low pressures. It is also established that many people with elevated IOP do not develop the disease. Successful surgical pressure reduction protects over two thirds of patients from progressing but a third continue to deteriorate although possibly at a slower rate.

It is clear that there must be other risk factors: age, myopia and race are among them. I would like to review the circulatory risk factors which have also been implicated. It should be pointed out that separating vascular factors from mechanical factors is artificial and may be counterproductive. The disease almost certainly involves an interplay of many factors. Nor is there a vascular factor but rather many circulatory factors some of which may in fact be brought about by the elevation of the IOP which is known to interfere with the axoplasmic flow. Some vascular factors may be secondary to the damage caused by the disease. There may be some vascular factors on the other hand that have no relationship to IOP at all and may in fact be the cause of the disease in some patients just as IOP elevation is causative in so many others.

Hemodynamic alterations of the circulation may be produced by alterations of the systemic blood pressure (BP) or the height of the IOP as well as by the composition and qualities of the blood itself. Organic obstructive changes of the small vessel wall are probably independent of the IOP level. However, faulty autoregulation may be modifying the tissue effects produced by fluctuations of the perfusion pressure. As in other circulations beds of the body more than one mechanism may be operative in the same patient, for instance a poststenotic dilatation of a blood vessel may diminish or abolish its ability to participate in autoregulation.

The local blood supply is dependent on: (1) perfusion pressure; (2) resistance of the blood vessels (tone); (3) composition of the blood.

Changes in the Hemodynamics of the Ocular Circulation

Almost 30 years ago it was shown that when vascular hypertension is treated and the perfusion pressure to the eye is reduced in stable glaucoma patients, there can nonetheless be a rapid progression of their visual field damage [1].

Gaffner and Goldman found that the experimental IOP elevation required to produce scotomas had to be greater the higher the BP of the individual [2].

Shock-like states were found to be followed by a clinical picture indistinguishable from normal tension glaucoma (NTG). These patients did not show progression of their field defects when observed over long periods of time. Unfortunately they constitute only a small group of all glaucoma patients [3]. They probably also belong to the group with large optic discs so that a large cup was present before any disease occurred. Pallor and the classical localised field defects were almost certainly produced by the infarction during the shock-like episode.

At that time it was also reported that most glaucoma patients had low diastolic perfusion pressures and those who did not often had a history of cardiovascular crises at which time their perfusion pressure would have been extraordinarily low. A low perfusion pressure can of course be produced by either a high IOP or a low BP or a lesser combination of both [4].

Silent myocardial infarction has been found more commmonly in glaucoma patients than in age-matched nonglaucomatous controls [5].

There are many reports showing that glaucoma patients, particularly those with normal IOPs, had low systemic and ophthalmic artery BPs. This has not been universally confirmed but there are good reasons for the discrepant findings [6-11].

Hayreh, Kaiser and Flammer, Graham and I, and others have shown that the BP in glaucoma patients, when monitored round the clock, is more likely to show arterial pressure dips, particularly at night, than are found in non-glaucomatous counterparts. We found that patients whose glaucomatous field defects are progressing have significantly more "dippers" than those whose disease is stable [12-15].

Tielsch found that, at diastolic perfusion pressures from 90 mm Hg down to about 40 mm Hg, there was no increase in the prevalence of glaucoma in his population study, but in those with diastolic perfusion pressures below 40 mm Hg the prevalence rose steeply. He suggested that the risk of having glaucoma rises as the perfusion pressure decreases [16]. Tielsch, reporting also from the Baltimore population survey, found that young people with high BP appeared to be protected from glaucomatous damage whereas elderly people with hypertension had more glaucoma than did normotensives individuals [16].

Vasospasm

Corbett et al. reported that almost 50% of their NTG patients had migraine much more frequently than expected [17]. Sossi and Anderson found that elevating the BP of monkeys with angiotensin failed to protect the optic nerve from elevated IOP, in fact the opposite was true. They postulated that this was due to the vasospasm produced by the drug which leaked through the choroidal capillaries and reached the prelaminar optic nerve at the site of the peripapillary choroidal crescents [18].

Flammer and coworkers showed that vasospasm in response to cold in the fingers was very common in NTG patients. Cooling the hand of such vasospastic individuals made their field defects worse. This could be reversed with nifedipine, a powerful calcium channel blocker [19]. In a cruder and less time consuming way we reported similar findings not only in NTG but in chronic open angle glaucoma (COAG) patients in general [20]. Flammer has recently extended his observations to show that NTG patients are supersensitive to intra-arterial endothelin injections.

Schulzer et al. reported on two distinct clusters of glaucoma patients. One cluster was predominantly vasospastic to cold and the other was largely nonvasospastic to cold but had abnormalities in the biochemical markers normally associated with microvascular disease. Each grouping contained both NTG and COAG patients. In the vasospastic group there was a relationship between the amount of field defect and the highest IOP in the eye, whereas in the other cluster there was no such relationship. These findings imply that there may be some glaucoma patients, independently of whether they have elevated or normal eye pressures, in whom the IOP is related to the disease and there are others in whom the IOP is much less related to the disease and in whom pressure reduction might possibly be expected to make less difference. The vasospastic tendency may interfere with autoregulation so that changes in perfusion pressure, whether due to elevated IOP or a BP drop, may not be compensated for, with damaging results [21].

The prevalence of localised vessel narrowing at the optic disc margin was described by Rader et al. in anterior ischemic optic neuropathies (AION) and COAG. We suggested that these vessels are vasospastic, which, taken together, may explain the leakage of vasoactive materials from the circulation through the choroidal circulation, which has no tight junctions, into the area of the peripapillary atrophy where the muscular coat of the vessels may be affected [22].

Vascular tone is finely balanced and controlled through the intact vascular endothelium. Basal release of nitric oxide produces vasodilatation. Prostacyclin is also an endothelial vasodilator. The endothelins, also produced by endothelium, are powerful vasoconstrictors which produce vasospasm when the endothelium becomes dysfunctional. Thromboxane A2, prostaglandin H2 and superoxide anions are also vasoconstrictors. Other causes for vasospasm are stress, cold, nicotine, Raynaud's disease and collagen diseases [23].

The deeper parts of the optic nerve are nourished by the short posterior ciliary vessels, which are effectively end arteries. Between them are the watershed zones which have a variable relationship to the optic nerve, but in many individuals they run through the nerve itself. A fall of the perfusion pressure, and/or a rise in the vascular tone, both of which decrease blood flow, may produce ischemic changes in the watershed areas, particularly when autoregulation is impaired, as has been reported in glaucomatous eyes [24, 25].

Magnetic resonance imaging of the brains of NTG patients and age matched controls reveals the presence of confluent, deep, white matter lesions in NTG patients. Such lesions are associated with ischemia in elderly patients and have been found with vasospastic disease and arteritis in younger patients [26, 27].

We, among others, showed that using transcranial ultrasound, the velocity in the ophthalmic artery diminished with age but was also significantly prolonged in glaucoma patients. In the absence of being able to measure the diameter of the vessel we could only infer that this had something to do with blood flow. Incidentally, we could demonstrate, using this technique, that smoking half a cigarette significantly altered the blood velocity in the ophthalmic artery. Again patients with progressive visual field defects were more likely to have slower velocities than those whose glaucoma appeared stable [28].

Several groups have been able to show changes in the velocity and resistivity in the central retinal artery (CRA), short posterior ciliary artery (SPCAs) using colour Doppler imaging [29-33]. In asymmetric glaucoma patients we found significant differences in the systolic and diastolic velocities of the CRAs between the two eyes when the asymmetry of the disease was most pronounced. Both the worse and the better eyes showed significant changes in the systolic and diastolic velocities and the resistivity index of the CRA compared to nonglaucomatous eyes of similar age. The SPCAs also showed those differences from controls in the systolic and diastolic velocities. Even the better eyes, which were judged by us to have quite normal fields and discs, showed these differences. This suggests but does not prove that some circulatory disturbances may precede rather than follow glaucomatous damage [34].

Pillunat and coworkers have presented evidence that at least some NTG patients must have vasospasm in the ciliary circulation which can be reversed with carbon dioxide or calcium channel blockers. Such findings may have some interesting therapeutic implications in the future [35, 36].

Harris and coworkers have recently also shown that various ß-blockers have different effects on the SPCAs and that the ß1-blockers may in fact decrease the resistivity in those vessels, possibly by abolishing vasospasm [37].

The vascular factors are only a part of the multifactorial disease currently known as the open angle glaucomas. Whether they are entirely causal in some individuals or merely modify the substrate for the other risk factors as well as the relationship of these factors to apoptosis and IOP has yet to be worked out.

References

1. Harrington DO (1959), The pathogenesis of the glaucoma field. Am J Ophthalmol 47:177-185
2. Gafner F, Goldmann H (1955) Experimentelle Untersuchungen uber den Zusamehang von Augenstegerung und Gesichtsfeldschadigungen. Ophthalmologica 130:357-377
3. Drance SM (1977) The visual field in low tension glaucoma and shock induced optic neuropathy. Arch Ophthalmol 95:1359-1361
4. Drance SM, Johnson DG (1968) Some studies on the circulation of patients with advanced chronic simple glaucoma.Canad J Ophthal 3:149-155
5. Kaiser HJ, Flammer J, Burckhardt D (1993) Silent myocardial ischemia in glaucoma patients. Ophthalmologica 207:6-8

6. Kaiser HJ, Flammer J, Graf T, Stumpftg D, (1993) Systemic blood pressure in glaucoma patients. Graefe's Arch Clin Exp Ophthalmol 231:677-680
7. Grammer E, (1995) Risk factors in glaucoma: clinical studies. In: Kriegelstein GK (ed) Glaucoma update, 5th ed. Kaden, Heidelberg, pp 14-31
8. Perasalo R, Raitta C, Low C (1990) Blood pressure a risk factor for nerve fiber loss in institutionalised geriatic glaucoma patients. Acta Ophthalmol 195:65-67
9. Sachsenweger R (1963) Der Eînfluss des Blutdruckes auf die prognose des Glaukoms. Klin, Monatsbl Augenheilk 142:625-633
10. Goldberg I, Hollows FC, Kaas MA, Becker B (1982) Systemic factors in patients with low tension glaucoma. Br J Ophthalmol 65:56-65
11. Drance SM (1973) Some factors involved in the production of low tension glaucoma. Arch Ophthalmol 89:45
12. Hayreh SS, Zimmerman MB, Podhajsky P, Alward WLM (1994) Nocturnal arterial hypotension and its role in optic nerve head ischaemic disorders Am J Ophthalmol 117:603-24
13. Kaiser HJ, Flammer J (1991) Systemic hypotension: risk factor for glaucomatous damage? Ophthalmologica 203:105-108
14. Graham SL, Drance SM, Wijsman K, Douglas GR, Mikelberg FS (1995) Ambulatory blood pressure monitoring in glaucoma- the nocturnal dip. Ophthalmology 102:61-69
15. Bechetoille A, Bresson-Dumont H (1995) Behaviour of systemic blood pressure in different types of glaucoma. In: Krieglstein GK (ed): Update to glaucoma 5. Kaden, Heidelberg, pp 32-36
16. Tielsch JM, Katz J, Sommer A, Quigley HA, Javitt JC (1995) Hypertension, perfusion pressure and primary open-angle glaucoma. Arch Ophthalmol 113:216-221
17. Corbett JJ, Phelps CD, Eslinger P, Montague PR (1985) The neurologic evaluation of patients with low tension glaucoma. Invest Ophthalmol Vis Sci 26:1101-1104
18. Sossi N, Anderson DR (1983) Blockage of axonal transport induced by elevation of IOP. Effect of arterial hypertension induced by angiotensin. Arch Ophthalmol l01:94-99
19. Flammer J, Guthauser U, Mahler M (1987) Do ocular vasospasm help cause low tension glaucoma? Doc Ophthalmol Proc Ser 49:397-399
20. Drance SM, Douglas GR, Wijsman K, Schulzer M (1988) Response of blood flow to warm and cold in normals and NTG patients. Am J Ophthalmol 105:35-39
21. Schulzer M, Drance SM, Carter CJ, Brooks DE, Douglas GR, Lau W (1990) Biostatistical evidence for two distinct populations with COAG. Br J Ophthalmol 74:196-200
22. Rader J, Feuer W, Anderson D (1994) Peripapillary vasoconstriction in the glaucomas and the anterior ischaemic optic neuropathies. Am J Ophthalmol 117:72-80
23. Luscher TF, Meyer P, Haefliger IO, Flammer J (1955) Endothelial mediators as regulators of the ophthalmic circulation. Drance SM, Anderson DR (eds) In: Optic nerve in glaucoma. Kugler, Amsterdam, pp 259-281
24. Hayreh SS (1990) In vivo choroidal circulation and its watershed zones. Eye 4:273-289
25. Hayreh SS (1989) Blood supply of the optic nerve in health and disease. In: Lambrou G, Greve E (eds) Ocular blood flow in glaucoma. Kugler, Amsterdam, pp 3-48.
26. Stroman GA, Stewart WC, Golnik KC, Cure JL, Olinger RE (1995) Magnetic resonance imaging in patients with LTG. Arch Ophthalmol 113:168-172
27. Chimovitz MI, Estes ML, Furlan AJ, Awad IA (1992) Further observations on the pathology of subcortical lesions identified on magnetic resonance imaging. Arch Neurol 49:747-752
28. Rojanapongpun P, Drance SM (1993) Ophthalmic flow velocity in glaucomatous and normal subjects. Brit J Ophthalmol 77:25-29
29. Augustyniak E, Swietliczko I, Aaslid R (1989) Ocena przedkosci przeplywu krwi i krzywej pulsacji w tetnicach rzeskowych tylnych w jaskrze. Klin Oczna: 91:3-6
30. Lieb WE, Cohen SM, Merton DA, Shields JA, Mitchell DG, Goldberg BB (1991) Color Doppler imaging of the eye and orbit. Technique and normal vascular anatomy. Arch Ophthalmol 109:527-32
31. Harris A, Williamson TH, Shoemaker JA, Sergott RC, Spaeth GL, Katz JL (1995) Reproducibility of colour Doppler imaging assessment of blood flow velocity in orbital vessels. J Glaucoma (in press)
32. Rankin SJA, Walman BE, Buckley AR, Drance SM (1995) Colour Doppler imaging of the optic nerve vasculature in glaucoma. Am J Ophthalmol 119:685-693
33. Galassi F, Nuzzaci G, Sodi A (1992) Colour Doppler imaging in the evaluation of optic nerve blood supply in normal and glaucomatous subjects. Int Ophthalmol 16:273-276
34. Nicolela M, Drance SM, Rankin SJA, Buekley AR, Walman BE (1996) Colour Doppler imaging in asymmetric glaucoma patients with unilateral visual field loss. Am J Ophthal 121:502-510
35. Pillunat LE, Lang GK, Harris A (1995) Ocular carbon dioxide reactivity and calcium channel blockers in NTG. In: Drance SM (ed) Update to glaucoma, ocular blood flow and drug treatment. Kugler, Amsterdam p 67

36. Netland PA, Grosskreutz CL, Feke GT, Hart LJ (1995) Colour Doppler ultrasound analysis of ocular circulation after topical calcium channel blocker. Am J Ophthal 119:694-700

37. Harris A, Spaeth GL, Sergott RC, Katz JL, Cantor LB, Martin BJ (1995) Retrobulbar arterial hemodynamic effects of betaxolol and timolol in NTG. Am J Ophthal 120:168-175

Ocular Blood Flow and Its Autoregulation

C. Bisantis

Institute of Ophthalmology, University of Padua, Via Giustiniani 2, 35100 Padua, Italy

Hemodynamics of Retinal Blood Flow

To completely assess the hemodynamic of the ocular circulation, information regarding many parameters is required. These parameters include: vessel length, vessel cross-sectional area; blood pressure; blood flow; pulsatile flow; vessel wall tension; resistance to flow; blood viscosity; turbulence; critical closing pressure; intra ocular pressure (IOP) [1].
The mean ocular perfusion pressure (MOPP) is the most important parameter in discussing ocular blood flow (OBF) characteristics.
This parameter is especially important when IOP is higher than normal or in glaucomatous eyes.
The formula to estimate MOPP is:
MOPP = 2/3 [DBP + 1/3 (SBP -DBP)] -IOP
where DPB is diastolic blood pressure and SBP is systolic blood pressure.
The OBF (or blood velocity x cross-sectional area), depends on MOPP and is estimated to be approximately 1 ml/min; only 2%-5% of total OBF supplies the retina [2].
The blood flow to the eye is mainly pulsatile, the mean pulsatile component of blood flow estimated to be approximately 0.724 ml/min [3]. The retinal circulation has a mean flow of 0.033 ml/min [4].
All vascular systems have some mechanism of blood flow autoregolation, which is the ability of an organ to maintain relatively constant blood flow despite changes in perfusion pressure.
The eye has unusual hemodynamic properties because its tissues are subjected to high IOP. For this reason the physiologic balance of OBF depends on the systemic blood pressure, ocular vascular resistance and IOP.
In the retina the role of the autonomic nervous system is uncertain. The mechanism of the responses of retinal vessels to hyperoxia or hypercapnia is also poorly understood. In the retina blood flow autoregolation is mediated by metabolites from retinal cells [1, 2, 5, 6]. By constrast, uveal tissue, autonomic receptors are clearly present and their active role is demonstrated by: (a) reduction of blood flow after sympathetic system stimulation; (b) increase in choroidal flow after cervical sympathectomy [6, 7].
Nonetheless in the retina, autoregolation of blood flow is very efficient and has been confirmed by numerous experiments. Significant reduction and increase of retinal blood flow (RBF) has been recorded after flickering light exposure, constant illumination or dark exposure. After 5 min of dark exposure, retinal arteriolar blood velocity increases 40%-55%, while flickering ligt increases RBF by 30%. Constant illumination vs dark exposure reduces RBF by 40%-55% [6, 8-15].
Hypoxia increases blood velocity by 38% and the diameter of arterioles and venules by 8.2% and 7.4%, respectively. Likewise, hyperoxia reduces blood velocity by 36% and the diameters of venules and arterioles by 10% and 5%-6% respectively [8, 16-19].
The RBF does not decrease until the IOP is about 34 mm Hg and does not increase until the IOP is lower than 10 mm Hg [8]. When IOP increases, perfusion of the eye continues until the IOP is 6 mm Hg below the perfusion pressure of the blood in the ophthalmic circulation [7, 8, 20]. The RBF is also regulated by increments of up to 40% during increases in systemic pressure [21].

The Choroidal Circulation

There are many differences between the responses of the retinal and choroidal circulations, the most evident being that choroidal blood flow (CBF) is reduced when ocular perfusion pressure is reduced while the RBF remains stable [6]. For example, during postural changes, despite alterations in perfusion pressure, retinal blood velocity remains stable [22, 23]. In the same situation choroidal autoregulation is not efficient: on assuming the supine position blood decreases by 27.5% in normal eyes and by even more in hypertensive and glaucomatous eyes [24]. Nevertheless an efficient regulation of CBF has been demonstrated in conditions of acute and chronic systemic hypertension [25-28]. The reactive vasoconstriction is this case is mediated by a very rich sympathetic plexus. However, an adequate choroidal vascular response to the increase in IOP is lacking, because choroidal vasodilatation is possible only in conditions of hypo or normal IOP [29]. Choroidal autoregulation occurs at IOPs of between 8 and 15 mm Hg [29, 30]. By contrast, the retinal circulation is able to maintain a constant blood flow at a range of IOPs (between 10 and 34 mm Hg) [8]. Optic nerve blood flow in not uniform in all capillary and post-capillary portions. The prelaminar region receives vessels from the retinal circulation, the laminar region from the choroidal circulation and the retrolaminar region from pial vessels. Blood flow is higher in the laminar portion, as with CBF, but in the prelaminar portions the flow significantly decreases [31].

In our opinion, another very important condition, not sufficiently stressed, for normal optic nerve head circulation and autoregolation is the morphology of the anastomotic circle of Haller-Zinn. Morphological variations in terms of form, position and branches exist among individuals and between the two eyes of the same individual [32].

Choroidal Blood Volume Regulation and Effect on Intraocular Pressure

All previous studies showed that the choroid is incapable of active autoregolation when the perfusion pressure gradient is decreased by raising IOP.

Is there an alternative way? That is, can choroidal blood volume regulation control variations of IOP?

Two simple considerations can help us to answer these two questions. First, the outflow from the choroid is higher than that of the anterior chamber. Second, small variations of volume in the choroidal compartment are able to have a large effect on IOP.

While the choroidal capillaries are very large compared to other capillaries, they also exhibit a wide range of sizes and show a direct connection between arteries and veins.

Vasoconstriction occurs actively when smooth muscle tone is active, and passively when intraluminal pressure is decreased or extraluminal pressure is increased. The first case induces a vascular constriction, the second case a vascular collapse.

Control of these mechanisms depends on transmural vessel pressure or better on parietal tension. The rule regulating parietal tension is La Place's law, which says that the parietal tension depends, above all, on vessel radius. Thus, under external and internal vascular pressures, small vessels have a parietal tension lower than that of larger vessels and each vessel has a critical closing pressure which depends on its radius. In others words, if the choroidal vascular bed is composed of vessels with very different diameters, regulation of critical closing pressure will be finer and more sophisticated and the volume control will be more efficient [33], without causing hypoxic damage due to the elevated CBF.

We believe that ocular hypertension induces a randomized critical closing pressure which

Table 1. Model of choroidal autoregulation of blood flow

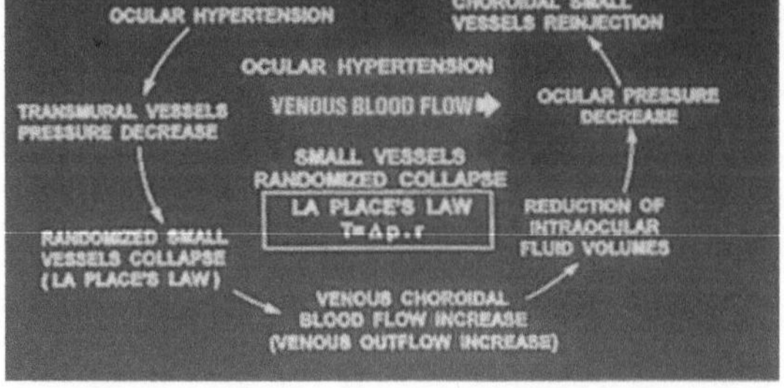

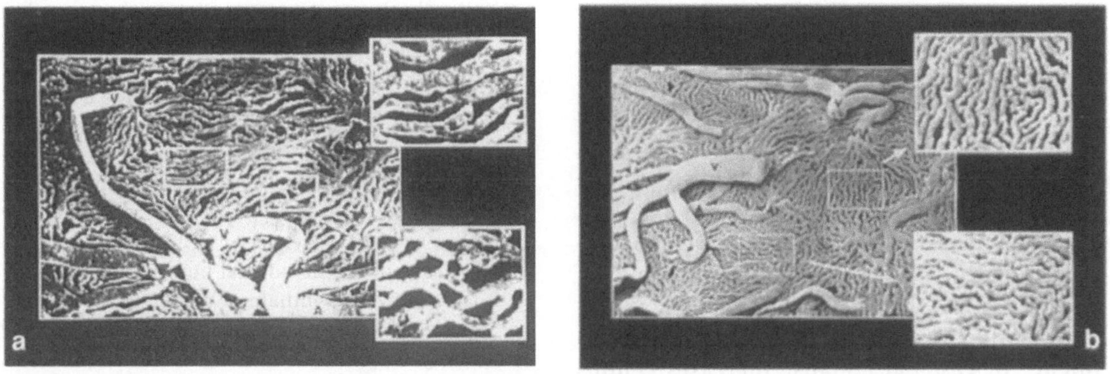

Fig. 1a, b. Corrosion vascular casts (**a**) and scanning electron microscopy (**b**) of human choroidal vasculature at the equator. In both **a** and **b**, evaluation of capillary diameters shows a constant difference in the vessel dimensions. (From [34])

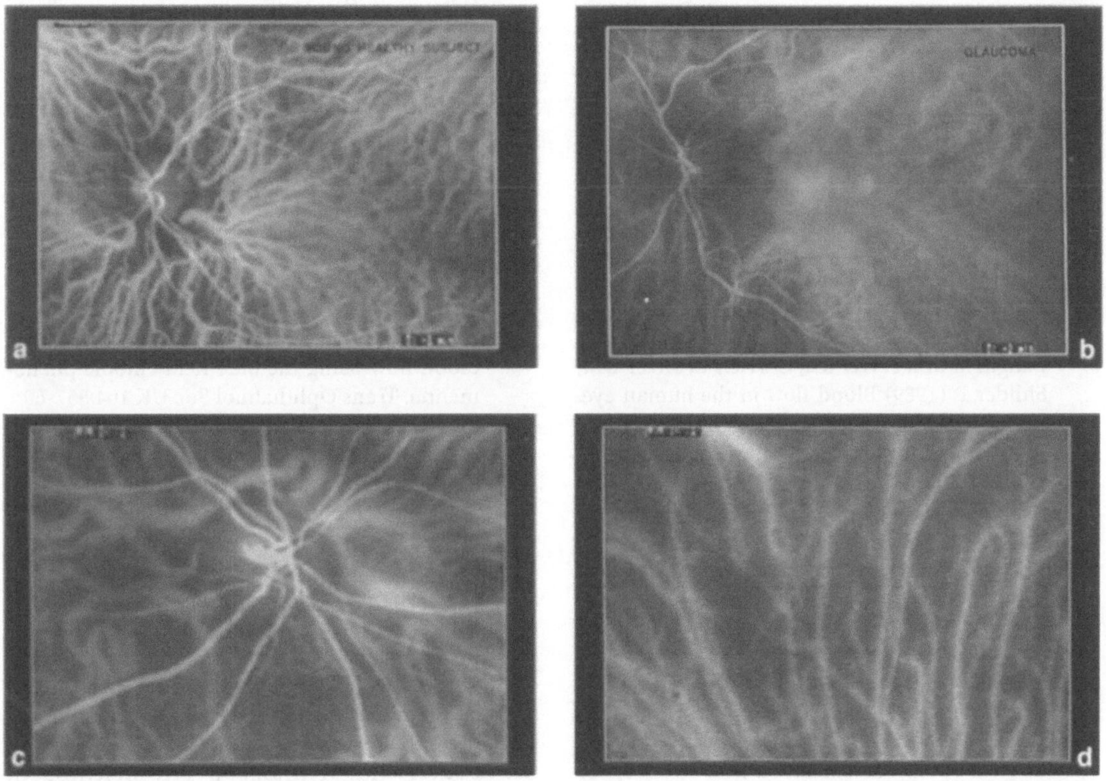

Fig. 2a-d. Choroidal vasculature; scanning laser ophthalmoscope examination of glaucomatous eyes. **a** Young healthy subject; **b-d** glaucomatous eyes, numerous areas of vascular exclusion (probably) representing areas of vascular collapse

increases venous outflow and reduces intraocular flow volumes [33]. Our model of choroidal blood volume regulation is summarized in Table 1.

This model is also valid for choroidal precapillaries and arterioles and is supported by our detailed analysis of choroidal vascular casts and by our recent study of CBF in glaucomatous eyes using the scanning laser ophthalmoscope (SLO). Vascular casts showed constant morphological differences in many vessels: precapillaries, arterioles, venules and capillaries (Fig. 1).

Our SLO studies, not yet statistically checked, show many areas of vascular exclusions, probably representing areas of vascular collapse (Fig. 2).

Summary

After reviewing current knowledge of the autoregulation of OBF in the retina, choroid and optic nerve head circulation, a mechanism of CBF compensation, when IOP increases, can be proposed.
This hypothesis is made possible by considering: high CBF, differences in the dimensions of the choroidal vessels, and La Place's law. During ocular hypertension, a randomized sequence of vascular collapse increases venous CBF with reduction of intraocular fluid volumes and decrease of ocular pressure. Analysis of the diameters of choroidal vessels (from vascular casts) and recent studies of glaucomatous eyes with the SLO may be considered the first data supporting this still controversial hypothesis.

References

1. Williamson TH, Harris A (1994) Ocular blood flow measurement. Br J Ophthalmol 78:939-945
2. Hill DW (1976) Measurement of retinal blood flow. Trans Ophthalmol Soc UK 96:199-201
3. Langham ME, Farrel RA, O'Brien U, Silver DM, Shilder P (1989) Blood flow in the human eye. Acta Ophthalmol Suppl 191:9-13
4. Riva CE, Grunwald JE, Sinclair SH, Petrig BL (1985) Blood velocity and volumetric flow rate in human retinal vessels. Invest Ophthalmol Vis Sci 26:1124-32
5. Williamson TH, Barr D, Baxter GM (1994) Understanding of the retinal circulation provided by an anomalous retinal vein. Br J Ophthalmol 78:798-9
6. Bill A, Sperber GO (1990) Central of retinal and choroidal blood flow. Eye 4:319-25
7. Weiter JJ, Schachar RA, Ernest JT (1973) Control of intraocular blood flow II effects of sympathetic tone. Invest Ophtalmol 12:332-4
8. Riva CE, Grunwald JE, Petrig BL, (1983) Reactivity of the human retinal circulation to darkness: a laser Doppler velocity study. Invest Ophthalmol Vis Sci 24:737-40
9. Linsenmaier RA (1986) Effects of light and darkness on oxygen distribution and consumption in the cat retina. J Gen Physiol 88:521-42
10. Linsenmeier RA, Braun RD (1992) Oxigen distribution and consumption in the cat retina during normoxia and hypoxemia. J Gen Physiol 99:177-97
11. Kiryi J, Asrami S, Shamidi M, Mori M, Zeimer R (1995) Local response of the primate retinal microcirculation to increased metabolic demand induced by flicker. Invest Ophthalmol Vis Sci 36:1240-46
12. Grunwald JE, Deleharty J (1992) Effect of topical carteol on the normal human retinal circulation. Invest Ophthalmol Vis Sci 33:1853-6
13. Medrano CJ, Fox DA (1993) Light-and pharmacologically-induced decreases in rat photoreceptor and inner retinal respiration. Invest Ophthalmol Vis Sci 34 (Suppl): 1279
14. Medrano CJ, Fox DA (1995) Oxygen consumption in the rat outer and inner retina: light- and pharmacologically induced inhibition. Exp Eye Res 61:273-84
15. Feke GT, Zuckerman R, Green GJ, Veiter JJ (1983) Response of human retinal blood flow to light and dark. Arvo Abstracts. Invest Ophthalmol Vis Sci 24:136
16. Tsacopoulos M, David NJ (1973) The effects of arterial pCO_2 on relative retinal blood flow in monkeys. Invest Ophthalmol 12:335-47
17. Hill DW (1989) Ocular and retinal blood flow. Acta Ophthalmol (Suppl) 191:15-8
18. Fallon TJ, Maxwell D, Kohner EM (1985) Measurement of autoregulation of retinal blood flow using the blue field entopic phenomenon. Trans Ophthalmol Soc UK 104:857-60
19. Marris A, Shoemaker JA, Burgoyne J, Weinland M, Cantor LB (1994) The acute effect of topical beta-adrenergic antagonists on normal perimacular haemodidynamics. J Glaucoma (in press)
20. Best M, Blumenthal M, Futterman HA, Galin MA (1969) Critical closure of intraocular blood vessels. Arch Ophthalmol 82:385-92
21. Robinson F, Riva CE, Grunwald JE, Petrig BL, Sinclair SH (1986) Retinal blood flow autoregulation in response to an acute increase in blood pressure. Invest Ophthalmol Vis Sci 27:722-6
22. Baxter GM, Williamson TH, McKillop G, Dutton GN (1992) Color Doppler ultrasound of orbital and optic nerve blood flow: effects of posture and timolol 0.5%. Invest Ophthalmol Vis Sci 33:604-10
23. Williamson TH, Baxter GM, Dutton GN (1993) Doppler velocimetry of the arterial vasculature of the optic nerve head and orbit. Eye 7:74-9
24. Trew DR, Smith SE (1991) Postural study in pulsative ocular blood flow. I ocular hypertension and normotension. Br J Ophthalmol 75: 66-70

Discussion

Question: Bonomi

To Dr. Van Buskirk. You induced vasoconstriction of the optic nerve vessels associated with an enlargement and deepening of the optic disk cup. Is this deepening of the cup associated with one of these findings: a block of assonal flow, a reduction of the number of fiber, or a ganglionar cell loss?

Question: Greve

Well, while he is going to the microphone, I have a question for him. What does he feel about the relation between this phenomenon and what we see in the clinic? There is a tendency, I would say, of the more vascular glaucomas not to have this concentric enlargement?
Do you see this as a glaucoma process or as a secondary process?

Answer: Van Buskirk

The first question had to do with the changes in ganglion cells that we described this morning. We haven't done a study, we are just beginning to develop this model in monkeys; it's more appropriate to do this study on monkeys because of the difference in the laminar region between the monkey and the rabbit. But we want to establish the model in the rabbit first, mainly for economic reasons. So far we have seen an enlargement and a deepening of the cup in a rabbit, but we have not carried the model beyond two months on monkeys, so we have not seen any clinical changes in the monkey as yet.
The enlargement of the cup appears to be diffuse, not focal so far in the rabbit, but really I don't know if the rabbit would apply to a chronical situation.

Question: Greve

I have one question for the last speaker. He mentioned a work, I believe, from the Swedish workers on the flow in the entire portion of the optic nerve head (you quoted Bill and co-workers). You said it is a very high flow like in the choroid. Do I recollect that correctly?

Answer: Bisantis

The flow in the entire portion is not so high because the perfusion is from the retina, and the retina has not a very high blood flow. The flow is relatively high in the laminar portion, not in the post laminar portion for a relative reduction of the blood and tissue relationship, because in the post laminar portion we have the myelinic component and this relatively reduces the amount of blood flow.

Question: Greve

The question I wanted to ask you is: do you think that the fact that these flows are similar in the laminar portion and in the choroid does mean that they are directly connected, how otherwise could one get the same high flows?

Answer: Bisantis

In the lamina the flow is directly connected with the circulation of the choroid because the derivation is from the short posterior ciliary arteries. It is not so high as the choroidal circulation, but it is higher than the prelaminar and rectrolaminar ones.

Question: Greve

Does this have anything to do with supply? Does it mean that it gets blood from the choroid?

Answer: Bisantis

The difference is in the number of vessels, because in the prelaminar region there are not so many vessels as in the choroidal region.

Question: Greve

Van Buskirk wanted to say something about that. An interesting point is where exactly does the blood come from. Many theories have been proposed, and this might be one long-awaited answer.

Answer: Van Buskirk

I tell you what I know about it. Our study suggested that the laminar area derives its blood from branches of the short posterior ciliary arteries.

There is very little, if any, significant communication between the choroid and the laminar region itself. The peripapillary area of the optic nerve has very few vessels; it acts as a watershed zone with branches that go to the choroid and to the optic nerve.

I suspect that flow differences could be explained by the differences in the characteristics of the capillaries in the region; the resistance of the capillary is probably higher in the lamina than in the choroid.

Answer: Quigley

It is not so important, I think, that both the optic nerve head and the choroid receive their blood supply from similar larger arteries, as it is more important that the internal nutrition supplied by the vasculature in each tissue should be studied. Your question, I think, was: can you measure the choroid and the optic nerve head blood flow by similar techniques? The techniques that are appropriate in one tissue are sometimes not appropriate in the other, for example the microsphere technique. What is known is that the optic nerve head does normally have other regulations, in the sense that to a certain level, when the eye pressure rises, the blood flow stays the same. Autoregulation normality is a major susceptibility factor in glaucoma patients that you have heard.

Answer: Bisantis

Also the individual variations of this region and the number of anastomotic systems must be considered. These are not always active and not always similar in a large number of patients.

Question: L. Quaranta

To Dr. Drance. Did you find a greater incidence of papillary hemorrhages in your normal tension glaucoma patients with a greater nocturnal dip of systemic blood pressure?

Answer: Drance

No, we haven't noticed it, but you know, you would notice what you are looking for and we have been occupied with other things in these patients and we haven't particularly looked at the disc during the period of pressure reduction. We are fairly certain that there is no difference between people who have dips and people who don't have dips in the ordinary incidence of the prevalence of hemorrhages in the disc, but your question was: do they arise sometimes during that period? I have no idea, I don't spend my time between 1 o'clock and 6 o'clock in the clinic.

DIAGNOSIS

Imaging Optic Nerve and Nerve Fiber Layer: Optical Coherence Tomography

J.S. Schuman

Glaucoma Service, New England Eye Center, 750 Washington Street, Boston, MA 02111, USA

First I would like to thank the president and the chairman, Professor Bucci who invited me to speak at this meeting. What I would like to discuss this afternoon is a new technology called optical coherence tomography, so I'd like to acknowledge my co-investigators: Tamar Pedut-Kloizman, Ellen Hertzmark, Jason Wilkins, Jeffery Coker, Adarsh Arya, Carmen Pullafito, Lise Pieroth of New England Eye Center, Michael Hee and James Fujimotó of MIT and Eric Swanson at Lincoln Laboratory.

Optical coherence tomography is a means of producing cross-sectional images of tissue using light. It is analogous to CAT scan which uses X-rays, MR imaging which uses spin resonance or ultrasound, but OCT uses light. The principle behind the device is interferometry; there is a superluminiscent diode as the source. Light from the diode is split to a reference arm and to the sample, and both go back to a detector where the signal is received. By using very low coherence light, the width of the signal envelope is limited, and that is how high resolution is achieved with this device. The resolution is in the order of 10 microns in tissue, the sensitivity is extremely high, the incident power on the eye is low well within the ANSI safety standards, it is completely non-contact and non-invasive, and it uses a reliable diode fiber optic system. Our instrument is connected to a slit lamp, although the one that we have is a prototype and future commercial instruments I understand will be integral to a fundus camera.

A number of possibilities exist for the application of OCT in both the anterior and posterior segment. In the anterior segment, OCT can be used for examining corneal thickness and surface profile, anterior chamber depth and the iris; unfortunately the angle structures are shadowed by the sclera and OCT probably is not a good instrument for looking in this area. On the prototype device, there are two galvenometrically driven mirrors, there is a 78D Volk lens, and a fiber optic carries the light from the superluminescent diode and light back to the detector. The OCT image is seen in real time and the infrared fundus image is used for aiming the OCT beam; both of these are displayed on separate monitors and displayed in real time. The OCT examination of the retina is similar to indirect slit lamp biomicroscopy. It uses a STET Volk lens, the patient fixates either on external light or on an internal fixation beam, and the fundus is visualized using infrared light, which is much more comfortable for the patient than visible light. It takes 2.5 seconds using a proprotype device to acquire an image; using a commercial device it is said to take less than 1 second. This is an example of an OCT through a macula. The arrow displays where the OCT was taken, and here you can see the layers of the retina and the foveal pit.

Initially, when we first began investigating this technology, we would simply put in a single probe-beam and receive a signal back; this is analogous to A-scan ultrasound. David Huang, who was a medical student at that time, had the idea of putting a series of these A-scans together, analogous to B-scan ultrasound, and that is how OCT began. We moved from measurements on a transected eye in a cup to in vivo measurement and found that there was an effect due to respiration and pulsation. An algorithm was developed that to process the image, so that the image that I showed you before becomes smooth as you see here on the right.

No depth information is lost using this processing algorithm, the information simply taken from an image like this and winds up to create an image which looks like this.

This is an OCT of the retina moving all the way from the macula across the optic nerve head. You see the foveal pit, and what's interesting here is that you can see the retinal nerve fiber layer, which is the red band here, thickening as you approach the optic disc.

We have found that circular scans are most useful in examining patients with glaucoma. We perform circular scans, around the optic nerve head. The optimal size of the circle that we have found to date is 3.37 mm. As you can see in these two circular scans, the nerve fiber layer is relatively thick close to the optic nerve head, and you can see the double hump pattern that was characterized in terms of nerve fiber layer height by Caprioli. As you move further away from the optic nerve head you can see the entire nerve fiber layer thin somewhat. We have looked at the reproducibility of measurements of nerve fiber layer thickness using OCT and we have found that reproducibility is on the order of 15 to 20 or 30 microns standard deviation.

I'd like to show you a couple of retinal images and then we will turn our attention to glaucoma. First let me show you a macular hole with OCT. This is a patient with a macular hole; this is the clinical photograph and here you can see the macular hole on OCT. You can see the rounded edges of the retina as it appears in the histology books, and the posterior vitreous face. You can measure the distance between the vitreous and the retina, the thickness of the retina, etc. This is a patient with vitreo-macular traction, and what's interesting here is the interface of the vitreous and the retina, and the foveal edema in this area. This patient following the scan had surgery and vision went from 20/200 to 20/40. Macular edema has a characteristic appearance by OCT depending on the type of macular edema. This is a patient with cystoid macular edema and you can see the cystic spaces in the fovea. This patient has a macular edema following a retinal artery occlusion. You can see the cherry red spot in the clinical photograph and the edema in the retina. This is a patient with diabetic macular edema, and you can see that it has a different appearance than the other types of macular edema that I have shown you. We have recently published a study that indicates that the thickness of the macula by OCT in diabetic macular edema correlates well with visual acuity.

Let's turn our attention now to glaucoma. As we know, the nerve fiber layer radiates in these arcuate bundles towards the optic nerve. This is a photo from Dr Quigley which shows the nerve fiber layer very nicely in this patient. OCT can be used for cross sectional imaging of the nerve fiber layer as I mentioned. This is different from other imaging technologies we are using in glaucoma. For instance, confocal scanning laser ophtalmoscopy creates coronal sections through the optic nerve. A series of 32 planes are taken through the optic nerve deeper and deeper into the eye. The nerve fiber analyzer, which is made by Laser Diagnostic Technologies, uses the different approach to quantify nerve fiber layer thickness; the principle is that of elipsometry. Polarized light is shown in the eye using the Nerve Fiber Analyzer, the nerve fiber layer is by birefringent and it rotates the axis of that polarized light, and the degree of rotation is then correlated with nerve fiber layer thickness using this device. Unfortunately, we know that there are other by birefringent structures in the eye. Some early studies with the nerve fiber analyzer have shown that there may be difficulty in picking up areas of focal defects with this device. More needs to be learned about the nerve fiber analyzer.

OCT, in contrast, produces cross-sectional images of the retina from which the nerve fiber layer thickness is quantitated directly. I mentioned that we are performing circular scans around the optic nerve and that this has produced the most valuable information in glaucoma. We can also perform radial scans through the optic nerve head which produces images that look like these. I'd like to show you few case reports on patients with glaucoma using OCT, and then tell you a little bit about our studies in the glaucomatous monkey model and about the pilot study which we reported fairly recently. This is a normal eye, normal optic nerve head, normal fiber layer, normal visual field and this is an OCT in this normal eye. The white line delimits the anterior boundary of the nerve fiber layer and the first blue line delimits the posterior boundary of the nerve fiber layer. The second blue line is the posterior boundary of the retina. This is a cross sectional image through the optic nerve head in this normal individual. The nerve fiber layer thicknesses are summarized here on the bottom by quadrant and by clock hour. This is an individual with glaucomatous cupping. I apologize for this clinical photo; the patient had some nuclear sclerotic cataract, but I think that you can see that there is a thinning of the neuroretinal rim inferotemporally in this individual, and this correlates with a superior arcuate visual field defect. This is the radial scan through the optic nerve head, and the circular scan around the optic nerve head. What's interesting in this individual is the thinning, especially inferiorly, of the nerve fiber layer, which correlates with the nerve fiber layer, with the neuroretinal rim thinning and the visual field defect that we saw.

This individual has a focal nerve fiber layer defect in this area here. Perhaps you can see it better on the red free photograph. This correlates with this inferior nasal defect on the visual field, and on the OCT there is a focal area of thinning. The superior quadrant mean nerve fiber layer thickness is 138 microns, but in the focal area of thinning is 110 microns. This is an individual with two focal defects. You can see a defect here, and a slit-likey defect superiorly. This correlates with the visual field that you see here, and this correlates with the OCT with thinning in this area correlating with this superior slit-like defect and in this area with this broader temporal defect.

This is an individual with end-stage glaucoma, a large cup, a marked visual field defect, and dramatic thinning of the nerve fiber layer. You can also see on the radial scan, the deep cup with steep margins of the optic nerve head.

This is a normal monkey eye and this a stereo disc photograph and a nerve fiber layer photograph from this normal monkey. This is the OCT in this normal monkey eye and a radial scan through the optic nerve head in the normal monkey eye. This is the control eye in that monkey; this is at the beginning of the study before glaucoma was introduced and that was about three or four months into the study after glaucoma has been induced. The monkey has been running pressures in the thirties to forties. You can see the marked cupping that has occurred and the changes in the position of the blood vessels from the beginning to the end of the study. This is a radial scan through the optic nerve head before glaucoma was induced and following several months of glaucoma. This is a nerve fiber layer photo from the beginning of the study before glaucoma was induced and after several months of glaucoma. You can see that the nerve fiber layer has deteriorated markedly over that former period; this is the OCT from the beginning of the study in the glaucomatous eye and towards the end of the study and you can see the marked thinning that has occurred in the nerve fiber layer by OCT. We looked at the change in the nerve fiber layer thickness over time. The triangle represents the control eye and the blue circles represent the study eye. You can see the thinning that occurs in the nerve fiber layer. This is overall and this is in the inferior quadrant, which we feel probably is the most sensitive area to look, and you can easily detect the difference between the glaucomatous and the control eye. This is a scan through a normal monkey eye, and the nerve fiber layer thickness is approximately 140 microns in this area. That correlates with position A, where the nerve fiber layer thickness is approximately 130 microns by histopathology; this is the same eye, same section.

We performed a study, which we published relatively recently, in which we looked at a number of eyes and we found that the mean fiber layer thickness in normal eyes was about 135 microns, and 108 microns in glaucomatous eyes: however, the inferior quadrant nerve fiber layer thickness seems to be somewhat more sensitive in differentiating between normal and glaucomatous eyes. Indeed, in normal eyes we found 165 microns for the inferior quadrant, and 125 microns in glaucoma, which is more than two standard deviations difference. As you can see in this pilot study, the number of normals was small. There was a significant difference between the means, but there was overlap between the two groups. We found that superior visual field defects were associated with significantly thinner inferior nerve fiber layer and inferior visual field defects were associated with thinner superior nerve fiber layer, as you would expect; however, cup to disc ratio was not significantly related to visual field defects. That's not looking at notching or focal thinning, but just cup to disc ratio. We did find a trend for neuroretinal rim area to be associated with field defects. We also found the nerve fiber layer thickness decreased with aging, even controlling for the diagnosis of glaucoma. Here you can see the data on a scatter plot with a regression line drawn showing the thinning of the nerve fiber layer over time. That's been shown clinically by Airaksinen and others, and using the nerve fiber layer analyzer by Kitazawa. This is the data for cup to disc ratio and aging and for neuroretinal rim area and aging, and it shows no relationship for these two parameters with aging.

In conclusion, we feel that OCT can measure nerve fiber layer thickness in normal and glaucomatous eyes; the inferior nerve fiber layer thickness seems to be the best predictor or differentiator of glaucoma and normals; OCT correlates well with conventional technologies including examination of the patient, visual field etc. We are now performing larger National Institute of Health sponsored cross-sectional and longitudinal studies in normal and glaucomatous eyes.

We have also recently concluded a longitudinal study in the glaucomatous monkey model, and we are correlating this data to histopathology. I have given you our data on reproducibility in humans.

Morphological Aspects in the Diagnosis and Pathogenesis of Glaucomatous Optic Neuropathy*

J.B. Jonas

Department of Ophthalmology and Eye Hospital, University Erlangen-Nürnberg, Schwabachanlage 6, 91054 Erlangen, Germany

Introduction

The optic disc, optic nerve head or optic papilla as it was originally termed by William Briggs (1650-1704) is the internal surface of the posterior scleral foramen through which the retinal ganglion cell axons leave the eye. This posterior scleral opening forms a truncated cone with a narrow neck internally (diameter 1.5 to 2.0 mm) and a broad base externally (diameter: 3.5 mm). The optic disc is divided into the intrapapillary region containing the optic cup and the neuroretinal rim, and the parapapillary region with the chorioretinal atrophy. The intrapapillary region is separated from the parapapillary region by the peripapillary scleral ring of Elschnig forming the wall of the optic disc. Important variables to describe the optic disc morphology are: 1) optic disc size; 2) optic disc form; 3) size and 4) shape of the neuroretinal rim; 5) optic cup size in relation to the optic disc area; 6) cup to disc ratios; 7) presence and location of splinter-shaped hemorrhages; 8) occurrence, size, configuration and location of the parapapillary chorioretinal atrophy; 9) diameter of the retinal vessels; and 10) visibility of the retinal nerve fiber layer.

Optic Disc Size

Similar to the size of the inner aperture of the scleral optic nerve canal, the area of the optic disc shows an interindividual variability of 1:7 in a normal population [1-3]. Based on the Gaussian-like distribution curve of the optic disc area, microdiscs and macrodiscs can be defined morphometrically: a microdisc as being smaller than the mean minus twofold standard deviation and a macrodisc as being larger than the mean plus twofold standard deviation. Beyond each of these limits only 2.3% of a standard population can be expected. The macrodiscs can further be divided 1) into primary macrodiscs that are constant in size after birth and that can be subclassified into the subgroup of asymptomatic primary macrodiscs without any morphologic or functional defects [4], and the subgroup of primary symptomatic macrodiscs with morphologic and functional defects such as optic disc pits [5] and "Morning-Glory-Syndrome" [6]; and 2) into acquired or secondary macrodiscs increasing in size postnatally and occuring in eyes with secondary macrophthalmus as is the case in high myopia and congenital glaucoma [7].
This interindividual optic disc size variability is morphogenetically and pathogenetically important. Morphogenetically, because eyes with large optic discs as compared to eyes with small optic nerve heads have 1) a larger neuroretinal rim area [2, 3, 8-10]; 2) more optic nerve fibers [11, 12]; 3) less nerve fiber crowding per mm^2 disc area [12]; 4) a higher count and a larger total area of lamina cribrosa pores [13]; 5) a higher ratio of interpore connective tissue area to total lamina cribrosa area [13]; 6) a higher count of cilioretinal arteries [14]; and 7) a

* Supported by Deutsche Forschungsgemeinschaft (Klinische Forschergruppe "Glaukome", grant number Na 55/6-2)

higher count of retinal photoreceptors [15] and retinal pigment epithelium cells [16] in combination with a larger retinal surface area [15].

The optic disc size variability is pathogenetically important because some optic nerve anomalies and diseases are correlated with the optic disc size: optic disc drusen [17, 18], pseudopapilledema [19, 20] and nonarteritic anterior ischemic optic neuropathy [21, 22] occur significantly more often in small optic discs while pits of the optic disc [5] and the Morning-Glory-Syndrome [6] are more common in large optic nerve heads. Eyes with arteritic anterior ischemic optic neuropathy [22], retinal vessel occlusions [23] and primary open-angle glaucoma [24] have normal-sized optic discs.

In glaucoma, the optic disc has been reported to be abnormally large in eyes with normal-pressure glaucoma [25-27] while another study suggested that this finding could at least partially be due to an artifact by the selection of patients [28]. Eyes with pseudoexfoliative glaucoma [25] and eyes with primary pigment dispersion glaucoma [29] have been reported to have a slightly smaller optic disc than normal eyes. For all three of these glaucoma types an artifact by the selection of patient has, however, not been ruled out yet. Eyes with primary open-angle glaucoma have a normal sized optic disc [24].

Within a range of - 5 to + 5 diopters of refractive error, the optic disc size is independent of the degree of ametropia [3]. In eyes with high myopia, it is significantly larger [7] and in eyes with marked hyperopia (> +5 D) it is significantly smaller than in eyes with a normal refractive error.

Similar to the optic disc area, the horizontal optic disc diameter also is not interindividually constant showing a variability of 1:2.9 [3]. In spite of that, the optic disc diameter has been taken as interindividual size unit to compare intraocular lesions such as malignant melanomas. For an even more exact investigation, therefore, the lesion similar to the optic disc should be measured in absolute size units that are millimeter with correction of the photographic magnification [30-35] instead of taking the interindividually variable disc diameter.

The optic disc size can be determined using optic disc photographs, plotting the outlines of the optic disc structures on paper and evaluating planimetrically the figure [3], or with the help of computerized semiautomatic optic disc analyzers such as laser scanning ophthalmoscopes [34].

As an alternative to these sophisticated and time consuming techniques, more simple methods exist [36-40]. For the latter, the horizontal and vertical disc diameters can be measured ophthalmoscopically using a standard Goldmann three mirror contact lens and a commercial slit lamp with adjustable length of the beam [38]. The values of the horizontal and vertical disc diameters have to be multiplied by a factor of 1.26 to receive the same results as by measuring the optic disc on photographs and correcting the ocular and camera magnification factor. Based on these direct measurements of the horizontal and vertical disc diameters, one calculates the optic disc area by applying the formula of an ellipse (area = $\pi/4$ times horizontal diameter times vertical diameter) [41]. The error for the ophthalmoscopic determination of the disc diameters is 6.4 ± 4.8% (mean ± SD). It is independent of the optic disc size and the refractive error for a range of -5 diopters to +5 diopters. The error for the calculation of the optic disc area by applying the formula of an ellipse and taken into account the horizontal and vertical disc diameters as measured upon ophthalmoscopy is 9.3 ± 6.7%.

Concerning the optic disc size, one has also to take into account that the optic disc area varies between the various ethnical groups. It is relatively small in Caucasians, medium sized in Mexicans and Asians, and relatively large in Afro-Americans [42-45].

Optic Disc Form

The optic disc has a slightly vertically oval form with the vertical diameter being about 10% larger than the horizontal one [3]. The disc form is not correlated with age, sex and right and left eye. For a myopic refractive error of less than -8 diopters, normal eyes and glaucoma eyes do not differ significantly ($p > 0.20$) in their slightly vertically oval optic disc shape [46]. Within the primary open-angle glaucoma group, the optic disc shape is not correlated with the neuroretinal rim area and the mean perimetric defect, neither interindividually nor in an intraindividual bilateral comparison [46]. In highly myopic eyes, besides being larger, the optic disc is significantly more ovally configurated, more obliquely orientated than in any other group [7].

In contrast to the size of the optic nerve head, the optic disc shape does not show a pronounced interindividual variability. As single variable, it is not markedly important for diagnosis and pathogenesis of glaucoma [46]. This is valid for eyes with a myopic refractive error of less than -8 diopters. In highly myopic eyes, the myopic stretching of the globe might lead to an abnormal optic disc shape in combination with a secondary enlargement of optic disc [47]. This may be important for the susceptibility to glaucomatous optic nerve fiber loss.

Neuroretinal Rim Size

As the intrapapillary extension of the retinal nerve fibers, the neuroretinal rim is one of the main targets in the intravital evaluation of the optic nerve. The neuroretinal rim size is not interindividually constant but shows similar to the optic disc and cup a considerably high variability. It is correlated with the optic disc area: the larger the disc, the larger the rim [2, 3, 8-10]. This correlation rim area/disc area corresponds with the positive correlation between optic disc size on one hand and optic nerve fiber count [11, 12] and count and summed area of the lamina cribrosa pores [13] on the other hand. It points towards a greater anatomic reserve capacity in eyes with large optic discs. In the scattergram of the correlation rim area to disc area [3] three subgroups of optic nerve heads are included: 1) in optic nerve heads with circular steep cupping the optic cup more than the neuroretinal rim enlarges with increasing optic disc area; 2) in optic discs with temporal flat sloping the neuroretinal rim more than the optic cup enlarges in relation to the optic disc; and 3) in discs without cupping the neuroretinal rim is identical in size and form with the optic disc. Possible reasons for the interindividual size variability of the rim are a different nerve fiber count, a different relation between embryologically formed and regressed retinal ganglion cell axons [4, 48], different density of nerve fibers within the optic disc, different lamina cribrosa architecture, different diameters of retinal ganglion cell axons, different proportion of glial cells on the whole intrapapillary tissue, and/or other factors.

The nerve fibers within the neuroretinal rim are retinotopically arranged [50, 51]. Axons from ganglion cells close to the optic disc lie more centrally in the optic disc while axons from cells in the retinal periphery lie at the optic nerve head margins. This corresponds to the nerve fiber distribution in the retinal nerve fiber layer [50, 51].

Neuroretinal Rim Shape

In normal eyes, the neuroretinal rim shows a characteristic configuration based on the vertically oval optic disc and the horizontally oval optic cup [3]: it is significantly broadest at the inferior disc pole, followed by the superior pole, the nasal disc area, and finally the temporal disc region. This form is correlated with 1) the diameter of the retinal artery and vein that are significantly wider in the inferior temporal arcade than in the superior temporal arcade [52]; 2) the visibility of the retinal nerve fiber bundles that are significantly more often better detectable in the inferior temporal region than in the superior temporal region [53, 54]; 3) the location of the foveola 0.53 ± 0.34 mm inferior to the optic disc center [53]; and 4) the morphology of the lamina cribrosa with the largest pores and relatively the least amount of interpore connective tissue in the inferior and superior regions as compared to the temporal and nasal sectors [13, 55].

Although the neuroretinal rim is broadest in the inferior part of the optic disc, the neuroretinal rim above a horizontal line drawn through the center of the foveola is larger than below this line. It is explainable by the location of the foveal centre temporal inferior to the optic disc. It corresponds to the higher differential light sensitivity in the inferior visual field than in the superior visual hemisphere.

In glaucoma, the rim loses area and changes its form [31, 56-63]. In cross-section and longitudinal studies, glaucomatous rim loss started in the temporal inferior disc region, followed by the temporal superior region, the temporal horizontal area, the nasal inferior region and finally the nasal superior region [58, 64].

It indicates that for an early diagnosis of glaucoma especially the temporal inferior and the temporal superior disc sectors should be checked for glaucomatous changes. One of the reasons for the sequence of disc sectors concerning the glaucomatous neuroretinal rim loss may be the anatomy of the lamina cribrosa with the larger pores and the less amount of interpore connective tissue in the inferior and superior disc regions than in the temporal and nasal disc areas [13, 55]. Taking into account the slightly ecentric location of the retinal vessel trunk in the nasal upper quadrant of the vertically oval optic disc [13], one can infer that the progressive sequence of rim loss in glaucoma may also be dependent upon the distance of the region to the retinal vessel trunk; the further away the region from the retinal vessel trunk, the more likely it is to be affected by rim loss [65]. As a corollary, glaucoma eyes with an atypical location of the retinal vessel trunk or an unsual optic disc form were found to exhibit an abnormal glaucomatous rim configuration.

Optic Cup Size in Relation to the Optic Disc Area

The intrapapillary region as the area inside of the peripapillary scleral ring consists of the neuroretinal rim and the optic cup. In normal eyes, the cup form is horizontally oval with the horizontal diameter being about 7.7% longer than the vertical diameter [3]. Parallel to the optic disc and the neuroretinal rim, also the optic cup shows a high interindividual variability [3, 4]. Similar to macrodiscs macrocups can be defined as being larger than the mean plus twofold standard deviations. The macrocups can be subdivided into: 1) primary macrocups that are also called pseudoglaucomatous but physiologic macrocups in primary macrodiscs [4]; and into 2) acquired or secondary macrocups that occur in normal sized eyes with glaucomatous optic nerve damage, and in eyes with secondary macrophthalmus due to congenital glaucoma.
The areas of the optic disc and optic cup are correlated with each other: the larger the optic disc, the larger the optic cup [2, 3]. In small optic discs cupping normally does not occur. In morphologic glaucoma diagnosis, this feature has to be taken into account because early glaucomatous optic nerve damage resulting in relatively low cup/disc ratios of 0.2 or 0.3 can be "hidden" in such small optic discs [66]. Glaucomatous eyes with small optic discs can have low cup/disc ratios but often show abnormalities in the parapapillary region [67, 68] including the retinal nerve fiber layer.
In contrast to nonglaucomatous optic nerve damage [69], the optic cup enlarges progressively in glaucoma due to the loss of neuroretinal rim [31, 56-63]. The cup increase is an important parameter in the differential diagnosis of eyes with glaucoma compared to eyes with nonglaucomatous optic nerve atrophy. Simultaneous to the cup enlargement in glaucoma, the cup depeens. This cup deepening depends on the height of intraocular pressure and varies between the different types of glaucoma [47].

Cup/Disc Ratios

Due to the vertically oval optic disc and the horizontally oval optic cup, the cup/disc ratios in normal eyes are horizontally significantly larger than vertically [3]. In less than 7% of normal eyes, the horizontal cup/disc ratio is smaller than the vertical one. It indicates that the quotient of the horizontal to vertical cup/disc ratio is normally smaller than 1.0 . It is important for the diagnosis of glaucoma, in which usually the vertical cup/disc ratio increases faster than the horizontal one leading to a quotient of the horizontal to vertical cup/disc ratio higher than 1.0 [24, 70].
As ratio of cup diameter to disc diameter, the cup/disc ratios depend on the optic disc and cup size that both show a considerably high interindividual variability and that both are correlated with each other. Eyes with small optic discs have small cups, and eyes with large optic nerve heads have large cups. Accordingly, cup/disc ratios ranging in a normal population from 0.0 to 0.84 are low in small optic nerve heads, and they are high in large optic discs [3]. An unusually high cup/disc ratio, therefore, can be physiologic in eyes with large optic nerve heads [4] while an average cup/disk ratio is uncommon in normal eyes with small optic discs. In the diagnosis of glaucomatous optic

nerve damage, this interindividual variability of cup/disc ratios and their dependence on the optic disc size has to be taken into account. Eyes with physiologically high cup/disc ratios in macrodiscs should not be overdiagnosed considered to be glaucomatous [4], and eyes with increased intraocular pressure, small optic nerve heads, and average or low cup/disc ratios should not be underdiagnosed regarded to be only "ocular hypertensive" without signs of glaucomatous optic nerve damage [66].

Optic Disc Hemorrhages

Splinter-shaped or flame-shaped hemorrhages at the border of the optic disc are a hallmark of glaucomatous optic nerve atrophy [71-75]. Very rarely found in normal eyes, these disc hemorrhages are detected in about 4% to 7% of glaucoma eyes. Their frequency increases from an early stage of glaucoma to a medium advanced stage and decreases again towards a very far advanced stage [75]. The disc hemorrhages are not found in disc regions or eyes without detectable neuroretinal rim [75]. In early glaucoma they are usually located in the temporal inferior or superior disc regions. They are found less often in secondary open-angle glaucoma and more frequently in normal-pressure glaucoma than in primary open-angle glaucoma [47, 75]. They are correlated with localized retinal nerve fiber layer defects, neuroretinal rim notches and circumscribed perimetrical loss [72, 74, 75]. They are visible about for 4 to 12 weeks after the initial bleeding [76]. After the same period, often a localized defect or a broadening of a localized retinal nerve fiber layer can be detected correlating with a circumscribed scotoma in the visual field [73]. Flame-shaped optic disc hemorrhages indicate the presence and progression of glaucoma. They can be helpful for the classification of the glaucoma type.

Parapapillary Chorioretinal Atrophy

In the parapapillary region the chorioretinal atrophy [67, 77-87] bordering the optic disc can be classified into two zones [67, 88, 89]. A peripheral zone (zone Alpha) is characterized by an irregular hypo- and hyperpigmentation and intimated thinning of the chorioretinal tissue layer. On its outer side it is adjacent to the retina, and on its inner side it is in touch with a zone characterized by visible sclera and visible large choroidal vessels (zone Beta), or with the peripapillary scleral ring, respectively. Features of the inner zone (zone Beta) are marked atrophy of the retinal pigment epithelium and of the choriocapillaris, good visibility of the large choroidal vessels and the sclera, thinning of the chorioretinal tissues, and round borders to the adjacent zone Alpha on its peripheral side and to the peripapillary scleral ring on its central side. If both zones are present, zone Beta is always closer to the optic disc than zone Alpha. The histologic equivalent of zone Beta is a complete loss of retinal pigment epithelium and of choriocapillaris, the ophthalmoscopic appearance of zone Alpha is caused by irregularities of the retinal pigment epithelium and the parapapillary choroid [87, 90, 91]. In normal eyes, both zones Alpha and Beta are largest and most frequent in the temporal horizontal sector, followed by the inferior temporal area and the superior temporal region. They are smallest and most rare in the nasal parapapillary area. Zone Alpha with a mean frequency of 83.9% is more common than zone Beta (mean frequency: 16.3%) [67]. Zones Alpha and Beta have to be differentiated from the scleral crescent in eyes with high myopia and from the inferior scleral crescent in eyes with "tilted optic discs".

Both zones are in normal eyes and eyes with nonglaucomatous descending optic nerve atrophy not significantly different in size, form and frequency [92], while in eyes with glaucomatous optic nerve atrophy both zones are significantly larger and zone Beta occurs more often than in the normal eyes. Size of both zones and frequency of zone Beta are significantly correlated with variables indicating the severity of the glaucomatous optic nerve damage such as neuroretinal rim loss, decrease of retinal vessel diameter, reduced visibility of the retinal nerve fiber bundles, and perimetric defects [67, 88, 89]. The location of the parapapillary chorioretinal atrophy is spatially correlated with the neuroretinal rim loss in the intrapapillary region. It is larger in that sector with the more marked rim loss. It is associated with shallow disc cupping, a high degree of fundus tessellation and only slightly elevated intraocular pressure [67]. In contrast to glaucomatous eyes, the parapapillary atrophy is normal in eyes with nonglaucomatous optic nerve atrophy including those eyes after nonarteritic anterior ischemic optic neuropathy [69, 92]. Evaluation of the parapapillary atrophy can therefore be helpful in the differential diagnosis of glaucomatous and nonglaucomatous optic nerve damage.

Diameter of Retinal Vessels

The diameter of retinal vessels is decreased in eyes with glaucomatous and nonglaucomatous optic nerve damage as compared with normal eyes [52, 92, 93]. It points at a secondary diminution of the vessel caliber due to the decreased count of optic nerve fibers and retinal ganglion cells. A small retinal vessel diameter can be taken as relative indicator of an optic nerve damage independently of a glaucomatous or a nonglaucomatous genesis. It is not pathognomonic for glaucoma.

Besides a general decrease of the diameter of the retinal arterioles, a focal narrowing of the retinal arterioles has recently been described [94, 95]. It was significantly and positively correlated with age in normal subjects. It occurs significantly more often and more pronounced in the eyes with optic neuropathies than in the normal eyes when matched for age. In glaucoma eyes, focal narrowing of the arterioles is significantly correlated with the degree of optic nerve damage. Besides a tendency towards a more marked vessel narrowing in eyes with normal-pressure glaucoma, focal narrowing of the retinal arterioles does not vary significantly between the various optic neuropathies when matched for neuroretinal rim area and visual field defect [95]. It is independent of an enlarged parapapillary chorioretinal atrophy. Similar to general constriction, focal narrowing of the retinal arterioles is found more frequently and more marked in eyes with glaucomatous or nonglaucomatous optic nerve damage than in normal eyes. As it is the case for the generalized reduction of the diameter of the retinal arterioles, focal narrowing is typical for optic nerve atrophy, but not pathognomonic for glaucoma.

Evaluation of the Retinal Nerve Fiber Layer

Normal Eyes

The retinal nerve fiber layer (RNFL) contains the retinal ganglion cell axons covered by astrocytes and bundled by processes of Müller cells [96]. Since it is part of the afferent visual pathway, its evaluation is essential for diagnosis of optic nerve anomalies and diseases. It can be assessed ophthalmoscopically or on wide-angle red-free photographs. For its ophthalmoscopical evaluation, it is helpful to use green light. In eyes with opaque media, a yellow lens coloration, and a low degree of pigmentation of the retinal pigment epithelium, the RNFL is worse visible than in eyes with clear media and deeply pigmented retinal pigment epithelium.

The retinal nerve fiber layer is composed of ganglion cell axons, astrocytes, retinal vessels, and Müller cell processes forming as their basal lamina the inner limiting membrane as vitreal covering of the nerve fiber layer. The ganglion cell axons leave their cell body in vitreal direction, pierce through the axons of those ganglion cells located more peripherally and bend towards the optic disc forming then the inner part of the nerve fiber layer. They are incompletely enveloped by astrocyte processes still allowing direct but functionally probably unimportant axon-axon contact. Axons from neighbouring ganglion cells are grouped into adjacent fiber bundles by elongated sheetlike processes of Müller cells with some exchange of axons between the bundles. Lateral dissemination of individual fibers is not extensive and a retinotopic organisation is preserved.

The axons of the ganglion cells nasally to optic disc run directly towards the optic disc while those of the ganglion cells in the temporal fundus describe an arcuate course around the fovea. By that they are divided into a superior temporal and inferior temporal group touching each other at the temporal raphe that extends from the foveola to the temporal periphery of the retina.

The nerve fiber layer thickness increases from the fundus periphery to the optic disc with regional differences. It is thickest at the vertical optic disc poles and thinner at the temporal and nasal optic disc borders [97-100]. This corresponds to: 1) the configuration of the neuroretinal rim that is significantly broadest at the inferior disc pole, followed by the superior disc pole, the nasal disc region, and finally the temporal disc border [3]; and 2) the ophthalmoscopic visibility of the retinal nerve fiber bundles that are significantly better detectable in the inferior and superior parapapillary areas than at the temporal and nasal optic disc borders [53, 54]. In the foveal region nerve fibers are absent.

The pattern of the fiber bundles can be detected as bright striations in the retinal reflex by clinical ophthalmoscopy and on red-free wide-angle fundus photographs. It is most obvious where the nerve fiber layer is thickest. The bright striations of the fiber bundles are offset by darker elongated processes of Müller cell origin surrounding the bundles. In normal eyes the retinal nerve fiber bundles are ophthalmoscopically significantly more often better detectable in the inferior temporal arcade than in the superior temporal arcade. This points to a higher accumulation of nerve fibers in the inferior temporal region corresponding to: 1) the form of the neuroretinal rim as described above; 2) the diameter of the retinal vessels that are significantly wider in the inferior temporal arcade than in the superior temporal arcade [52]; and 3) the location of the foveola about 0.53 + 0.34 mm inferior to the optic disc center [53].

With a diameter of about 20 μm the nerve fiber bundles are larger than the spatial resolution of the eye limited by diffraction of the pupil and chromatic and spheric aberration of cornea and lens. The nerve fibers themselves with a mean diameter of 1 μm are considerablely smaller than the ocular spatial resolution and can thus not be detected ophthalmoscopically. It explains why in advanced optic nerve atrophy a nerve fiber layer can not be seen ophthalmoscopically although nerve fibers and visual function may still partially be preserved.

The diameter of the nerve fibers is smaller in the temporal parapapillary region than in the nasal region or at the vertical optic disc poles. Nerve fibers of the superior temporal or inferior temporal arcade sampled in the peripapillary region contain relatively more small fibers than when sampled in a greater distance from the disc. Axon bundles of the papillomacular area sampled near the optic disc contain relatively large fibers than close to the foveola. This corresponds to: 1) the presumed higher density of Beta ganglion cells in the fovea and higher density of Alpha ganglion cells in the fundus periphery; and 2) the distribution of the nerve fiber diameter in the retrobulbar portion of the optic nerve in the temporal part of which the nerve fiber diameter is significantly smaller than in its nasal region.

Astrocytes and Müller cells as neuroglial system surround the nerve fibers and provide a structural framework supporting the neural elements. The Müller cells occupy nearly all intercellular retinal space and form as their basal lamina the inner limiting membrane. The astrocyte processes envelop all nerve fibers giving structural and nutritional support, and in combination with the pericytes they cover the retinal capillaries isolating the retinal ganglion cells and their axons from the retinal blood flow. This complex of astrocyte and Müller cell channels, established early in embryogenesis, may play some role in the development and orientation of axons as they grow from the ganglion cells toward the optic papilla.

The large retinal blood vessels, arterioles and venoles lie in the superficial part of the nerve fiber layer. They are partially covered by nerve fibers causing blurred imaging. In nerve fiber loss the vessels lose their nerve fiber covering and are more sharply demarcated. A clear outlining of the retinal blood vessels can thus be taken as hint for optic nerve damage. Within the superior temporal and inferior temporal arcade the arterioles are runnning in the center of the main nerve fiber bundle striation while the course of the venoles often located in the periphery of the fiber bundle striation is more irregular.

In normal eyes, visibility of the RNFL is regionally uneven distributed [53, 54]. Dividing the fundus into eight regions, the nerve fiber bundles are best visible in the temporal inferior sector, followed by the temporal superior area, the nasal superior region and finally the nasal inferior sector. It is least visible in the superior, inferior, temporal horizontal and nasal horizontal regions. Correspondingly, the retinal artery diameter is significantly widest at the temporal inferior disc border, followed the temporal superior disc region, the nasal superior area and finally the nasal inferior disc region. This is in agreement with the configuration of the neuroretinal rim that is broadest at the temporal inferior disc border, followed the temporal superior disc region. The sectors' sequence concerning the best visibility of the RNFL correlates with the sectors' sequence in respect to rim configuration and retinal artery caliber. Physiologically, it points towards an anatomical and nutritional relationship. Visibility of the RNFL decreases with age [53, 54]. This correlates with an age-related reduction of the optic nerve fiber count with an annual loss of about 4.000 to 5.000 fibers/year out of an original population of presumably 1.5 million optic nerve fibers [12, 101-103]. These features of the normal RNFL are important for diagnosis of RNFL changes secondary to optic nerve damage in the diseased eye.

Glaucoma

By definition, glaucomatous optic nerve atrophy is associated with an optic nerve fiber loss and thus decreased visibility of the RNFL. This nerve fiber loss can occur in a diffuse way or in form of localized defects [104-108].

Diffuse Retinal Nerve Fiber Layer Loss

The diffuse loss in the visibility of the RNFL is more difficult to be detected than localized defects. It is helpful to determine the sectors' sequence with regard to the best visibility of the RNFL [53, 54]. If the RNFL is much better visible in the temporal superior region than in the temporal inferior sector, a loss of retinal nerve fibers might have occurred in the inferior temporal area. It is also useful to estimate how sharply the retinal vessels can be seen.
Normally, they are partially covered by some nerve fibers crossing them on their way to the optic disc. This results in an unsharp imaging of the retinal vessels. In eyes with nerve fiber loss, the vessels are uncovered and more clearly visible.

Localized Retinal Nerve Fiber Layer Loss

The localized RNFL-defects are defined as wedge-shaped areas with their basis often reaching the temporal horizontal fundus raphe and with their tip touching the optic disc border [104-108]. Ophthalmoscopically and on red-free photographs, they appear darker than the surrounding retina. Since they are not present in normal eyes, they signify an abnormality. They can occur in many optic nerve diseases such as optic disc drusen, tumors of the pituitary gland and the glaucoma. They should not be confounded with slit-like or fusiform pseudodefects, which fail to fan out from the disc to periphery. These are of no diagnostic significance since they are encountered in many normal eyes.
In glaucoma the localized RNFL-defects are most frequently detected in the temporal inferior region followed by the temporal superior fundus area. In cross-section studies they are found in about 20% of the eyes examined. Their frequency increases significantly from an "early" glaucoma stage to a subgroup with medium advanced glaucomatous damage and decreased again to a stage with marked glaucomatous changes [108]. They can be proceeded by optic disc hemorrhages about six to eight weeks earlier [72, 73]. They correspond with localized deep scotomata in the visual field and with neuroretinal rim notches. Within the glaucoma group, localised RNFL-defects occur most often ($P<0.05$) in normal pressure glaucoma, followed by primary open-angle glaucoma and finally secondary open-angle glaucoma [74, 108]. They are positively associated with disc haemorrhages [73, 75]. Since they are usually not present in normal eyes, the localized RNFL defects have a high specificity to indicate an optic nerve damage. Being present also in eyes with slight neuroretinal rim loss, they are helpful in the diagnosis of early glaucoma [107]. The association between localised RNFL-defects and disc haemorrhages and the varying frequency of disc hemorrhages and localised RNFL-defects in different types of glaucoma is diagnostically and pathogenetically [109] important.

Differences in the Appearance of the Optic Disc between Various Types of the Glaucomas

Primary open-angle glaucoma

Eyes with high myopia (refractive error >-8 diopters) ("highly myopic type of primary open-angle glaucoma"): secondary macrodiscs with elliptical form, flat and concentric cupping, relatively low frequency of disc hemorrhages and localized RNFL defects, large parapapillary atrophy, diffuse nerve fiber loss, normal or almost intraocular pressure readings. Diffuse type of glaucomatous optic nerve damage.

Eyes with normal or only moderately elevated intraocular pressure and marked fundus tessellation ("senile sclerotic" or better "atrophic" type of primary open-angle glaucoma): normal optic disc size and shape, shallow concentric cupping, relatively low frequency of disc hemorrhages and localized retinal nerve fiber layer defects, large parapapillary atrophy, diffuse nerve fiber loss, diffuse visual field loss; normal or almost intraocular pressure readings. Diffuse type of glaucomatous optic nerve damage.

Eyes with normal intraocular pressure, a normal refractive error and no marked fundus tessellation ("focal type of primary open-angle glaucoma"): optic disc with presumably normal size and with normal shape, deep and steep cupping, parapapillary atrophy equal in size compared to eyes with primary open-angle glaucoma, relatively high frequency of disc hemorrhages, localized RNFL defects and circumscribed perimetric defects. Focally accentuated type of glaucomatous optic nerve damage.

Eyes with primary open-angle glaucoma and patient age < 40 years ("juvenile type of primary open-angle glaucoma"; "barotraumatic type of primary open-angle glaucoma"): normal-sized and normal-shaped optic disc, deep and steep disc cupping, relatively low frequency of neuroretinal rim notches, disc hemorrhages and localized retinal nerve fiber layer defects, small parapapillary atrophy, highly elevated intraocular pressure. Diffuse type of glaucomatous optic nerve damage.

Secondary open-angle glaucoma

- Due to primary melanin dispersion syndrome ("pigmentary glaucoma"): abnormally small optic discs [29]
- due to pseudoexfoliation syndrome ("pseudoexfoliative glaucoma"): optic disc size probably slightly smaller than in primary open-angle glaucoma [25].

Optic Disc Morphology in Ocular Hypertensive Eyes

In ocular hypertensive eyes as compared to the normal eyes, significant differences can be detected for a smaller area and an abnormal shape of the neuroretinal rim, larger zones α and β of the parapapillary chorioretinal atrophy, a decreased visibility of the RNFL and a higher frequency of localized nerve fiber layer defects [68]. The variables most useful to indicate an optic nerve damage are an abnormal shape of the neuroretinal rim and a decreased visibility of the nerve fiber layer. The most specific variable is the presence of localized retinal nerve fiber layer defects. Evaluation of these variables is helpful for the early diagnosis of glaucoma.

References

1. Franceschetti A, Bock RH (1950) Megalopapilla: A new congenital anomaly. Am J Ophthalmol 33:227-235
2. Bengtsson B (1976) The variation and covariation of cup and disc diameters. Acta Ophthalmol 54:804-818
3. Jonas JB, Gusek GC, Naumann GOH (1988) Optic disc, cup and neuroretinal rim size, configuration, and correlations in normal eyes. Invest Ophthalmol Vis Sci 29:1151-1158; Correction: Invest Ophthalmol Vis Sci (1992); 33:474-475
4. Jonas JB, Zäch FM, Gusek GC, Naumann GOH (1989) Pseudoglaucomatous physiologic large cups. Am J Ophthalmol 107:137-144
5. Jonas JB, Naumann GOH (1987) Papillengruben in großen Papillae nervi optici. Papillometrische Charakteristika in 15 Augen. Klin Monatsbl Augenheilkd 191:287-291
6. Jonas JB, Koniszewski G, Naumann GOH (1989) "Morning-Glory-Syndrome" bzw. "Handmannsche Anomalie" in kongenitalen Makropapillen. Extremvariante "konfluierender Papillengruben"?. Klin Monatsbl Augenheilkd 195:371-374
7. Jonas JB, Gusek GC, Naumann GOH (1988) Optic disk morphometry in high myopia. Graefe's Arch Clin Exp Ophthalmol 226:587-590
8. Betz Ph, Camps Fr, Collignon-Brach C, Weekers R (1981) Photographie stéréoscopique et photogrammétrie de l'excavation physiologique de la papille. J Fr Ophtalmol 4:193-203
9. Caprioli J, Miller JM (1987) Optic disc rim area

is related to disc size in normal subjects. Arch Ophthalmol 105:1683-1685
10. Britton RJ, Drance SM, Schulzer MD, Douglas GR, Mawson DK (1987) The area of the neuroretinal rim of the optic nerve in normal eyes. Am J Ophthalmol 103:497-504
11. Quigley HA, Coleman AL, Dorman-Pease ME (1991) Larger optic nerve heads have more nerve fibers in normal monkey eyes. Arch Ophthalmol 109:1441-1443
12. Jonas JB, Schmidt AM, Müller-Bergh JA, Schlötzer-Schrehardt UM, Naumann GOH (1992) Human optic nerve fiber count and optic disc size. Invest Ophthalmol Vis Sci 33:2012-2018.
13. Jonas JB, Mardin CY, Schlötzer-Schrehardt U, Naumann GOH (1991) Morphometry of the human lamina cribrosa surface. Invest Ophthalmol Vis Sci 32:401-405
14. Jonas JB, Guggenmoos-Holzmann I, Naumann GOH (1988) Cilioretinal arteries in large optic discs. Ophthalmic Res 20:269-274
15. Panda-Jonas S, Jonas JB, Jakobczyk M, Schneider U (1994) Retinal photoreceptor count, retinal surface area, and optic disc size in normal human eyes. Ophthalmology 101:519-523
16. Panda-Jonas S, Jonas JB, Jakobczyk-Zmija M (1996) Retinal pigment epithelium cell count, density and correlations in normal human eyes. Am J Ophthalmol 121:181-189
17. Spencer WH (1978) Drusen of the optic disc and aberrant axoplasmatic flow. The XXXIV Edward Jackson Memorial Lecture. Am J Ophthalmol 85:1-12
18. Jonas JB, Gusek GC, Guggenmoos-Holzmann I, Naumann GOH (1987) Optic nerve head drusen associated with abnormally small optic discs. Int Ophthalmol 11:79-82
19. Rosenberg MA, Savino PJ, Glaser JA (1979) A clinical analysis of pseudopapilledema. I. Population, laterality, acuity, refractive error, ophthalmoscopic characteristics, and coincident disease. Arch Ophthalmol 97:65-70
20. Jonas JB, Gusek GC, Guggenmoos-Holzmann I, Naumann GOH (1988) Pseudopapilledema associated with abnormally small optic discs. Acta Ophthalmol 66:190-193
21. Beck RW, Savino PJ, Repka MX, Schatz NJ, Sergott RC (1984) Optic disc structure in anterior ischemic optic neuropathy. Ophthalmology 91:1334-1337
22. Jonas JB, Gusek GC, Naumann GOH (1988) Anterior ischemic optic neuropathy:nonarteritic form in small and giant cell arteritis in normal sized optic discs. Int Ophthalmol 12:119-125
23. Gusek GC, Jonas JB, Naumann GOH (1990) Retinale Gefäßverschlüsse sind unabhängig von der Papillengröße. Klin Monatsbl Augenheilkd 197:14-17
24. Jonas JB, Gusek GC, Naumann GOH (1988) Optic disc morphometry in chronic primary open-angle glaucoma. I. Morphometric intrapapillary characteristics. Graefe's Arch Clin Exp Ophthalmol 226:522-530
25. Tuulonen A, Airaksinen PJ (1992) Optic disc size in exfoliative, primary open-angle and low-tension glaucoma. Arch Ophthalmol 110:211-213
26. Burk ROW, Rohrschneider K, Noac H, Völcker HE (1992) Are large optic nerve heads susceptible to glaucomatous damage at normal intraocular pressure? Graefe's Arch Clin Exp Ophthalmol 230:552-560
27. Jonas JB (1992) Size of glaucomatous optic discs. Ger J Opthalmol 1:41-44
28. Jonas JB, Stürmer J, Papastathopoulos KI, Meier-Gibbons F, Dichtl A (1995) Optic disc size and optic nerve damage in normal-pressure glaucoma. Br J Ophthalmol 79:1102-1105
29. Jonas JB, Dichtl A (1995) Optic disc size in pigmentary glaucoma. AAO-Abstract. Ophthalmology 102 (Suppl.):136
30. Littmann H (1982) Zur Bestimmung der wahren Größe eines Objektes auf dem Hintergrund des lebenden Auges. Klin Monatsbl Augenheilkd 180:286-289
31. Betz Ph, Camps F, Collignon-Brach J, Lavergne G, Weekers R (1982) Biometric study of the disc cup in open-angle glaucoma. Graefe's Arch Clin Exp Ophthalmol 218:70-74
32. Airaksinen PJ, Drance SM (1985) Neuroretinal rim area and retinal nerve fiber layer in glaucoma. Arch Ophthalmol 103:203-204
33. Caprioli J, Klingbeil U, Sears M, Pope B (1986) Reproducibility of optic disc measurements with computerized analysis of stereoscopic video images. Arch Opthalmol 104:1035-1039
34. Burk ROW, Rohrschneider K, Takamoto T, Völcker HE, Schwartz B (1993) Laser scanning tomography and stereophotogrammetry in three-dimensional optic disc analysis. Grafe's Arch Clin Exp Ophthalmol 231:193-198
35. Funk J (1991) Early detection of glaucoma by longitudinal monitoring of the optic disc structure. Graefe's Arch Clin Exp Ophthalmol 229:57-61
36. Montgomery D (1991) Measurement of optic disc and neuroretinal rim areas in normal and glaucomatous eyes. Ophthalmology 98:50-59
37. Spencer AF, Vernon SA (1994) Optic disc measurement with the Zeiss four mirror contact lens. Br J Ophthalmol 78:775-780
38. Jonas JB, Papastathopoulos KI (1995) Ophthalmoscopic measurement of the optic disc. Ophthalmology 102:1102-1106
39. Gross P, Drance SM (1995) Comparison of sim-

ple ophthalmoscopic and planimetric measurement of glaucomatous neuroretinal rim. J Glaucoma 4:314-316
40. Spencer F, Vernon SA (1996) Repeatability and reproducibility of optic disc measurements with the Zeiss 4-mirror contact lens. Ophthalmology 103:163-167
41. Jonas JB, Königsreuther KA, Montgomery DMI (1994) Calculation of the optic disc and cup area by the minimal and maximal diameters (Brief Report). Br J Ophthalmol 78:510
42. Beck RW, Messner DK, Musch DC, Martonyi CL, Lichter PR (1985) Is there a racial difference in physiologic cup size? Ophthalmology 92:873-876
43. Chi T, Ritch R, Stickler D, Pitman B, Tsai C, Hsieh FY (1989) Racial differences in optic nerve head parameters. Arch Ophthalmol 107:836-839
44. Mansour AM (1989) Racial variation of optic disc size. ARVO Abstract. Invest Ophthalmol Vis Sci (Suppl) 30:367
45. Varma R, Tielsch JM, Quigley HA, Hilton SC, Katz J, Spaeth GL, Sommer A (1994) Race-, age-, gender-, and refractive error-related differences in the normal optic disc. Arch Ophthalmol 112:1068-1076
46. Jonas JB, Papastathopoulos KI (1996) Optic disc shape in glaucoma. Graefe's Arch Clin Exp Ophthalmol 1996 (in press)
47. Jonas JB, Xu L (1993) Optic disc morphology in different types of glaucoma. ARVO-Abstract. Invest Ophthalmol Vis Sci 34:761
48. Rajic P, Riley KP (1983) Overproduction and elimination of retinal axons in the fetal rhesus monkey. Science 219:1441-1444
49. Provis JM, van Driel D, Billson FA, Russel P (1985) Human fetal optic nerve: overproduction and elimination of retinal axons during development. J Comp Neurol 238:92-110
50. Radius RL, Anderson DR (1979) The course of axons through the retina and the optic nerve head. Arch Ophthalmol 97:1154-1158
51. Wolff E, Penman GG (1950) The position occupied by the peripheral retinal fibre in the nerve-fibre layer and at the optic nerve head. Acta XVI Concilium Ophthalmologicum 1:625-635
52. Jonas JB, Nguyen XN, Naumann GOH (1989) Parapapillary retinal vessel diameter in normal and glaucoma eyes. I. Morphometric data. Invest Ophthalmol Vis Sci 30:1599-1603
53. Jonas JB, Nguyen NX, Naumann GOH (1989) The retinal nerve fiber layer in normal eyes. Ophthalmology 96:627-632
54. Jonas JB, Schiro D (1993) Normal retinal nerve fiber layer visibility correlated to rim width and vessel caliber. Graefe's Arch Clin Exp Ophthalmol 231:207-211
55. Radius RL, Gonzales M (1981) Anatomy of the lamina cribrosa in human eyes. Arch Ophthalmol 99:2159-2162
56. Airaksinen PJ, Drance SM, Schulzer M (1985) Neuroretinal rim area in early glaucoma. Am J Ophthalmol 99:1-4
57. Caprioli J, Miller JM, Sears M (1987) Quantitative evaluation of the optic nerve head in patients with unilateral visual field loss from primary open-angle glaucoma. Ophthalmology 94:1484-1487
58. Tuulonen A, Airaksinen PJ (1991) Initial glaucomatous optic disk and retinal nerve fiber layer abnormalities and the mode of their progression. Am J Ophthalmol 111:485-490
59. Airaksinen PJ, Tuulonen A, Alanko HI (1992) Rate and progression of neuroretinal rim area decrease in ocular hypertension and glaucoma. Arch Ophthalmol 110:210-226
60. Caprioli J (1992) Discrimination between normal and glaucomatous eyes. Invest Ophthalmol Vis Sci 33:153-159
61. Tuulonen A, Airaksinen PJ, Schwartz B, Alanko HI, Juvala PA (1992) Neuroretinal rim area measurements by confuguration and pallor in ocular hypertension and glaucoma. Ophthalmology 99:1111-1116
62. Tuulonen A (1993) The morphological pattern of early glaucomatous damage. Curr Opinion Ophthalmology 4:29-34
63. Zeyen TG, Caprioli J (1993) Progression of disc and field damage in early glaucoma. Arch Ophthalmol 111:62-65
64. Jonas JB, Fernández M, Stürmer J (1993) Pattern of glaucomatous neuroretinal rim loss. Ophthalmology; 100:63-67
65. Jonas JB, Fernández MC (1994) Shape of the neuroretinal rim and position of the central retinal vessels in glaucoma. Br J Ophthalmol 78:99-102
66. Jonas JB, Fernández MC, Naumann GOH (1990) Glaucomatous optic nerve damage in small discs with low cup/disk ratios. Ophthalmology 97:1211-1215
67. Jonas JB, Fernández MC, Naumann GOH (1992) Glaucomatous parapapillary chorioretinal atrophy: occurrence and correlations. Arch Ophthalmol 110:214-222
68. Jonas JB, Königsreuther KA (1994) Optic disk appearance in ocular hypertensive eyes. Am J Ophthalmol 117:732-740
69. Jonas JB, Xu L (1993) Optic disc morphology in eyes after nonarteritic anterior ischemic optic neuropathy. Invest Ophthalmol Vis Sci 34:2260-2265
70. Jonas JB, Gusek GC, Naumann GOH (1988) Optic disc morphometry in chronic primary open-angle glaucoma. II. Correlation of the intrapapillary parameters to visual field indices. Graefe's Arch Clin Exp Ophthalmol

226:531-538
71. Drance SM, Fairclough M, Butler DM, Kottler MS (1977) The importance of disc hemorrhage in the prognosis of chronic open-angle glaucoma. Arch Ophthalmol 95:226-228
72. Airaksinen PJ, Mustonen E, Alanko HI (1981) Optic disc haemorrhages - An analysis of stereophotographs and clinical data of 112 patients. Arch Ophthalmol 99:1795-1801
73. Airaksinen PJ, Heijl A (1982) Visual field and retinal nerve fiber layer in early glaucoma after optic disc haemorrhage. Acta Ophthalmol 61:186-194
74. Kitazawa Y, Shirato S, Yamamoto T (1986) Optic disc hemorrhage in low-tension glaucoma. Ophthalmology 93:853-857
75. Jonas JB, Xu L (1994) Optic disc hemorrhages in glaucoma. Am J Ophthalmol 118:1-8
76. Heijl A (1986) Frequent disc photography and computerized perimetry in eyes with optic disc hemorrhage. Acta Ophthalmol 64:274
77. Bücklers M (1929) Anatomische Untersuchung über die Beziehung zwischen der senilen und myopischen circumpapillären Aderhautatrophie. Unter Beifügen eines Falles von hochgradiger Anisometropie. Arch für Ophthalmol 121:243-283
78. Primrose J (1971) The incidence of the peripapillary halo glaucomatosus. Trans Ophthalmol Soc UK 89:585-588
79. Hayreh SS (1969) Blood supply of the optic nerve head and its role in optic atrophy, glaucoma and oedema of the optic disc. Brit J Ophthalmol 53:721-748
80. Wilensky JT, Kolker AE (1976) Peripapillary changes in glaucoma. Am J Ophthalmol 81:341-345
81. Anderson DR (1983) Correlation of the peripapillary damage with the disc anatomy and field abnormalities in glaucoma. Doc Ophthalmol Proc Ser 35:1-10
82. Heijl A, Samander C (1985) Peripapillary atrophy and glaucomatous visual field defects. Doc Ophthalmol Proc Ser 42:403-407
83. Airaksinen PJ, Juvala PA, Tuulonen A, Alanko AI, Valkonen R, Tuohino A (1987) Change of peripapillary atrophy in glaucoma. In: Krieglstein GK (ed) Glaucoma Update III. Springer-Verlag, Berlin-Heidelberg, pp 97-102
84. Nevarez J, Rockwood EJ, Anderson DR (1988) The configuration of peripapillary tissue in unilateral glaucoma. Arch Ophthalmol 106:901-903
85. Rockwood EJ, Anderson DR (1988) Acquired peripapillary changes and progression in glaucoma. Graefe's Arch Clin Exp Ophthalmol. 226:510-515
86. Buus DR, Anderson DR (1989) Peripapillary crescents and halos in normal-tension glaucoma and ocular hypertension. Ophthalmology. 96:16-19
87. Fantes FE, Anderson DR (1989) Clinical histologic correlation of human peripapillary anatomy. Ophthalmology 96:20-25
88. Jonas JB, Nguyen NX, Gusek GC, Naumann GOH (1989) Parapapillary chorio-retinal atrophy in normal and glaucoma eyes. I. Morphometric data. Invest Ophthalmol Vis Sci 30:908-918
89. Jonas JB, Naumann GOH (1989) Parapapillary chorio-retinal atrophy in normal and glaucoma eyes. II. Correlations. Invest Ophthalmol Vis Sci 30:919-926
90. Jonas JB, Königsreuther KA, Naumann GOH (1992) Optic disc histomorphometry in normal eyes and eyes with secondary angle-closure glaucoma. II. Parapapillary region. Graefe's Arch Clin Exp Ophthalmol 230:134-139
91. Kubota T, Jonas JB, Naumann GOH (1993) Direct clinico-histological correlation of parapapillary chorioretinal atrophy. Br J Ophthalmol 77:103-106
92. Jonas JB, Fernández MC, Naumann GOH (1991) Parapapillary atrophy and retinal vessel caliber in nonglaucomatous optic nerve damage. Invest Ophthalmol Vis Sci 32:2942-2947
93. Frisén L, Claesson M (1984) Narrowing of the retinal arterioles in descending optic atrophy. A quantitative clinical study. Ophthalmology 91:1342-1346
94. Rader J, Feuer J, Anderson DR (1994) Peripapillary vasoconstriction in the glaucomas and the anterior ischemic optic neuropathy. Am J Ophthalmol 117:72-80
95. Papastathopoulos KI, Jonas JB (1995) Focal narrowing of retinal arterioles in optic nerve atrophy. Ophthalmology 102:1706-1711
96. Jonas JB, Dichtl A (1996) Evaluation of the retinal nerve fiber layer. Surv of Ophthalmol 40:369-378
97. Radius RL (1980) Thickness of the retinal nerve fiber layer in primate eyes. Arch Ophthalmol 98:1625-1629
98. Quigley HA, Addicks EM (1982) Quantitative studies of retinal nerve fiber layer defects. Arch Ophthalmol 100:807-814
99. Takamoto T, Schwartz B (1989) Photogrammetic measurement of the nerve fiber layer thickness. Ophthalmology 96:1315-1319
100. Schwartz B, Takamoto T (1992) Retinal nerve fiber layer thickness and its functional correlations with the visual field. Bull Soc Belge Ophthalmol 244:64-72
101. Oppel O (1963) Mikroskopische Untersuchung über die Anzahl und Kaliber der markhaltigen Nervenfasern im Fasciculus opticus des menschen. Graefe's Arch Clin Exp Ophthalmol 166:18-19
102. Balazsi AG, Rootman J, Drance SM, Schulzer M,

Douglas GR (1984) The effect of age on the nerve fiber population of the human optic nerve. Am J Ophthalmol 97:760-766
103. Mikelberg FS, Drance SM, Schulzer M, Yidegiligne HM, Weis MM (1989) The normal human optic nerve. Axon count and axon diameter distribution. Ophthalmology 96:1325-1328
104. Airaksinen PJ, Drance SM, Douglas GR, Mawson DK, Nieminen H (1984) Diffuse and localized nerve fiber loss in glaucoma. Am J Ophthalmol 98:566-571
105. Airaksinen PJ, Lakowski R, Drance SM, Price M (1986) Color vision and retinal nerve fiber layer in early glaucoma. Am J Ophthalmol 101:208-213
106. Quigley HA Katz J, Derick RJ, Gilbert D, Sommer A (1992) An evaluation of optic disc and nerve fiber layer examinations in monitoring progression of early glaucoma damage. Ophthalmology 99:19-28
107. Tuulonen A, Lehtola J, Airaksinen PJ (1993) Nerve fiber layer defects with normal visual fields. Ophthalmology 100:587-598
108. Jonas JB, Schiro D (1994) Localized wedge shaped defects of the retinal nerve fiber layer in glaucoma. Br J Ophthalmol 78:285-290
109. Drance SM (1988) Mechanisms of optic nerve damage in glaucoma. Fortschr Ophthalmol 85:611-613
110. Spaeth GL, Hitchings RA, Silavingam E (1976) The optic disc in glaucoma: pathogenetic correlation of five patterns of cupping in chronic open-angle glaucoma. Trans Am Acad Ophthalmol Otolaryngol 81:Op-217-223
111. Drance SM, Airaksinen PJ, Price M, Schulzer M, Douglas GR, Tansley BW (1986) The correlation of functional and structural measurements in glaucoma patients and normal subjects. Am J Ophthalmol 102:612-616
112. Geijssen HC, Greve EL (1987) The spectrum of primary open-angle glaucoma I: senile sclerotic glaucoma versus high tension glaucoma. Ophthalmic Surgery 18:207-213
113. Geijssen C (1991) Studies on normal pressure glaucoma. Kugler Publications, Amstelveen, Netherlands
114. Spaeth GL (1992) Development of glaucomatous changes of the optic nerve. In: Varma R, Spaeth GL (eds) The optic nerve in glaucoma. Lippincott Co, Philadelphia p 79
115. Caprioli J (1993) Correlation between disc appearance and type of glaucoma. In: Varma R, Spaeth GL (eds) The optic nerve in glaucoma. Lippincott Co, Philadelphia, pp 91-98
116. Spaeth GL (1994) A new classification of glaucoma including focal glaucoma. Surv Ophthalmol 38 (Suppl.) S9-S17

Sensivity and Specificity of Diagnostic Parameters of Glaucoma

N. Orzalesi, S. Miglior, and L. Rossetti

Eye Clinic of the University of Milan, S. Paolo Hospital, Via di Rudinì 8, 20142 Milan, Italy

Introduction

Glaucoma is defined by the occurrence of optic nerve atrophy and visual field changes in the presence of increased intraocular pressure (IOP) (primary open angle glaucoma, POAG) or normal IOP (low tension glaucoma, LTG).
Several diagnostic parameters are used in the clinical setting in order to better evaluate glaucomatous eyes and eyes at risk for glaucoma: IOP (once a day assessment, diurnal curve, etc.), visual field testing (kinetic, static, computerized, blue on yellow, high pass, etc.), optic disc evaluation (ophthalmoscopy, photography, tomography, etc.), and retinal nerve fiber layer evaluation (red-free photography, scanning laser ophthalmoscopy, polarimetry, etc.). The assessment of colour vision, contrast sensitivity and electroretinographic activity [1] as well as a series of provocative tests may also be used, but their diagnostic validity is less relevant.
Although all of these diagnostic parameters may be taken into account in the clinical setting, it is well known that not all of them may give the same result: positive (i.e., the patient has glaucoma), or negative (i.e., the patient does not have glaucoma). The most common situation in a "glaucoma suspect" patient is that only a subset of the diagnostic procedures is positive. Such a situation may also occur in the case of a totally normal patient (when one would expect only negative results to be obtained) or in the case of a glaucomatous patient (when one would expect only positive results to be obtained). Such a limitation holds in the various stages of glaucoma either when examining a patient for the first time or when monitoring the same patient in order to detect changes related to the progression of the disease.
Given the clinical relevance of functional damage, visual field defects, particularly those assessed by means of central threshold computerized perimetry, are usually considered as the gold standard (i.e., the reference parameter) for the diagnosis of glaucoma (Table 1).

Table 1. Statistical definitions

Gold standard	Ideally, the most precise indicator of the disease (e.g., biopsy). In most cases, the diagnostic test, which more precisely indicates the presence of the disease, commonly used to assess sensitivity and specificity of other diagnostic procedures.
Sensitivity	The proportion of true positives correctly identified by the test.
Specificity	The proportion of true negatives correctly identified by the test.
Validity, accuracy or diagnostic precision	The proportion of true positives plus true negatives correctly identified by the test.
Cut off	Threshold value of the measured diagnostic parameter (e.g., tonometry) which separates normals from abnormals.

Sensitivity and specificity of the diagnostic parameters in detecting glaucoma refer to visual field assessment and may vary with the stage of the disease. However, the use of standard visual field assessment procedures can lead to misconceptions regarding the utility of new procedures. In fact, when visual field assessment is used as the gold standard and compared to new tests, it is assumed that the standard should have a higher sensitivity and specificity than the new procedures. However a new test may classify the eyes differently, because it may correctly identify some of the false positives and false negatives missed by the gold standard. However, identifying a proportion of glaucoma suspects as "abnormal" does not imply that the new test is more sensitive than the gold standard, as only conversion to glaucoma in the course of a prolonged follow-up will allow the assumption of increased sensitivity of the new test to be confirmed [2].

Actually, the aim of much of the medical research in the field of glaucoma has been to improve the methods of early diagnosis, and advanced technology has allowed the development of new, often highly sophisticated, tools for this purpose. Before discussing the value of all these tests, we must remember that the sensitivity and specificity of any diagnostic parameter vary along with the cutoff point used to separate normal from diseased people. The choice of a cutoff is not a statistical decision, but should be made according to the relative costs (not necessarily financial) associated with false positive and false negative test results. This in turn will be related to the clinical implications that will follow a positive test and whether the test is a screening test or a diagnostic test (to be used for diagnosis and follow-up). A practical approach to determine the cutoff value which fits with the highest sensitivity and specificity is to plot the sensitivity vs. specificity for each possible cutoff. The curve thus obtained is known as a receiver operating characteristic (ROC) curve. The area under the curve is used as a score (SS) for the global separation ability (i.e., clinical validity) of the diagnostic test. The theoretical maximum of SS is 1 if the curve reaches the upper left corner of the diagram (sensitivity and specificity = 1) (Fig. 1).

Another important issue, particularly when dealing with early diagnosis, is related to the validation of new diagnostic parameters. Some of these are highly sophisticated methods that have been designed to "catch" the smallest amount of difference between healthy and abnormal patients. When judging the value of such tests one should always consider the methodological variability of the test (repeatability and reproducibility) and the actual clinical relevance of the test results.

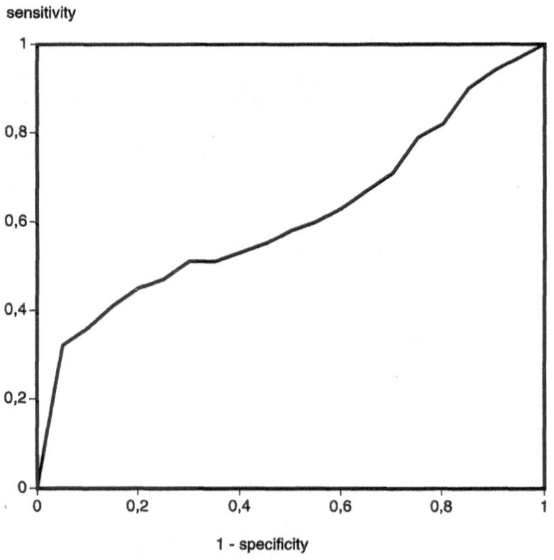

Fig. 1. Receiver operating characteristics curve for rim/disc area ratio in the diagnosis of glaucoma

If the detection of glaucoma in the advanced phases only seldom represents a diagnostic problem, the assessment of the clinical validity of available methods in monitoring the disease may be crucial.

The aim of this report is to review the clinical validity of the most important diagnostic parameters and procedures in the assessment of glaucoma, both in the early and more advanced stages, and in the detection of progression. The statistical definitions adopted in the text are listed in Table 1.

Intraocular Pressure Measurement

Evaluation of IOP has traditionally been the cornerstone for diagnosis and follow-up of the disease. Although IOP is the most important known risk factor for developing glaucoma, its role in the disease is still debated. In fact, there is not a clear threshold value of IOP that is indicative of pathologic changes and, eventually, glaucoma. While glaucomatous changes are directly associated with markedly increased IOP (close to central retinal diastolic pressure), for IOP values ranging from 20 to 30 mm Hg a direct linear relationship between pressure levels and visual dysfunction has not been convincingly demonstrated, and most patients

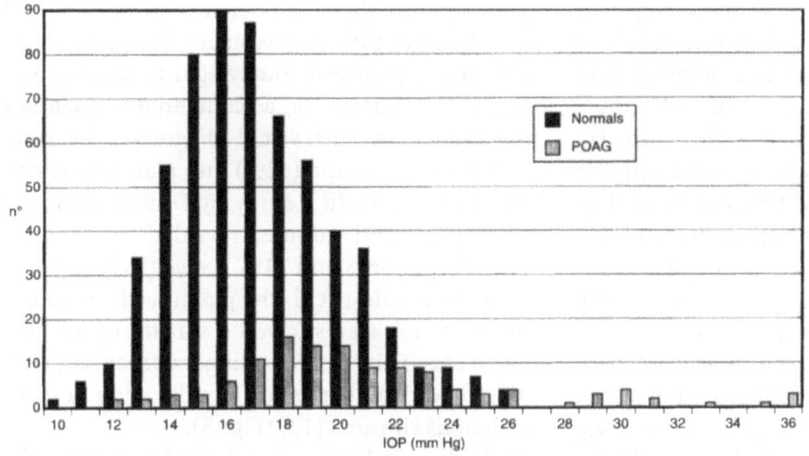

Fig. 2. Distribution of IOP in normal and glaucomatous patients. The overlap in pressure levels between the two groups is so great that tonometry is diagnostically almost of no value in all but the most extreme cases

with glaucoma have IOP levels in that range. To further complicate the assessment of the relationship between IOP and visual loss in glaucoma, there are the "incomplete syndromes", that is the LTGs in which typical glaucomatous visual field and disc damage appear with normal (or lower than normal) IOP levels, and the "ocular hypertensives" with elevated IOPs and absolutely normal fields and discs (Fig. 2).

A number of epidemiologic studies have shown that elevated IOP is an important risk factor for developing glaucoma and that the prevalence of the disease tended to increase with the height of the screening IOP value, particularly at levels above 30 mm Hg (relative risk = 39.0). Although the risk of glaucoma was low at lower IOP levels, the vast majority of all cases in the population (included the cases with glaucoma) had "low" IOP (< 21 mm Hg).

Data from most large-scale epidemiologic studies [3, 4] indicated that at least half of glaucomatous eyes had a screening IOP below 21 mm Hg. Using the data from those large-scale epidemiologic studies and assuming a prevalence of the disease in the Western adult population of about 0.5% and of ocular hypertension of 7.5%, it is possible to calculate a rough estimate of the sensitivity and specificity of the IOP measurement as a screening test for the diagnosis of glaucoma, adopting the conventionally accepted cutoff value for IOP of 21 mm Hg [4]. Sensitivity is low, approximately 50%, and in a hypothetical screening with a single tonometric measurement one is likely to overlook about half of the "true glaucomas". This is confirmed by recent data from the Baltimore Eye Survey, indicating that the sensitivity of IOP to detect glaucoma was about 40% for a cutoff of 20.5 mm Hg [5]. By contrast, at this cutoff, specificity of tonometric measurement is high (about 90%); in fact, within the entire adult population enrolled in the screening, a value of IOP ≤ 21 mm Hg is strongly indicative of a normal condition, and the probability of being normal given a normal value of IOP is very high. Nevertheless, the diagnostic yield of IOP measurement, after full clinical diagnostic work-up in all the patients with a positive test result, again is very low, around 3-4%. This is true because within an adult population an IOP > 21 mm Hg is a relatively frequent condition compared to having glaucoma and, although incidence of glaucoma among ocular hypertensives is about 15 times that observed among normotensives [4], a large number of patients with IOP > 21 mm Hg need to be completely and properly examined in order to diagnose a relatively small number of glaucoma cases.

Monitoring IOP provides more information for the diagnosis of the disease than does one tonometric measurement. A large-scale epidemiologic study in the USA showed that in glaucomatous eyes the IOP tended to rise on follow-up, in contrast with nonglaucomatous eyes in which the IOP was as likely to rise as to fall [3]. Screening with at least two tonometric measurements seemed to improve the performance of the test in detecting glaucoma, although, overall, sensitivity remained low.

Other important issues are whether the IOP levels are specific and sensitive indicators for monitoring the course of the disease and whether the assessment of reduction of IOP is of value for preventing further visual loss. There are data from retrospective studies indicating that there is a clear relationship between levels of IOP under treatment and the rate of visual field loss over time. In particular, the rate of annual field loss in the group with IOP > 22 mm Hg was reported to be double as compared with the group in which IOP ranged between 14 and 16 mm Hg [6]. However, other authors focusing on the same clinical question failed to find a significant association between mean level of IOP and rate of visual field damage [7]. These kinds of studies might be subjected to a number of systematic errors that could considerably affect their results and conclusions. Only a large-scale randomized clinical trial will allow establishment of the clinical validity of IOP measurement as a proper surrogate for assessment of visual function [8].

Optic Disc Evaluation

Optic disc evaluation is an objective procedure, which is not negatively affected by variable performances of the patient (as may happen in the case of visual field testing), allows the detection of extremely typical structural changes (the pattern of glaucomatous cupping is almost unique) and may be quantitatively performed and recorded by means of several modern instruments with manual or automatic procedures. A series of new diagnostic parameters have been developed to better discriminate between normal and glaucomatous optic discs [9]. For this reasons optic disc evaluation is a major step in the diagnosis of glaucoma.

As far as sensitivity and specificity in detecting glaucomatous damage is concerned, optic disc evaluation has shown a generally limited sensitivity and specificity in discriminating between normal and glaucomatous eyes in cross-sectional studies. This is explained by the marked overlap of optic disc planimetric measurements, cup/disc ratio (c/d), rim area, rim area/disc area ratio, etc., between normal and glaucomatous eyes. The only parameter which showed a high SS as calculated by means of ROC curves were the maximum vertical c/d (SS = 0.96), and rim area in the vertical direction (SS = 0.86) as calculated by the Optic Nerve Head Analyzer (ONHA) [10]. In a study by O'Connor et al., the qualitative evaluation of stereoscopic color optic disc photographs showed a sensitivity of 72% and specificity of 87% in measuring the presence or absence of glaucomatous visual field loss (diagnostic precision 82%) as compared to quantitative evaluations such as c/d (diagnostic precision = 59%), cup volume (62%) and planimetric rim area (65%) [11]. In a study by Drance et al., the vertical c/d and rim area revealed a diagnostic precision of 86% and 71%, respectively [1]. In a study by Orzalesi et al., the planimetric measurement of rim area showed a sensitivity of 31% and a specificity of 96% using a nomogram with 95% prediction bands for identification of glaucomatous rim area [12] (Fig. 3).

Optic disc evaluation is extremely useful in the detection of glaucoma onset or progression (particularly in the early stages of the disease). Studies of human specimens showed that a certain number of retinal nerve fibers (RNFs) are lost before the onset of detectable visual field defects [13]. Sommer et al. observed the presence of retinal nerve fiber layer defects 6 years before field loss in 60% of their patients with ocular hypertension at baseline [14]. As a good clinical correlation between progressive RNF loss and progressive morphometric optic disc changes in glaucoma has been observed [15, 16], a decrease in rim disc area over time may be assumed to be an estimate of progressive RNF atrophy. Odberg and Riise, in reporting the results of the first prospective study of sequential optic disc stereophotography, confirmed the impression that, in the earliest stages of the disease, a decrease in the neuroretinal rim area of the disc may be observed before the occurrence of visual field defects [17]. Quigley et al. showed that qualitative optic disc changes preceded visual field loss in seven of 37 (19%) ocular hypertensive (OHT) patients at baseline who converted to POAG during a follow-up of 5 years [16].

Optic disc evaluation by means of planimetry and visual field testing have different degrees of sensitivity in detecting progressive structural and functional changes according to the stage of the disease. Only a few studies have quantitatively compared the rates of disc [18] and visual field changes among patients at high risk of developing glaucoma and patients with glaucoma [19, 20]. Their results indicate that measurable optic disc changes precede visual field loss in the early glaucomatous stages. Zeyen and Caprioli and Miglior et al. documented the higher sensitivity of optic disc planimetry with

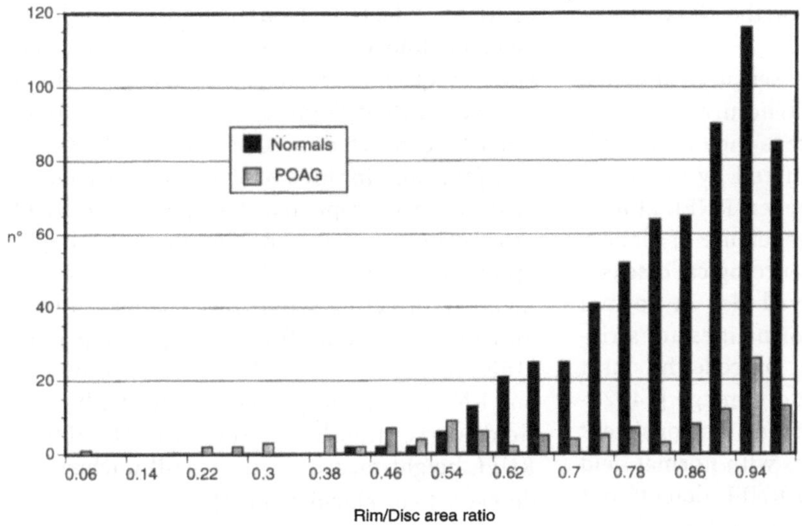

Fig. 3. Distribution of rim/disc area ratio in normal and glaucomatous patients. Note that values greater than 0.42 are consistent both with normality and glaucoma

respect to standard visual field examination in detecting early changes in the follow-up of patients at "high risk" for glaucoma [21, 22]. In the same study, however, Miglior et al. showed a lower sensitivity of optic disc planimetry with respect to visual field testing in detecting progressive changes in the advanced stages of POAG [22]. These results are in agreement with a study of Caprioli, which reported a higher relative rate of disc-to-field change (0.065 mm^2/dB^2) in the early stages of POAG than in the more advanced stages (0.0012 mm^2/dB^2), the difference being statistically significant [23].

When comparing the sensitivity of color stereo-photograph evaluation with planimetry in the assessment of optic disc progressive changes, Caprioli documented a higher sensitivity of the former compared to the latter and a good correlation between the qualitative examination and visual field testing. Caprioli noticed that "evaluation by manual stereoplanimetry detected change in eyes with primarily diffuse structural damage not detected by the other qualitative method employed, and often before visual field loss occurred. Each may contribute to the identification of early damage depending on the stage of disease and the characteristics of individual patients" [23].

Other diagnostic parameters may be evaluated at the level of the optic disc: optic disc hemorrhages and parapapillary atrophy. The former are highly specific for glaucoma: Diehl et al. reported a prevalence of 0%, 0.44% and 2.44% in a total of 1123 normal, OHT and POAG patients. Although the low prevalence of disc hemorrhage in an unselected population limits its usefulness as a screening tool for glaucoma, it should be stressed that, 1 year following disc hemorrhage, the OHT eyes had an increased rate of retinal nerve fiber layer (RNFL) atrophy and conversion to initial visual field loss [24]. Parapapillary atrophy is commonly associated with glaucomatous eyes, compared to OHT and normal eyes. Moreover, it is greater in glaucomatous eyes than in OHT and normal eyes [25]. However, at present, the data on its diagnostic precision are not conclusive.

Confocal laser systems, which allow tomography of the optic disc to be performed, are still under examination in order to assess the reproducibility of the measurements of several diagnostic parameters. Quantitative data about sensitivity and specificity are lacking at the moment. However, it is possible to foresee for these systems (Heidelberg Retinal Tomograph and Scanning Laser Tomograph), the same limited sensitivity and specificity with respect to visual field evaluation in cross sectional studies, but possibly an increased sensitivity in detecting progressive glaucomatous changes [9].

Retinal Nerve Fiber Layer Examination

Retinal nerve fiber layer (RNFL) qualitative examination is usually performed on black and white, red-free photographs or by means of argon-blue scanning laser ophthalmoscopy. RNFL height may be measured by means of the ON-

HA, the Imagenet system, or the Nerve Fiber Analyzer (polarimeter).

RNFL examination is highly sensitive in detecting early glaucomatous structural changes. These changes usually precede the onset of visual field defects (as evaluated by means of standard perimetry). However, RNFL abnormalities are not an exclusive feature of glaucoma, but can occur also in neurological diseases [25-28] and may be observed also in normal eyes [14, 29-31]. RNFL abnormalities are strictly associated with and may precede the onset of glaucomatous visual field damage [14, 29-35]. RNFL defects are observed in a consistent number of hypertensive eyes with normal field indices [36, 37]. Localized RNFL defects not associated with central 30° visual field abnormalities actually present a depression of retinal sensitivity which may be revealed only by programs with 1° resolution [37], or by fundus perimetry [39, 40], thus indicating that RNF loss corresponds to visual field abnormalities. The subtle slit-like RNFL defects, also observed in a consistent proportion of normal eyes, whose specificity for the detection of early glaucoma is highly questionable [14, 29-31], are probably no more considered as an abnormal RNFL pattern. In fact, a recent study reported that localized RNFL defects have been observed only in less than 1% of eyes with normal IOP and field indices [37]. Airaksinen et al. and Miglior et al. showed a clear correlation between the RNFL pattern (normal, slit, wedge and diffuse defects) and the results of standard threshold perimetry and the global visual field indices [41, 42]. Miglior et al. reported a sensitivity of 100% and specificity of 80.2% of RNFL defects, assessed by means of scanning laser ophthalmoscopy, in detecting glaucomatous or normal visual field indices in a study carried out on POAG and OHT patients [36]. O'Connor et al., in a cross-sectional study carried out on healthy, OHT and POAG patients, documented a sensitivity and specificity of 70% and 77% for RNFL defects (assessed by means of black and white red-free photographs), and a sensitivity and specificity of 74% and 63% for quantitative RNFL height measurements (performed by ONHA), in detecting the presence or absence of glaucomatous visual field loss [11].

The sensitivity and specificity of RNFL examination have been evaluated also in longitudinal studies. Hoyt et al. described first the presence of RNFL defects in 14 patients who developed glaucomatous visual field loss 5 years later [43]. Quigley et al. could detect progressive RNFL changes in 18 of 37 (49%) OHT patients at baseline who converted to POAG during a follow-up of 5 years and in three of 37 (8%) OHT controls [16]. Caprioli reported that qualitative RNFL evaluation was less sensitive than qualitative optic disc evaluation and RNFL height measurements in detecting progressive changes in OHT and POAG patients followed up to 3.3 years (15% and 13.2% vs 7.2%). However, only disc and RNFL evaluation well correlated with visual field worsening, hence the clinical value of RNFL height measurement is still unclear and deserves to be elucidated [23].

Visual Field Examination

Visual field examination represents the fundamental diagnostic procedure in the management of POAG. As stated in the Introduction, the standard computerized threshold evaluation of the central 30° of the visual field is the gold standard parameter of POAG. Many possible analyses of the field plot help in classifying the visual field as glaucomatous or normal: single points evaluation, hemifield comparison, cluster analysis, global field indices, cumulative curves, etc. Automated suprathreshold visual field examination (full field 120 program of the Humphrey field analyzer) has also shown a higher sensitivity (for a specificity of 90%) in screening for glaucoma in a population-based survey than IOP measurement and vertical c/d assessment (52%, 39% and 45%, respectively) [5]. Moreover, new perimetric techniques have been recently introduced in clinical practice in order to improve the diagnostic precision of field examination.

Short wavelength automated perimetry (blue on yellow, B-Y) seems the most promising technique for field examination in glaucoma, given its high sensitivity. Wild et al., in a cross-sectional study, showed that B-Y perimetry identified visual field loss earlier than did standard perimetry (5 of 27 OHT patients had B-Y focal abnormality and a normal field, whereas 11 of 24 POAG patients demonstrated greater B-Y loss than the corresponding standard field)[44]. Sample and Weinreb, in a longitudinal study (range 6-26 months) on 21 POAG patients, reported that color visual fields may indicate significant progressive change in visual function before it is apparent on standard visual fields [45]. The results of two longitudinal studies, performed on OHT and POAG patients followed up to 5 years, are in agreement with the previously reported investigations: "B-Y perimetry deficits are an early indicator of glaucomatous damage and are predictive of impending glaucomatous visual field loss for standard perimetry. B-Y perimetry is effective in predicting which patients with early glaucomatous visual field loss are most likely to have progressive loss" [46, 47].

High-pass resolution perimetry (ring perimetry) is an alternative perimetric technique which allows a field test to be performed in short time and, at least theoretically, an estimate of the underlying ganglion cell population to be provided. Several clinical studies have indicated that ring perimetry is less sensitive, yet more specific, than standard perimetry when comparing eyes that have glaucoma and normal eyes [48]. Sample et al. reported that, although ring perimetry was comparable to standard perimetry in detecting glaucomatous visual field defects, it was no more sensitive in detecting field abnormalities among glaucoma suspects [49]. However, a recent study by Martinez et al. showed that, when using a more accurate approach in analyzing the standard visual field, such as the glaucoma hemifield test, ring and standard perimetry had the same levels of both sensitivity in identifying glaucoma eyes as being outside the normal limits (56%) and specificity (94% vs 100%), but ring perimetry could identify 32% of OHT eyes as being outside normal limits (vs the 8% of standard perimetry) [2].

As far as sensitivity and specificity of visual field testing in the follow-up are concerned, a recent study by Birch et al. reported different performances of three statistical packages of the Humphrey perimeter (Statpac linear regression analysis, Glaucoma change probability program and Progressor program) in detecting progression of field loss, none of them correlated well with the clinical impression of the course of the disease [50].

Conclusions

The structural and functional parameters reviewed here represent the "strongest weapons" in the hands of the ophthalmologist for the diagnostic management of POAG.

Tonometry is a valid method to identify patients at high risk for glaucoma, but unfortunately it fails in detecting LTG patients. The sensitivity of tonometry may be increased by means of repeated diurnal measurements, although it has been suggested that a single IOP measurement is highly predictive of the mean value of a diurnal curve [51]. Furthermore, although its characteristic of "soft" diagnostic parameter, tonometry is crucial in evaluating the hypotensive efficacy of therapy. It should be stressed, however, that the sensitivity and specificity of tonometry in detecting a real progression of glaucoma (surrogate diagnostic parameter) have to be still determined [8].

An accurate examination of the posterior segment of the eye is probably the most sensitive approach to the detection of early glaucomatous damage and its progression. At this stage, in fact, RNFL defects may be often detected in the presence of normal visual fields. Furthermore, qualitative and quantitative progressive optic disc changes may precede the onset or progression of field loss. Moreover it is the only diagnostic procedure which allows the ophthalmologist to suspect or identify LTG patients in the clinical setting.

An accurate visual field test is probably the most sensitive technique to monitor progression in the advanced stages of glaucoma. At this stage, only a few number of ganglion fibers and a limited amount of disc rim tissue may be observed, and any further structural alterations (which indeed may induce significant visual field loss) is hardly detectable with qualitative or quantitative examinations. Moreover, the sensitivity and specificity of visual field testing in the early stages of glaucoma will probably increase with the introduction of B-Y and ring perimetry, which have been shown to improve the diagnostic precision in this stage of the disease.

However, the sensitivity and specificity in detecting early and progressive glaucomatous changes may be significantly improved only by taking into account the results of a series of diagnostic procedures, thus allowing a complete overview of both structural and functional parameters to be obtained.

References

1. Drance SM, Airaksinen PJ, Price M, Schulzer M, Douglas GR, Tansley B (1987) The use of psycophysical, structural, and electrodiagnostic parameters to identify glaucomatous damage. Graefe's Arch Clin Exp Ophthalmol 225:365-8
2. Martinez GA, Sample PA, Weinreb RN (1995) Comparison of high-pass resolution perimetry and standard automated perimetry in glaucoma. Am J Ophthalmol 119:195-201
3. Sommer A, Tielsch JM, Katz J, Quigley HA, Gottsch JD, Javitt J, Singh K, Baltimore Eye Survey Research Group (1991) Relationship between intraocular pressure and primary open angle glaucoma among white and black Americans. The Baltimore Eye Survey. Arch Ophthalmol 109:1090-5
4. Sponsel WE (1989) Tonometry in question: can visual screening tests play a more decisive role in glaucoma diagnosis and management? Surv Ophthalmol 33 (suppl):291-300
5. Katz J, Tielsch JM, Quigley HA, Javitt J, Witt K, Sommer A (1993) Automated suprathreshold screening for glaucoma: the Baltimore Eye Survey. Invest Ophthalmol Vis Sci, 34:3271-7
6. Vogel R, Crick RP, Newsome RB, Shipley M, Blackmore H, Bulpit CJ (1990) Association between intraocular pressure and loss of visual field in chronic simple glaucoma. Br J Ophthalmol 74:3-6
7. Niesel P, Flammer J (1980) Correlations between IOP, visual field and visual acuity based on 11-years observations of treated chronic glaucoma. Int Ophthalmol 3:31-4
8. Rossetti L, Marchetti I, Orzalesi N, Scorpiglione N, Torri V, Liberati A (1993) Randomized clinical trials on medical treatment of glaucoma. Are they appropriate to guide clinical practice? Arch Ophthalmol 111:96-103
9. Cioffi GA (1993) Optic nerve head analysis in the 1990s. Glaucoma 2:77-9
10. Damms T, Dannheim F (1993) Sensitivity and specificity of optic disc parameters in chronic glaucoma. Invest Ophthalmol Vis Sci 34:2246-50
11. O'Connor DJ, Zeyen T, Caprioli J (1993) Comparison of methods to detect glaucomatous optic nerve damage. Ophthalmology, 100:1498-503
12. Orzalesi N, Miglior S, Brigatti L, Bottoni F (1991) Manual morphometry in normal and glaucomatous eyes. In: Bonomi L, Orzalesi N (eds) Glaucoma concepts in evolution. Kugler, Amsterdam, pp 51-69
13. Quigley HA, Addicks EM, Green VR (1982) Optic nerve damage in human glaucoma. III. Quantitative correlation of nerve fiber loss and visual field defects in glaucoma, ischemic neuropathy, papilledema, and toxic neuropathy. Arch Ophthalmol 100:135-146
14. Sommer A, Katz J, Quigley HA, Miller NR, Robin AL, Richter RC, Witt KA (1991) Clinically detectable nerve fiber layer atrophy precedes the onset of glaucomatous field loss. Arch Ophthalmol 109:77-83
15. Tuulonen A, Airaksinen PJ (1991) Initial glaucomatous optic disc and retinal nerve fiber layer abnormalities and their progression. Am J Ophthalmol 111:485-90
16. Quigley HA, Katz J, Derick RJ, Gilbert D, Sommer A (1992) An evaluation of optic disc and nerve fiber layer examinations in monitoring progression of early glaucoma damage. Ophthalmology 99:19-28
17. Odberg T, Riise D (1985) Early diagnosis of glaucoma: the value of successive stereophotography of the optic disc. Acta Ophthalmol 63:257-68
18. Airaksinen PJ, Tuulonen A, Alanko HI (1992) Rate and pattern of neuroretinal rim area decrease in ocular hypertension and glaucoma. Arch Ophthalmol 110:206-210
19. Harbin TS Jr, Podos SM, Kolker AE, Becker B (1976) Visual field progression in open angle glaucoma patients presenting with monocular field loss. Trans Am Acad Ophthalmol Otolaryngol 81:253-7
20. Kass MA, Kolker AE, Becker B (1976) Prognostic factors in glaucomatous visual field loss. Arch Ophthalmol 94:1274-6
21. Zeyen TG, Caprioli J (1993) Progression of disc and field damage in early glaucoma. Arch Ophthalmol 111:62-5
22. Miglior S, Brigatti L, Lonati C, Rossetti L, Pierrottet C, Orzalesi N (1996) Correlation between the progression of optic disc and visual field changes in glaucoma. Curr Eye Res 15:145-149
23. Caprioli J (1994) Clinical evaluation of the optic nerve in glaucoma. Tr Am Ophth Soc 92:589-641
24. Diehl DLC, Quigley HA, Miller NR, Sommer A, Burney EN (1990) Prevalence and significance of optic disc hemorrhage in a longitudinal study of glaucoma Arch Ophthalmol 108:545-50
25. Jonas JB, Fernandez MC, Naumann GOH (1992) Glaucomatous parapapillary atrophy. Occurrence and correlations. Arch Ophthalmol 110:214-22
26. Schiro D, Jonas JB (1994) Localized retinal nerve fiber layer defects in nonglaucomatous optic nerve atrophy. Graefe's Arch Clin Exp Ophthalmol 232:759-60
27. Tsai CS, Ritch R, Schwartz B, Lee SS, Miller NR, Chi T, Hsieh FY (1991) Optic nerve head and

nerve fiber layer in Alzheimer's disease. Arch Ophthalmol 109:199-204
28. Mac Fadyen DJ, Drance SM, Douglas GR, Airaksinen PJ, Mawson DK, Paty DW (1988) The retinal nerve fiber layer, neuroretinal rim area and visual evoked potentials in MS. Neurology 38:1353-8
29. Quigley HA, Miller NR, George T (1980) Clinical evaluation of nerve fiber layer atrophy as an indicator of glaucomatous optic nerve damage. Arch Ophthalmol 98:1564-71
30. Sommer A, Quigley HA, Robin AL, Miller NR, Katz J, Arkell S (1984) Evaluation of nerve fiber layer assessment. Arch Ophthalmol 102:1766-71
31. Quigley H.A. (1986) Examination of the retinal nerve fiber layer in the recognition of early glaucoma damage. Trans Am Ophthalmol Soc 84:-920-66
32. Hoyt WF, Newman NM (1972) The earliest observable defect in glaucoma? Lancet 1:692-3
33. Sommer A, Miller NR, Pollack I, Maumanee AE, George T (1977) The nerve fiber layer in the diagnosis of glaucoma . Arch Ophthalmol 95:2149-56
34. Airaksinen PJ, Drance SM, Douglas GR, Mawson DK, Nieminen H (1984) Diffuse and localized nerve fiber loss in glaucoma. Am J Ophthalmol 98:566-71
35. Quigley HA, Enger C, Katz J, Sommer A, Scott R, Gilbert D (1994) Risk factors for the development of visual field loss in ocular hypertension. Arch Ophthalmol 112:644-9
36. Miglior S, Rossetti L, Brigatti L, Bujtar E, Orzalesi N (1994) Reproducibility of retinal nerve fiber layer evaluation by dynamic scanning laser ophthalmoscopy. Am J Ophthalmol 118:16-23
37. Jonas JB, Konigsreuther KA (1994) Optic disc appearance in ocular hypertensive eyes. Am J Ophthalmol 117:732-40
38. Tuulonen A, Lethola J, Airaksinen PJ (1993) Nerve fiber layer defects with normal visual fields. Do normal optic disc and normal visual field indicate absence of glaucomatous abnormality? Ophthalmology 100:587-98
39. Stuermer J, Schroedel C, Rappl W (1991) Scanning laser ophthalmoscope for static fundus perimetry in glaucomatous nerve fiber bundles defects. In: Mills RP, Heijl A (eds) Perimetry update 1990-91. Kugler, Amsterdam, pp 85-92
40. Orzalesi N, Miglior S, Lonati C, Rossetti L (1995) Microperimetry of localized retinal nerve fiber layer defects. Invest Ophthalmol Vis Sci, 36 (ARVO suppl):170
41. Airaksinen PJ, Drance SM, Douglas GR, Schulzer M, Wijsman K (1985) Visual field and retinal nerve fiber layer comparisons in glaucoma. Arch Ophthalmol 103:205-7
42. Miglior S, Bujtar E, Brigatti L, Lonati C, Rossetti L, Pierrottet C, Orzalesi N (1994) Sensitivity and specificity of visual field indices and optic disc morphometry in the assessment of glaucomatous RNFL defects. Invest Ophthalmol Vis Sci 35 (ARVO suppl):2186
43. Hoyt WF, Frisen L, Newman NM (1973) Funduscopy of nerve fiber layer defects in glaucoma. Invest Ophthalmol Vis Sci 12:814-29
44. Wild JM, Moss ID, Whitaker D, O'Neill EC (1995) The statistical interpretation of Blue-on Yellow visual field loss. Invest Ophthalmol Vis Sci 36:1398-410
45. Sample AP, Weinreb RN (1992) Progressive color visual field loss in glaucoma. Invest Ophthalmol Vis Sci 33:2068-71
46. Johnson CA, Adams AJ, Casson EJ, Brandt JD (1993) Blue-on-Yellow perimetry can predict the development of glaucomatous visual field loss. Arch Ophthalmol 111:645-50
47. Johnson CA, Adams AJ, Casson EJ, Brandt JD (1993) Progression of early glaucomatous visual field loss as detected by Blue-on-Yellow and standard White-on-White automated perimetry. Arch Ophthalmol 111:651-6
48. Frisen L (1993) High-pass resolution perimetry: a clinical review. Doc Ophthalmol 83:1-25
49. Sample PA, Ahn DS, Lee PC, Weinreb R (1992) High-pass resolution perimetry in eyes with ocular hypertension and primary open angle glaucoma. Am J Ophthalmol 113:309-16
50. Birch MK, Wishart PK, O'Donnell NP (1995) Determining progressive visual field loss in serial Humphrey visual fields. Ophthalmology 102:1227-35
51. Phelps CD, Woolson RF, Kolker AE, Becker B (1974) Diurnal variation in intraocular pressure. Am J Ophthalmol 77:367-72

Early Visual Field Defects in Glaucoma: A Study of Eyes Developing Field Loss

A. Heijl and B. Bengtsson

Dept. of Ophthalmology, Malmö University Hospital, 20502 Malmö, Sweden

Introduction

Visual field defects may not be the first sign of glaucoma, but field loss is a hard diagnostic sign and therefore usually and correctly used to differentiate between ocular hypertension and glaucoma. Identification of visual field loss in a patient with previously normal fields usually entails a change of management. It is therefore clinically important to be able to recognize early glaucomatous field defects.

The view of what constitutes typical early glaucomatous field loss has not remained unchanged over time. Fifty years ago the earliest visual defects were considered to be enlargement of the blind spot, baring of the blind spot and contractions. Over time it has become clear that blind spot disturbances are of no consequence for the diagnosis of glaucoma, but scotomas in the central field and nasal constrictions have remained diagnostically important. Much of our present knowledge was acquired by the very thorough work of Aulhorn and Harms [1] with manual static perimetry. The usage of automated static threshold perimetry has also resulted in increasing knowledge, e.g., that early glaucomatous visual field loss is characterized by large variability with relative shallow defects and a gradual onset [2, 3]. Automation of perimetry has correctly focused interest on the central 30° field.

Early glaucomatous visual field defects can be defined in different ways. The most conventional definition would be the earliest visual field defects that occur during the course of the disease. Such information can be retrieved by analyzing data from patients developing glaucomatous visual field defects while being followed. Here we report the result of such a retrospective analysis of patients developing field loss while being followed.

Materials and Methods

We identified all patients in our department who had been followed for 5 years or more and who had been subjected to five or more Humphrey threshold field tests. A total of 530 patients fulfilled these criteria. We printed visual field series of those patients, including grey scale maps; Statpac glaucoma change probability maps [4] and regression analyses [5] for both eyes of all patients.

The visual field series of each individual eye was then evaluated, searching for series showing initially normal results followed by progressive field loss. Grey scale printouts and change probability maps were used in this evaluation. Fields from 74 patients were identified in this way. One eye was randomly selected from each of those patients in whom both eyes showed such progressive loss. The corresponding patient records were retrieved; eyes without glaucoma and eyes with concomitant disease that could affect the visual field were excluded.

A second evaluation of the visual fields was then performed using grey scales and probability maps. This time the fields were masked both for sequence and for patient. Then, eyes were excluded that did not show convincing conversion from normal to glaucomatous status. A total of 37 eyes of 37 patients (12 men and 25 women) then remained for analysis;

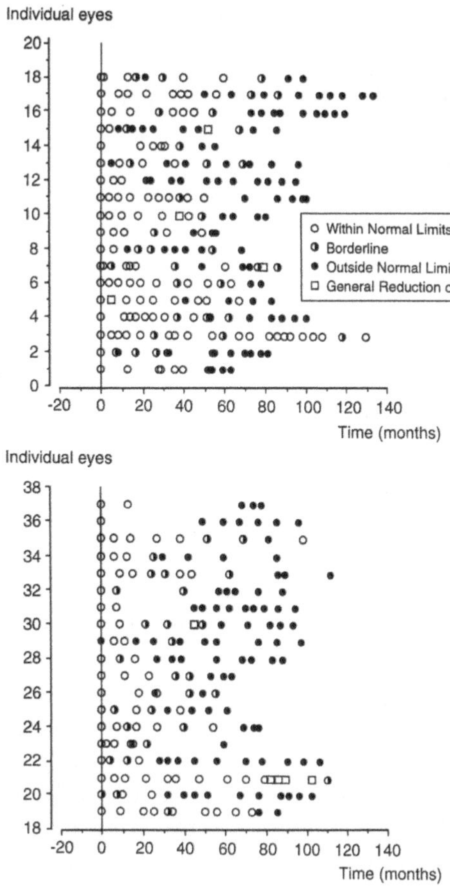

Fig. 1. Glaucoma hemifield test results in visual field series of patients developing glaucomatous visual field defects. Each line represents the tests of one patient plotted over time

their mean age was 66 years at the time of the initial field test (range 27 - 80 years).

All visual fields were classified as normal, suspect or pathological according to the glaucoma hemifield test (GHT) [6]. The results of this test were plotted for each eye over time (Fig. 1). "Conversion time", i.e. the time from definitely normal to definitely glaucomatous field status, was then calculated. This was defined as the time interval from the last of at least three (earlier) consecutive normal fields to the first of at least three (later) consecutive abnormal fields. In 23 visual field series this was the case, and at least three normal consecutive fields and at least three pathological consecutive fields were available. We also studied global field indices, mean deviation (MD) and pattern deviation (PSD) [5] at the time of the first definitely glaucomatous field defect.

Results

A typical, gradual development of field loss, in which definite defects were preceded by nondefinite defects in the same area, were seen in most eyes (Fig. 1). An example of grey scale printouts can be seen in Fig. 2.

The distribution of conversion times is shown in Fig. 3. The time interval varied from 1 year up to a little more than 6 years; the average time was 3.5 years.

The distributions of the global visual field indices MD and PSD at the time of the first stable glaucomatous visual field defect are shown in Fig. 4A and 4B, respectively. A large percentage of the fields actually had field index values within normal limits.

Discussion

Although the series is small, it is derived from a very large clinical database and may therefore allow some conclusions. The results clearly show that the earliest glaucomatous field defects are very variable. This has previously been reported by Werner and Drance [2], who found increased

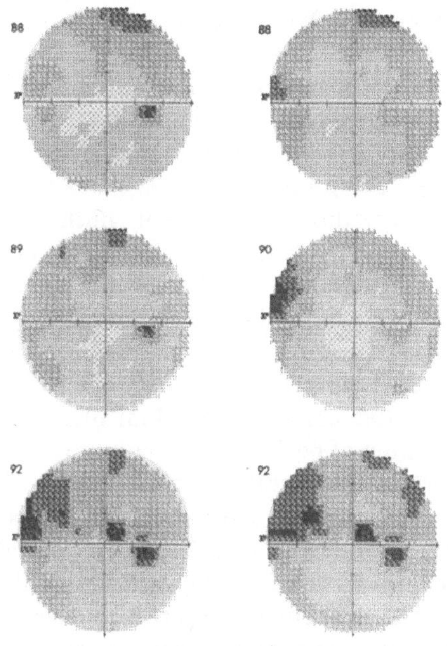

Fig. 2. Grey scale printouts from one eye developing glaucomatous visual field defects. It is obvious that variable and shallow field defects preceded definite field loss by several years

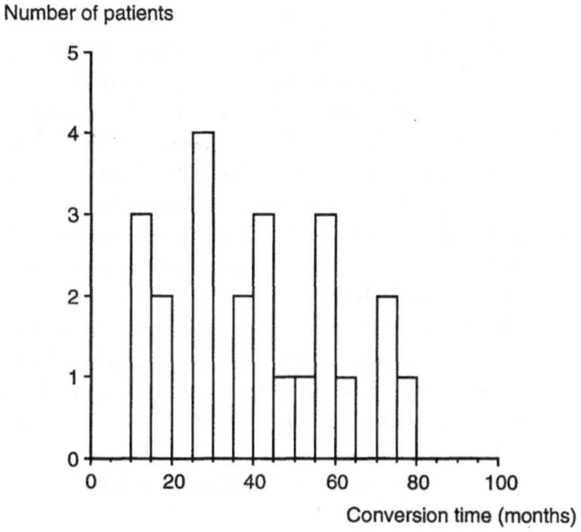

Fig. 3. The frequency distribution of "conversion time", i.e. the time interval from definitely normal to definitely glaucomatous visual field status

early disturbances in the area where definite glaucomatous field defects later appeared. Their observations were based on manual perimetry. It is well known that computerized static perimetry detects glaucomatous field loss at a considerably earlier stage than do manual techniques [7-9] and an analysis using computerized static perimetry – nowadays the standard of clinical care – is therefore well motivated. The fact that the fields in our analysis were obtained with computerized perimetry and that the field analysis was based on an objective expert system, the GHT, eliminates most examination and interpretation bias, giving increased credibility to the results.

From a clinical point of view the conversion time demonstrated by us is disturbingly high, since preferred practice patterns in patients with glaucoma/suspect glaucoma are very much influenced by visual field status.

The long time intervals between clearly normal and clearly abnormal could be used to argue that frequent visual field examinations are inefficient. On the other hand, the results clearly show an early diagnosis can be made if the results of *several consecutive* examinations are taken into account, instead of only the most recent one. Such analyses can benefit from tests administered at relatively short time intervals.

There is a need for other psychophysical methods that could help identify functional glaucomatous damage earlier than standard computerized static perimetry using white stimuli on a white background. Blue-on-yellow perimetry and motion detection perimetry are methods which seem to hold such promise [10-12]. However, blue-on-yellow interpatient variability is larger than that of conventional white-on-white threshold perimetry [13]. This increased variability results in wider normal limits for blue-on-yellow perimetry, which in turn may lead to

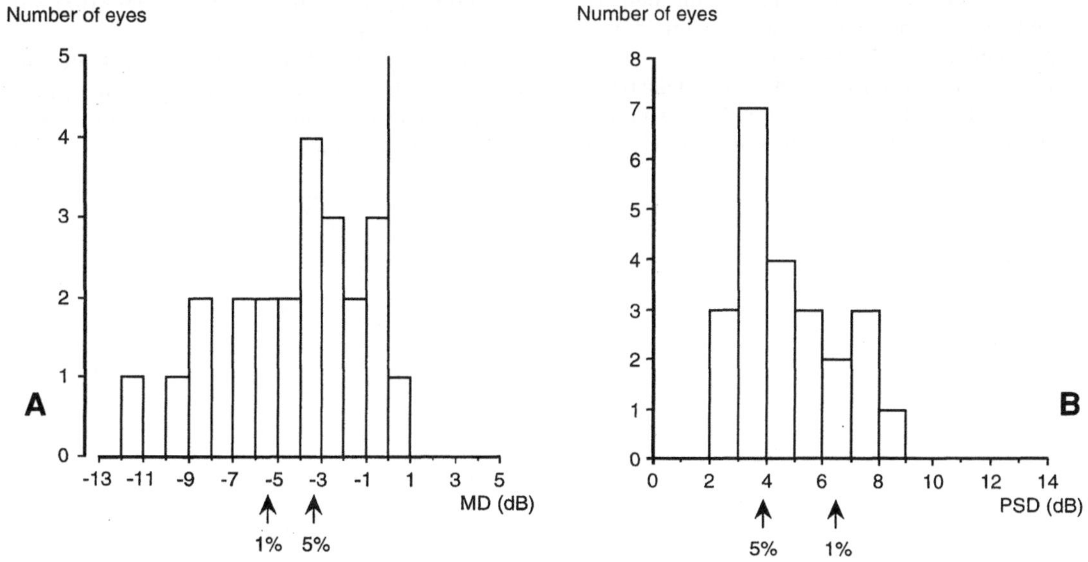

Fig. 4A, B. Frequency distributions of visual field indices MD (A) and PSD (B) at the time of first stable glaucomatous visual field defects. Significance limits for pathology at 5% and 1% levels are marked with *arrows*. Many eyes reached the stage of first stable glaucomatous visual field defects while index values still were normal

even longer conversion times from normal to glaucomatous field status. This is a factor worth studying and considering when establishing the best routine clinical practices.

It is hardly surprising that the visual field indices MD and PSD often were within normal limits at the time of the first stable field defect. These indices are not the most effective indicators of early detection of glaucomatous visual field defects [14] and are more suitable for follow-up.

We conclude that glaucomatous visual field defects appear gradually. The slow conversion from definitely normal to definitely abnormal may have implications for recommended visual field test intervals in clinical practice. The time interval from definitely normal to definitely glaucomatous varied from approximately 1 year to 6 years. However, early perimetric diagnosis is therefore improved if one can take into account several recently plotted fields instead of only the results of only one test.

References

1. Aulhorn E, Harms H (1967) Early visual field defects in glaucoma. In Glaucoma Symposium Tutzing Castle, Karger, Basel pp 151-186
2. Werner EB, Drance SM (1977) Early visual field disturbances in glaucoma. Arch Ophthalmol 95:1173-1175
3. Heijl Anders (1993) Perimetric point density and detection of glaucomatous visual field loss. Acta Ophthalmol 71: 445-450
4. Heijl A, Lindgren G, Lindgren A, Olsson J, Åsman P, Myers S, Patella M (1991) Extended statistical package for evaluation of single and multiple fields in glaucoma: Statpac 2. In Mills RP, Heijl A (eds) Perimetry update 1990/1991, 1991:303-315. Kugler & Gedini, Amsterdam
5. Heijl A, Lindgren G, Olsson J (1986) A package for the statistical analysis of visual fields. In EL Greve and A Heijl (eds) Doc Ophthalmol Proc Ser 49, pp 153-168. Dr Junks, Dordrecht
6. Åsman P, Heijl A (1992) Glaucoma hemifield test: automatic visual field evaluation. Arch Ophthalmol 110:812-819
7. Heijl A (1976) Automatic perimetry in visual field screening. A clinical study. Albrecht v Graefes Arch Klin Exp Ophthalmol 200: 21-37
8. Spahr J, Fankhauser F, Jenni A, Bebie H (1978) Praktische Erfahrungen mit dem automatischen Perimeter Octopus. Klin Mbl Augenheilk 172:470-477
9. Dyster-Aas K, Heijl A, Lundquist L (1980) Computerized visual field screening in the management of patients with ocular hypertension. Acta Ophthalmol 58: 918-928
10. Johnsson CA, Adams AJ, Casson EJ, Brandt JD (1993) Blue-on yellow can predict the development of glaucomatous visual loss. Arch Ophthalmol 111:645-650
11. Sample PA, Weinreb RN (1992) Progressive color visual field loss in glaucoma. Invest Ophthalmol 33: 2068-2071
12. Baez KA, McNaught AI, Dowler JG, Poinoosawmy D, Fitzke FW, Hitchings RA (1995) Motion detection threshold and field progression in normal tension glaucoma. Brit J Ophthalmol 79:125-128
13. Wild JM, Moss ID, Whitaker D, O'Neill EC (1995) The statistical interpretation of blue-on-yellow visual field loss. Invest Ophthalmol 36:1398-1410
14. Katz J, Sommer A, Gaasterland DE, Anderson DR (1991) Comparison of analytic algorithms for detecting glaucomatous visual field loss. Arch Ophthalmol 109:1684-1689

Clinical and Computerized Evaluation of the Retinal Nerve Fiber Layer

P. J. Airaksinen and A. Tuulonen

Department of Ophthalmology, University of Oulu, 90220 Oulu, Finland

Anatomy of the Retinal Nerve Fiber Layer

Retinal nerve fiber layer (RNFL) abnormalities in patients with glaucoma were first reported by Hoyt et al. in 1973 [1]. The first observable changes were thin, slit-like defects or grooves in the arcuate area of the RNFL. In further progressed cases wedge-shaped localized defects developed.

Healthy RNFL appears as regularly oriented striations, which are formed by axon bundles and compartmentalized in tunnels formed by Mueller's cell processes.

The RNFL is thickest in the peripapillary area, particularly upper and lower temporally where it can be as thick as 300 μm [2]. Nerve fibers originate from ganglion cells in the peripheral retina and converge into the chorioscleral canal making up the majority of the tissue in the optic nerve head.

The axon bundles curve around the macula in a pattern which determines the typical appearance of glaucomatous arcuate visual field defects.

The retinotopic organization of the nerve fibers is probably such that the more peripherally originated fibers are situated deep in the retina, closer to the pigment epithelium.

The more proximally originating fibers lay more superficially in the retina, closer to the vitreous.

In the optic nerve head the superficial nerve fiber bundles are located centrally whereas the more peripherally originating fibers are located closer to the edge of the chorioscleral canal.

Clinical Examination

In a routine clinical examination it is possible to observe the peripapillary RNFL with white light or, even better, with green light. The opaque, slightly silvery appearance of the nerve fiber bundles is easily detectable.

For RNFL observation photographic techniques are the most sensitive. We use low sensitivity, high resolution, black-and-white Kodak Tmax 100 film and a narrow band interference filter with 495 nm wavelength and with 92% transmittance at its peak wavelength [3]. Blue light is reflected back to the camera from the nerve fiber bundles, which therefore come out prominently white in the photographs. In defective areas with few or no axon bundles no light is reflected back to the camera but the blue light is absorbed into the underlying pigment epithelium.

Therefore such areas appear clearly darker than the surroundings [4, 5].

Clinical Observations

In previous publications we have reported that semi-quantitative estimates of the RNFL are highly correlated with visual field indices of light sensitivity perimetry and also with neuroretinal rim area measurements of the optic disc [6, 7]. In another study [8] we carried out multivariate analyses in order to find the combination of variables that would best separate healthy individuals from patients with glaucoma. One of the models included the following variables: vertical cup-disc ratio, diffuse RNFL score, and localized RNFL score. This combination correctly identified 98% of normals and 84% of patients with glaucoma. The finding was of particular interest since the model includes only optic disc and RNFL data without any psychophysical or electrophysiological measurements.

In order to determine the type of the first observable structural abnormalities in the fundus, we conducted a follow-up study of ocular hypertensive patients with an average follow-up period of 9.7 (5-15) years [9]. During the follow-up 38% of the patients developed glaucomatous abnormalities.

In 70% of cases RNFL and optic disc abnormalities were observed simultaneously. In approximately half of the cases the abnormalities were of the diffuse type, in which generalized reduction of axons is associated with generalized enlargement of the optic cup and diffuse thinning of the RNFL.

Computerized Analysis of the Retinal Nerve Fiber Layer

Until quite recently it has not been possible to quantify optic disc and RNFL findings with easy to use computerized instruments. This has clearly been a disadvantage and has stressed the value of visual field examination in glaucoma. However, the advent of digital imaging in ophthalmology [10] as well as scanning laser ophthalmoscopy [11] have made new developments possible.

Heidelberg Retina Tomograph

New and interesting instruments have been recently produced for quantitative analysis of the optic disc and the nerve fiber layer. One of them is the Heidelberg Retina Tomograph (HRT). It is a confocal laser scanning microscope that produces accurate topographic measurements of the optic disc structures with high reproducibility. The HRT reconstructs the three-dimensional optic disc topography on the basis of 32 optical section images [12-15].

It has become quite obvious that, in order to become clinically useful, including follow-up studies, a well defined and stable reference level is important for the proper performance of optic disc measurements. In our manual measurement technique the inner edge of the scleral ring is used as a reference plane both for optic disc and neuroretinal rim determination [16, 17]. Unlike the surface of the RNFL, the scleral ring forms a reference plane which most probably does not change with progressive glaucomatous damage [18].

With this reference level it is possible in the HRT to combine the RNFL height information with the neuroretinal rim area measurements and arrive at a new parameter, the neuroretinal rim volume. Preliminary results show that this parameter is independent of optic disc size and may be sensitive in separating normals from patients with glaucoma (unpublished data).

Nerve Fiber Analyzer

Although grading systems have been developed to classify nerve fiber layer abnormalities [19-21], the information given by nerve fiber layer photography remains qualitative in nature. The Nerve Fiber Analyzer is a new instrument for quantitation of the RNFL [22-26]. It is a confocal scanning laser ophthalmoscope in which the measurement technique is based on the assumption that the nerve fiber layer has birefringent properties. The change in the polarization state, called retardation, can be quantified by determining the phase shift between polarization of light returning from the eye with the known state of polarization of the illuminating laser beam. The retardation is linearly related to the histopathologic measurements of the RNFL in monkey and human eyes. Both the retardation measurements and retinal height measurements show a typical double-hump pattern of the RNFL. The coefficient of variation of the measurements ranges from 3.7% to 13.5%.

Optical Coherence Tomography

The latest instrument for quantitative measurements of the RNFL is Optical Coherence Tomograph (OCT) [27, 28]. The OCT is a noninvasive, noncontact instrument for imaging of the fundus. It is based on a low coherence interferometer (Michelson) and utilizes a superluminescent diode near infrared light (830 nm). The OCT has a scanning optical beam and it measures the round trip travel time of light reflected from the fundus. It creates a true cross-sectional image of the intraocular structures in micron scale resolution. Our preliminary results demonstrate that this instrument is capable of demonstrating and measuring generalized and localized RNFL abnormalities.

References

1. Hoyt WF, Frisen L, Newman NM (1973) Funduscopy of nerve fiber layer defects in glaucoma. Invest Ophthalmol 12: 814
2. Quigley HA, Addicks EM (1982) Quantitative studies of retinal nerve fiber layer defects. Arch Ophthalmol 100:807
3. Airaksinen PJ, Nieminen H (1985) Retinal nerve fiber layer photography in glaucoma. Ophthalmology 92:877-879
4. Leone M, Rolle T, Ferraris U (1986) Analisi della densità delle fibre nervose retiniche mediante fotografia aneritra in soggetti normali e glaucomatosi. Boll Oculist 65, suppl 6:49-53
5. Bottoni F, Gonnella P (1986) Esame delle fibre nervose retiniche (RNFL) e glaucoma cronico semplice. Boll Oculist 65, suppl 6:295-299
6. Airaksinen PJ, Drance SM, Douglas GR, Mawson DK (1984) Diffuse and localized nerve fiber loss in glaucoma. Am J Ophthalmol 98:566-571
7. Airaksinen PJ, Drance SM, Schulzer M (1985) Neuroretinal rim area in early glaucoma. Am J Ophthalmol 99:1-4
8. Drance SM, Airaksinen PJ, Price M, Schulzer, Douglas GR, Tansley BW (1986) Correlation of functional and structural measurements in glaucoma patients and normal subjects. Am J Ophthalmol 102:612-616
9. Tuulonen A, Airaksinen PJ (1991) Development and progression of glaucomatous abnormalities in ocular hypertensive patients converting into glaucoma. Am J Ophthalmol 111:485-490
10. Alanko HI, Nieminen H, Hyytinen P, Tuulonen A, Airaksinen PJ (1994) Digital imaging network for ophthalmic photography. Ophthalmology 101, 9A:144
11. Miglior S, Rossetti L, Lonati C, Orzalesi N (1995) Reproducibility of optic disc morphometry by scanning laser ophthalmoscopy. Invest Ophthalmol 36:S970
12. Zinser G, Wijnaendts-van-Resandt R W, Ihrig C (1988) Confocal laser scanning microscopy for ophthalmology. SPIE 1028:127-132
13. Burk ROB, Rohrschneider K, Noack H, Völcker HE (1991) Volumetric optic disc analysis by laser scanning tomography. Klin Monatsbl Augenheilkd 198: 522-529
14. Burk ROB, Rohrschneider K, Noack H, Völcker HE (1992) Are large optic nerve heads susceptible to glaucomatous damage at normal intraocular pressure? A three-dimensional study by laser scanning tomography. Graefe's Arch Clin Exp Ophthalmol 230:552-560
15. Rohrschneider K, Burk ROW, Kruse FE, Völcker HE (1994) Reproducibility of the optic nerve head topography with a new laser tomographic scanning device. Ophthalmology 101:1044-1049
16. Airaksinen PJ, Drance SM, Schulzer M (1985) Neuroretinal rim area in early glaucoma. Am J Ophthalmol 99:1-4
17. Jonas JB, Robert Y, Airaksinen PJ (1988) Definitionsentwurf der intra-und parapapillären Parameter für die 'Biomorphometrie des Nervus Optikus'. Klin Monatsbl Augenheilkd 192:621
18. Tuulonen A (1993) The morphological pattern of early glaucomatous damage. Curr Opin Ophthalmol 4; II:29-34
19. Airaksinen PJ, Drance SM, Douglas GR, Mawson DK, Nieminen H (1984) Diffuse and localized nerve fibre loss in glaucoma. Am J Ophthalmol 98:566-571
20. Jonas JB, Nguyen NX, Naumann GOH (1989) The retinal nerve fiber layer in normal eyes. Ophthalmology 96:627-632
21. Quigley HA, Reacher M, Katz J, Strahlman E, Gilbert D, Scott R (1993) Quantitative grading of nerve fiber layer photographs. Ophthalmology 100:1800-1807
22. Weinreb RN, Shakiba S, Zangwill L (1995) Scanning laser polarimetry to measure the nerve fiber layer of normal and glaucomatous eyes. Am J Ophthalmol 119:627-636
23. Weinreb RN, Shakiba S, Garden V, Zangwill L (1995) Comparison of scanning laser polarimetry with nerve fiber layer photography and retinal height measurements. In: Kriegelstein GK (ed) Glaucoma update. V. Kaden, Heidelberg, pp 140-148
24. Weinreb RN, Shakiba S, Sample PA, Shahrokni S, van Horn S, Garden V, Asawapphureekorn S, Zangwill L (1995) Association between quantitative nerve fiber layer measurement and visual field loss in glaucoma. Am J Ophthalmol 120:-732-738
25. Swanson WH, Lynn JR, Fellman RL, Starita RJ, Schumann SP, Nusinowitz S (1995) Interoperator variability in images obtained by laser polarimetry of the nerve fiber layer. J Glaucoma 4:414-418
26. Chi QM, Tomita G, Inazumi K, Hayakawa T, Ido T, Kitazawa Y (1995) Evaluation of the effect of aging on the retinal nerve fiber layer thickness using scanning laser polarimetry. J Glaucoma 4:406-413
27. Huang D, Lin CP, Schuman JS, Stinson WG, Chang W, Hee MR, Flotte T, Gregory K, Puliafito C, Fujimoto JG (1991) Optical coherence tomography. Science 254:1178-1181

28. Schuman JS, Hee MR, Puliafito CA, Pedut-Kloizman T, Lin AP, Herzmark E, Izatt JA, Swanson EA, Fujimoto JG (1995) Quantitation of nerve fiber layer thickness in normal and glaucomatous eyes using optical coherence tomography. A pilot study. Arch Ophthalmol 113:586-596

Use of Provoked-Response Tests in Glaucoma: An Update

C.A. Quaranta and L. Quaranta

Department of Ophthalmology, University of Brescia, Spedali Civili of Brescia, Piazzale Spedali Civili 1, 25121 Brescia, Italy

Introduction

The usefulness of provoked-response tests (PRTs) needs to be carefully revaluated on the basis of the concept that glaucoma is the result of an aberration of hydrodynamics and hemodynamics. There are two main types of PRTs, the first of which studies modifications in hydrodynamics. This group of PRTs is used essentially in the diagnosis and management of angle closure glaucomas, but at present the role of hydrodynamic PRT has been greatly reduced by the advent of new and sophisticated technologies. The second type of PRTs is related strictly to the study of ocular hemodynamics and allows identification of abnormal modifications of the autoregulatory system.

In this review, we will discuss this second group of provocative tests, with special attention to the problems related to the differential diagnosis of normal pressure glaucoma (NPG) and burned-out glaucoma (BOG).

We define BOG as a particular form of primary open angle glaucoma characterized by normal intraocular pressure (IOP) but with pathologic alterations of the optic nerve head and visual field. In these cases, the absence of progression of anatomic and functional damage suggests that IOP was elevated in the past but, by some unknown mechanism, returned to normal. In such a case it is very hard to differentiate BOG from NPG.

The ideal PRT would have strong theoretical support: (1) be easy and quick to perform; (2) be highly reproducible and sensitive; (3) have high specificity; and (4) define a feature that would aid in the diagnosis and management of the disease. At present, none of the available PRTs has all these characteristics. But, by using a combination of more than one of PRT, it is possible to obtain important clinical information to make a correct diagnosis and to optimize the management of each individual case.

When analyzing the results of PRTs, it must be kept in mind that every glaucoma patient is a unique individual and each test that we perform has to be interpreted strictly on the basis of the clinical evidence.

Herein we will review an important aspect of PRTs in the diagnosis and management of glaucomas: the differential diagnosis of BOG and NPG.

Provoked-Response Tests for Burned-Out Glaucoma and Normal Pressure Glaucoma

The main aim of this group of tests is to differentiate between these two forms of glaucoma. Although differentiation of NPG from BOG is not easy, some help can be provided by certain PRTs that we will discuss here.

Response to Cold and Warmth Test

Proposed in 1986 by Gasser et al. [1] and re-evaluated by Drance and colleagues [2], this test is designed to investigate the response of the vascular system in NPG to a vasoconstrictive stimulus. The test is performed by measuring blood flow within a finger, by means of a laser Doppler flow meter, before and after immersion of the hand in cold water (4 °C) for 10 s. This test has shown that patients with

NPG not only have an increased vasoconstrictive response after cold water submersion when compared with normal subjects, but also that blood flow in the finger was reduced before submersion when compared to normal subjects and to patients with primary open angle glaucoma. The limits of the test are poor reproducibility and lack of sensitivity. As a matter of fact, a recent study conducted by Usi and Iwata [3] did not confirm the results of Gasser or of Drance. The cold test does allow differentiation between NPG with vasospasm and BOG, in which vasospasm is rarely observed. However, it is evident from the different behaviours of primary open-angle glaucoma and NPG that the latter disease is a distinct entity directly related to vascular abnormalities.

Pressure Compliance Test of the Optic Nerve Head

Proposed by Pillunat, Stodtmeister and Wilmanns [4] in 1987, the pressure compliance test of the optic nerve head evaluates changes in amplitude of the visual evoked potential (VEP) during artificially induced incremental increases in IOP by using a scleral cup system. In the original investigation, 20 eyes of 20 normal subjects and 11 eyes of 14 NPG patients were studied. The trajectory of VEPs and IOPs showed a plateau in the decrease of VEP amplitude at IOPs of 30-60 mm Hg, but a linear decay of the VEP amplitude to an IOP of 90 mm Hg. In NPG eyes, there was no plateau and the VEP amplitude diminished linearly to an IOP of 60 mm Hg. This suggests that NPG patients lack or have an abnormality of the autoregulatory system that should maintain adequate perfusion. This particular test has thus provided important insight into the pathogenesis of NPG and, moreover, allows differentiation of patients with true NPG from those with BOG. As a matter of fact, in eyes with BOG the VEP/IOP trajectory is similar to that in normal subjects.

CO_2 Test

CO_2 is a potent vasodilating agent that affects particularly the cerebral and retinal microvasculature. The idea of using CO_2 breathing to determine the vascular implications in glaucoma was first broached by Bietti in the early 1960s [personal communication] and was later investigated by Pillunat and colleagues [5, 6], who evaluated the effect of 20% CO_2 breathing on visual performance by means of computerized perimetry and who assessed blood flow velocities by means of color Doppler imaging. Both studies revealed that 70% of NPG patients had improved visual performance and increased blood flow velocities in the orbital vessels following CO_2 breathing (responders), while 30% of the patients had no change (non-responders). On the basis of these results it seems that this test is able to differentiate NPG from BOG, rather than differentiating NPG with vasospasm, as interpreted by the authors. Regardless of this personal objection to the interpretation of their data, this test is of great interest in the diagnosis and study of the pathogenesis of NPG and BOG.

Pulsatile Ocular Blood Flow/IOP Trajectory

Proposed by Quaranta [7] in 1994, this PRT is able to differentiate the behaviour of the pulsatile ocular blood flow (PBF) trajectory in eyes with NPG from that of eyes with BOG. The test consists of measuring PBF by means of both the ocular blood flow system of Langham and the scleral cup system, under basal conditions and after experimentally induced increases in IOP of 5 and 10 mm Hg.

The results obtained on a sample of 20 eyes of 20 patients with NPG and on 25 eyes of 25 healthy volunteers showed that PBF under basal conditions is slightly, but significantly, reduced in eyes with NPG compared with normal eyes. The differences in behaviour of PBF trajectory are evidenced when the IOP is artificially increased by only 5 and 10 mm Hg. As a matter of fact, after an IOP increase of 5 mm Hg, there was a decrease in PBF of about 27% in the NPG group and 12% in the normal group. After an IOP increase of 10 mm Hg, the PBF decreased by about 52% and 22% in the NPG and normal groups, respectively. On the basis of this experimental evidence, it seems that in NPG eyes there is a deficiency of the autoregulatory system. Furthermore, this behaviour of the PBF trajectory is typical of NPG. In 15 eyes with BOG that were studied in a similar manner, Quaranta [personal communication] found that the behaviour of the trajectory was similar to that of the normal group.

Similar results were obtained by Trew and Smith [8, 9], who evaluated the PBF/IOP trajectory in response to postural changes (erect and supine) in normal subjects and in patients with NPG.

Conclusions

From a review of the literature, it is apparent that there is no uniformity of results on PRT and the differential diagnosis of BOG and NPG. Several tests have been proposed for such a purpose, but none of these tests have the characteristics that an optimal PRT should have. Furthermore, the majority of these tests are not easy to perform or interpret, so their use remains confined to the laboratory and they have little, if any, clinical impact.

In conclusion, although several different techniques have been proposed and applied clinically, at present the differential diagnosis of BOG and NPG remains a major clinical challenge. However, the integration of PRT results and clinical features can help the clinician to make a correct decision regarding diagnosis and management.

References

1. Gasser P, Flammer J, Guthauser U, Niesel P, Mahler F, Linder HR (1986) Bedeutung des Vasospastichen Syndroms in der Augenheilkunde. Klin Monatsbl Augenheilk 188:398-399
2. Drance SM, Douglas GR, Wijsman K, Schulzer M, Britton RJ (1988) Response of blood flow to warm and cold in normal and low-tension glaucoma patients. Am J Ophthalmol 105:35-39
3. Ususi T, Iwata K (1992) Finger blood flow in patients with low tension glaucoma and primary open-angle glaucoma. Br J Ophthalmol 76:2-4
4. Pillunat LE, Stodtmeister R, Wilmanns I (1987) Pressure compliance of the optic nerve head in low tension glaucoma. Br J Ophthalmol 71:181-187
5. Pillunat LE, Lang GK, Harris A (1994) The visual response to increased ocular blood flow in normal pressure glaucoma. Surv Ophthalmol 38:S139-S148
6. Pillunat LE, Lang GK (1992) Ocular carbondioxide reactivity in normal tension glaucoma. Invest Ophthalmol Vis Sci (Suppl) 33:1279
7. Quaranta L, Manni G, Donato F, Bucci MG (1994) The effect of increased intraocular pressure on pulsatile ocular blood flow in low tension glaucoma. Surv Ophthalmol 38:S177 S182
8. Trew DR, Smith SE (1991) Postural studies in pulsatile ocular blood flow: I. Ocular hypertension and normaltension. Br J Ophthalmol 75:66-70
9. Trew DR, Smith SE (1991) Postural studies in pulsatile ocular blood flow: II. Chronic open angle glaucoma. Br J Ophthalmol 75:71-75

Discussion

Question: De Natale

I wish to ask Dr. Schuman how much his technique is influenced by the opacity of the diottric structures, and also what is the specificity and sensitivity of this technique?

Answer: Schuman

The first part of the question was the effect of the media on imaging with OCT. Dense opacity such as posterior sub-cupping cataract can block the view of the fundus, and so imaging is difficult or impossible in that situation. When the cornea is completely opaque, again it would be difficult if not impossible to perform the examination. I cannot answer your question on sensitivity and specificity because the number of eyes that have been investigated is still small. I think that future studies will be able to answer that question, but I cannot answer it at this point.

Question: Carli

To Dr. Hejil. Do you prefer the 30-2 or 24-2 programme to detect an early glaucomatous damage? Do you think it would be appropriate to use regional indexes (according to Weber) for a localized damage in the analysis of the visual field?

Answer: Hejil

First, the very practical question of 24-2 versus 30-2. I don't think that you can find much more using 30-2 than 24-2. It's almost the same, but sometimes the extra points present in the 30-2 pattern can confirm what you have in the small 24-2 pattern. That is as far as I can go, I suppose, that 24-2 is more disturbed by non-specific errors. I think that for the non-expert user 24-2 fields sometimes can actually be easier to interpret. About your second question on localized loss versus diffuse loss, I think diagnosis should be based on changes in shape of the hill of vision and not on changes in height. One way might be to use pattern deviation maps in that step back programme or the glaucoma hemifield test which completely ignores the general height of the field. I agree with your question that it is in a clinical setting where we have a concurrence of cataract and glaucoma in maybe 1/3 to 1/2 of the patients. It's rather more helpful to look at the pattern or the shape of the visual field instead of at the height of the field or the volume of the hill of vision.

Question: Giuliano

To Dr. Airaksinen. Do you use the photographic or laser technique to study the nerve fiber layer, and what do you think of this type of evaluation in the early diagnosis of glaucoma?

Answer: Airaksinen

You mean in our everyday clinical routine work, so I understood your question. Of course, we use nerval imaging in all glaucoma suspects and in patients with glaucoma. Of course, they are more valuable in the very early stages or if you want to follow ocular hypertensives who do not show abnormalities yet. The further the glaucoma is progressive, the more valuable becomes the visual field and the less valuable are nerve fibres observation and optic disc observation. Actually, we of course make all examinations at the same time: optic disc stereo photographs or images, digital images at the moment, nerve fibres images and the visual fields, even if the visual fields are normal, because we feel that it's good to keep the patients active. We use all these information in the clinical setting, and we try to collect a lot of data in order to make clinical decisions. I hope I gave an answer to your question.

MEDICAL THERAPY

Diagnosing and Redefining Glaucoma*

R. N. Weinreb, A. Anton, and P. A. Sample

Glaucoma Center/0946, University of California, San Diego, 9500 Gilman Drive, La Jolla, CA 92093-0946, USA

Introduction

Patients with high intraocular pressure, but without measurable standard visual field loss or observable change in the appearance of the optic disc, are called ocular hypertensives despite the fact that they may have other progressive functional loss. It is likely that many of these eyes have glaucoma. In other words, certain types of functional, and also probably structural loss, may occur substantially sooner than shown by standard examining techniques. To state this unequivocally, one needs to know whether these eyes have a progressive optic neuropathy which, if left untreated, will eventually mimic glaucoma as defined by standard testing. To achieve this, it is necessary to correlate structural and functional tests, both standard and new.

As retinal ganglion cells and their axons are damaged, there is likely to be cellular dysfunction, a biologic response to injury or aging. It seems unlikely that clinically detectable structural change, which is largely dependent on cell death, always precedes cell dysfunction. This suggests that functional change, if it can be measured, should be an early, if not the first, indicator of abnormality in many eyes. The magnitude and character of ganglion cell dysfunction should most likely dictate the optimal test to detect abnormal function. Physiological and morphological studies can help guide the development of these tests, and psychophysics may uncover them by assessing a variety of functions to determine which is most sensitive to glaucomatous change.

Functional testing performed in clinical practice, which consists largely of standard visual fields, does not appear to be either optimal or sufficiently sensitive to detect early functional damage in many individuals. Quigley and coll. reported histological evidence that shows that a substantial loss of optic nerve axons can occur before the standard visual field is affected [1]. Our results, and those of others, with short wavelength automated perimetry (SWAP) are consistent with these findings [2-4]. A high percentage of ocular hypertensive eyes with normal standard visual fields show abnormal visual function when measured with SWAP or other functional tests. However, these deficits seem to encompass both magnocellular and parvocellular pathways, and not to be specific for solely either one.

Testing of specific magnocellular or parvocellular functions may be useful, particularly if loss of one or the other function predominates at certain stages of the glaucomatous process. Two illustrative cases will highlight this issue.

Case Reports

Case 1

A 69 year old female was evaluated in September 1991 with intraocular pressure of OD: 30 mm Hg and OS: 32 mm Hg. Optic discs

* Supported in part by grants from Foundation of Research (A.A) and National Eye Institute EZ08208 (PS)

appeared normal (Fig. 1). Standard achromatic perimetry was within normal limits (Fig. 2A). However, SWAP was abnormal (outside the 99.5% confidence limits) (Fig. 2B). In May 1992 intraocular pressure was OO: 28 mm Hg and no change was detected in the appearance of the optic disc. Both standard perimetry and SWAP were outside normal limits (Fig. 3). In December 1995 both standard perimetry and SWAP were outside normal limits, and the pattern deviation plot showed an initial inferior arcuate defect on standard field testing (Fig. 4) in the same location as detected with SWAP 4 years earlier.

Case 2

A 75 year old male with intraocular pressures OD: 24 mm Hg and OS: 20 mm Hg in May 1990. Optic discs appeared normal (Fig. 5). Visual field indices and glaucoma hemifield test evaluated with standard perimetry were within normal limits, but SWAP was abnormal (outside 99.5% confidence limit) (Fig. 6). Annual standard visual fields were within normal limits for 4 years, but in November 1993 SWAP showed an inferior nasal step (Fig. 7). In September 1994 an inferior nasal step was detected by standard perimetry (Fig. 8). Both the corrected pattern standard deviation and the glaucoma hemifield test were outside normal limits.

Various new functional tests are being assessed as the most sensitive and specific for diagnosing glaucoma. To determine which of them individually or in combination can best signal glaucoma will be an important step. To do this, one cannot simply compare the percentage of eyes that are abnormal on a given task with those abnormal on standard visual fields. Standard fields are already part of the diagnosis and are normal in suspect eyes by definition. It is useful to compare a new test with an established one because the pathologic population and its separation from normals are well defined. However, this can limit the validation of the new test if the established one is not as sensitive as other available diagnostic methods. Obviously, if an established test is the basis for diagnosis, it will appear more sensitive and specific than any test measured against it. An abnormality on a new test of visual function may not be indicative of glaucomatous damage. SWAP may have improved sensitivity because it

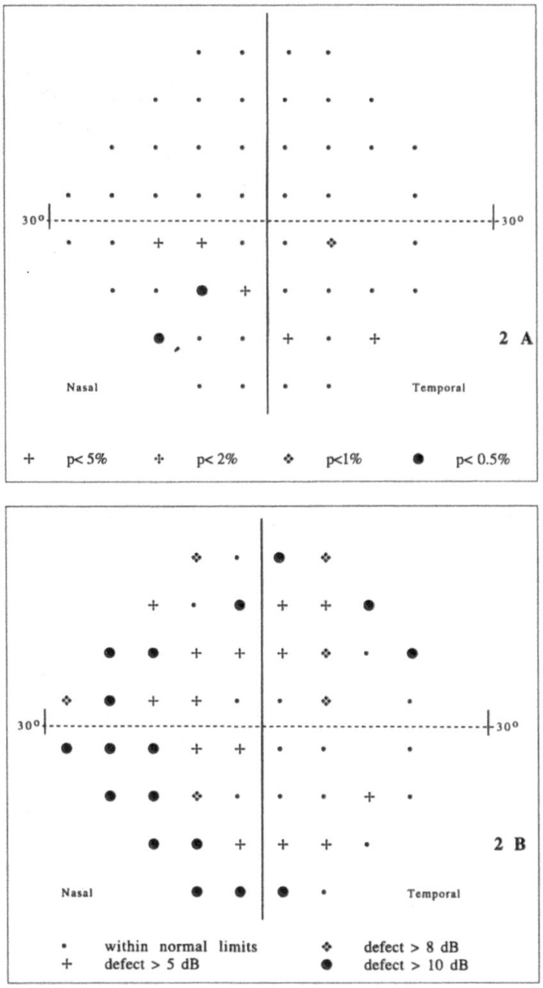

Fig. 2A, B. Visual fields in September 1991. Standard field (**A**) showed some defective points in the inferior hemifield, but the indices were within normal limits (MD: + 0.07 dB and CPSD: 1.06 dB) with borderline GHT. SWAP (**B**) detected superior and inferior arcuate defects and GHT showed generalized depression (case1)

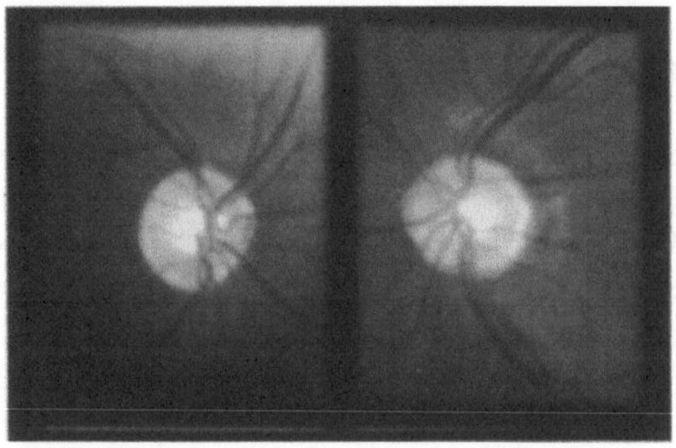

Fig. 1. Optic disc photographs (left and right eyes) in September 1991 appeared normal (case 1)

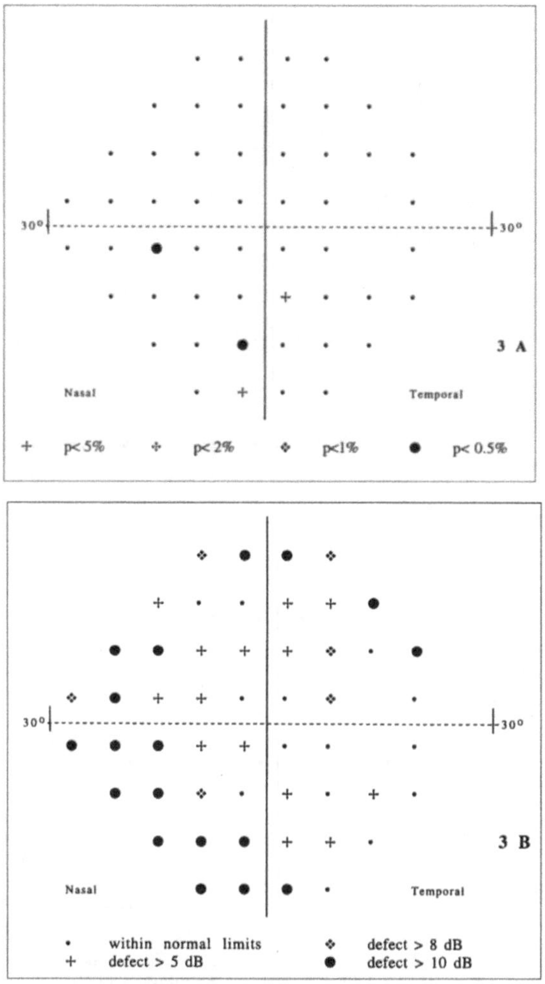

Fig. 3A, B. Visual fields in May 1992. Standard field (A) showed some defective points in the inferior hemifield (MD: + 1.97 dB, CPSD: 2.32 dB and outside 95% limits) and the GHT was borderline. SWAP (B) demonstrated the superior and inferior arcuate defects already detected a year before and the GHT was outside normal limits

is directed at measuring an isolated visual function. It has been used to follow-up ocular hypertensive eyes until their conversion to glaucoma. This type of prospective longitudinal information is necessary to evaluate any functional test.

To redefine glaucoma and recognize it at an earlier stage with new functional or structural tests, one needs to compare measures of functional loss with measures of the structural changes associated with glaucomatous optic neuropathy. It is possible that structural abnormality can be detected first in some eyes, and vice versa. For example, retinal nerve fiber layer

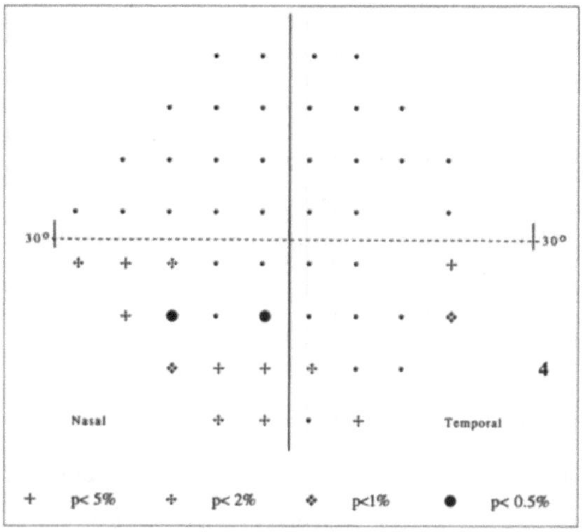

Fig. 4. Standard visual field in December 1995 showed a cluster of 13 defective locations in the inferior hemifield which formed an arcuate defect and nasal step (MD: –1.01 dB, CPSD: 2.11 dB and outside 95% limits) and the GHT was outside normal limits. The SWAP performed in 1995 is not shown

defects may precede the onset of standard visual field loss in glaucoma by several years. As structural and functional testing appear to complement each other, it is likely nevertheless that structural testing will continue to be used in conjunction with functional testing to diagnose glaucoma or detect changes in the individual patient. With time, these comparisons should lead to a better understanding of the process of glaucoma and allow us to identify the pertinent information from function, structure, and epidemiological factors that will best diagnose glaucoma and indicate glaucomatous progression. For now, we can conclude that a normal standard visual field and a normal optic disc appearance do not necessarily indicate the absence of glaucomatous abnormality.

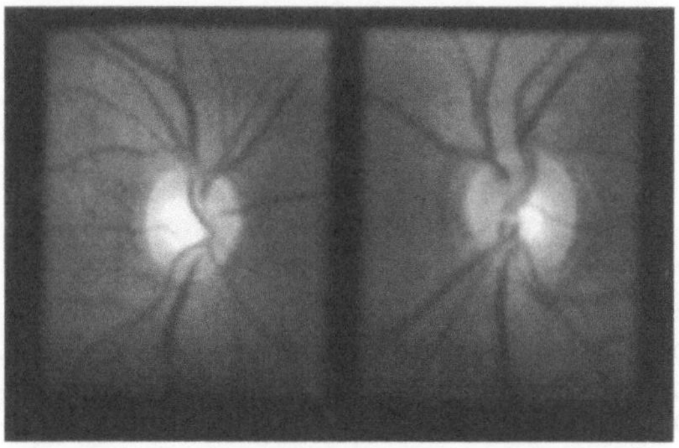

Fig. 5. Optic disc photographs (left and right eyes) in appeared normal in May 1990 (case 2)

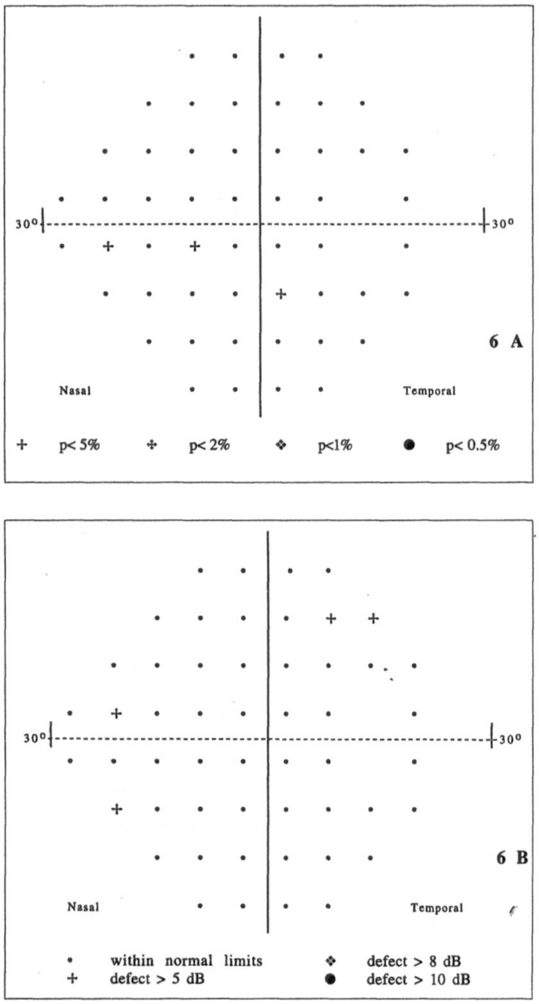

Fig. 6A, B. Visual fields in May 1990. Standard field (**A**) showed three defective points in the inferior hemifield, but the indices (MD: -1.19 dB, CPSD: 0.05 dB) and GHT were within normal limits. SWAP (**B**) detected four defective points and the GHT was outside normal limits (case 2)

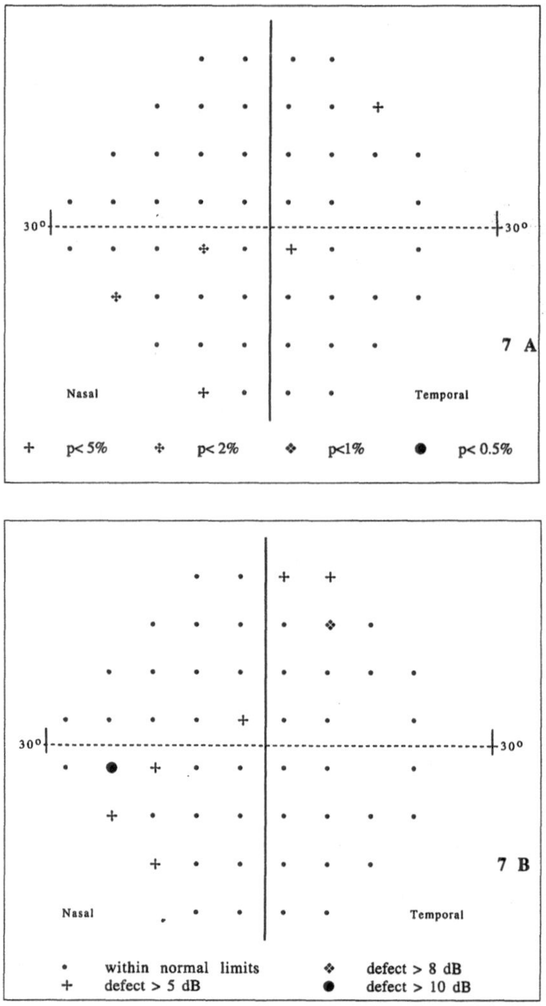

Fig. 7A, B. November 1993 visual fields. Standard field (**A**) showed five defective points, but the indices (MD: -0.37 dB, CPSD: 0.00 dB) and GHT were within normal limits. SWAP (**B**) detected an inferior nasal defect and a cluster of three defective points in the superior hemifidd. The GHT was borderline (case 2)

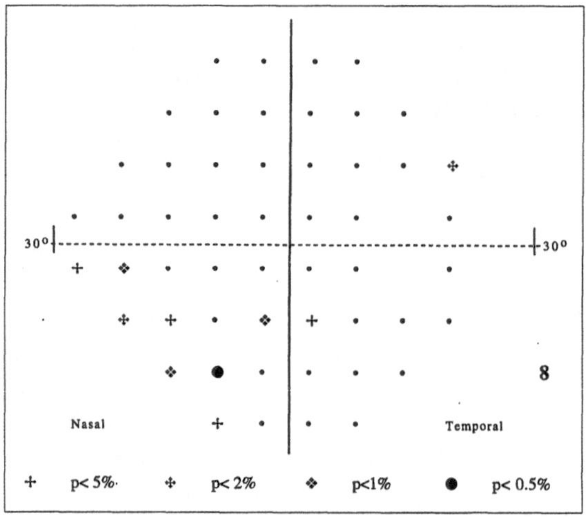

Fig. 8. September 1994 standard visual field showed a cluster of nine defective locations in the inferior hemifield which formed an initial arcuate defect and nasal step (MD: -2.19 dB, CPSD: 2.63 dB and outside 95% limits) and the GHT was borderline. The SWAP performed in 1994 is not shown because it was done with a new version for which the normative database is still not available (case 2)

References

1. Quigley HA, Dunkelberger GR, Green WR (1989) Studies of retinal ganglion cell atrophy correlated with automated perimetry in human eyes with glaucoma. Am J Ophthalmol 107:453-464
2. Sample PA, Weinreb RN (1990) Color perimetry for assessment of primary open-angle glaucoma. Invest Ophthalmol Vis Sci 31:1869-1875
3. Sample PA, Taylor JDN, Martinez GA, Lusky M, Weinreb RN (1993) Short-wavelength color visual fields in glaucoma suspects at risk. Am J Ophthalmol 115:225-233
4. Johnson CA, Adams AJ, Casson EJ, Brandt JD (1993) Blue-on-Yellow perimetry can predict the development of glaucomatous visual field loss. Arch Ophthalmol 111:645-650

When to Start Ocular Hypotensive Therapy?

G.K. Krieglstein

University Eye Clinic, Joseph-Stelzmann-Strasse 9, D-50924 Köln, Germany

Introduction

Tons of literature and many symposia full of controversies have been devoted to this issue. Repeated consideration is warranted by therapeutics and diagnostic tests. The grey zone between the precursors and the manifest disease becomes more and more transparent and we feel more confident in our decision making on when to start ocular hypotensive therapy. However, we are still far away of establishing a cookbook guideline or a rule of thumb for this question. The steps forward are small but they are identifiable and applicable to the care of our patients. The following brief review tries to substantiate this statement.

The problem

The decision to treat elevated intraocular pressure or normal pressure associated with various risk factors to develop glaucoma crucially depends on a careful consideration of prevalent risk factors of glaucoma versus the risk/benefit ratio of lifelong treatment with emphasis on the side effects of medications, costs of medications and consequences for the quality of life. A decision has to be found including a well informed patient promising adequate compliance in therapy and follow-up. The probability of loss of visual function for an individual patient is closely related to the composition of various risk factors which comprise the overall risk. The question, when to start ocular hypotensive therapy therefore goes along with the analysis of risk factors.

The pros and cons of intraocular pressure as the major risk factor

The disputable role of IOP for the development of glaucoma becomes evident in the cross national differences of the prevalence of different forms of glaucoma. In the western industrialized world open-angle glaucoma is at least five times more frequent than ocular hypertension. Whereas in Japan normal pressure glaucoma is three times more frequent than chronic open-angle glaucoma and even more frequent than ocular hypertension. Fifty percent of all glaucomas in Greenland are angle-closure glaucomas.

Is there a genetic background which modifies the pathogenetic significance of IOP? For this reason we do not rely on IOP alone for glaucoma screening, optic disc and visual field has to be included and the screening programs targeted on groups with verified risk factors. The role of IOP is even more confusing when considering temporal transitions from ocular hypertension to normal or from normal to normal tension glaucoma. Prospective population based studies showed that in about twenty percent of glaucoma patients initial damage to the optic nerve happened at IOP levels below 22 mm Hg. This again signals the 'dilemma' of IOP in the development of glaucoma. Elevated or even normal intraocular pressure as a pathogenetic key factor is obviously modified by perfusion parameters of the optic disk, by its mechanical compliance or even by an abnormal neuronal vulnerability. Fortunately IOP reduction makes sense for all of these components of pathogenesis of glaucoma.

If the relative risk to develop a visual field defect at IOP's below 16 mm Hg is defined to be 1, the risk for IOP's between 16 and 19 mm Hg would be already 1.7 (Armaly et al., 1980, modified by A. Sommer). This tells us, that even within normal IOP ranges the IOP related relative risk of developing a visual field defect rises. If a pressure range of 21-25 mm Hg is considered to constitute a relative risk for developing a visual field defect as 1, pressures over 30 mm Hg cause a relative risk of 15.3 (David et al., 1977, modified by A. Sommer). The risk of glaucomatous optic nerve damage is related to IOP beginning of even in the lower normal range and increasing linearly into the twenties. The slope of the regression line is modified by the presence or absence of other risk factors. There is no bellshaped, exponential correlation that could indicate a special crucial pressure range as a turning point in the pressure related glaucoma risk.

The subentity of normal tension glaucoma is often quoted for minor significance of intraocular pressure in the development of glaucoma. However, even in normal tension glaucoma IOP may be decisive. The IOP's are not 'normal' in these glaucomas, they are primarily grouped in the upper normal range and we do find the higher IOP in the eye with more advanced damage in asymmetric, bilateral cases.

For further confusion IOP can be erroneously interpreted to be normal: when there are unidentified IOP peaks outside the office hours, when there are abnormal postural responses of IOP, when there are 'normative' IOP rises (with an individual having IOP's in the low tens and having 22 mm Hg years later, probably comprising an IOP rise of 12 mm Hg within the normal range). There may be tonometric errors or IOP reduction by systemic medication. What makes IOP suspicious of glaucoma? When there are intermittent high IOP's which cause a broad range of fluctuations, sometimes more than 10 mm Hg, when there are abnormal postural responses, e.g. high IOP in the morning at bed time in the supine patient. No doubt, IOP is the major risk factor, if one is not aware of others we have to rely on it. Schulzer et al. (1990) identified two clusters of patients in his prospective study. In the first cluster there was a good correlation of IOP and field loss, in the second cluster there was a poor correlation of IOP and field loss, both clusters indicating either the predominance of IOP or the predominance of vascular risk factors.

Vascular risk factors relevant for the initiation of therapy

A series of ocular and systemic vascular risk factors is well known to facilitate the process of glaucomatous damage to the optic nerve. Among other ocular, vascular risk factors, the role of peripapillary hemorrhages, peripapillary atrophy, papillary venostasis, and arteritic neuronal lesions are well known. Systemic vascular disorders can dramatically contribute to the disease process as severe hypotony, migraine, peripheral angiospastic symptoms, diabetes, hypercoagulability, bradyarrhythmia, arrhythmia, and history of cardiovascular shock. With respect to its significance for development of glaucoma peripapillary hemorrhages are best investigated. These splinterlike bleedings may precede retinal nerve fiber layer defects, visual field defects, angiographic filling defects of the optic disk and rim notches of the disk, all in a time scale of years.

The information of the optic nerve head

After IOP and the consideration of ocular and systemic risk factors the appearance of the optic disk is one of the decisive remaining aspects for the decision when to start ocular hypotensive therapy. Optic disks with large C/D-ratios are prone to develop glaucomatous damage earlier at a given IOP level, than optic disks with a small C/D-ratio. Asymmetry of cupping especially in conjunction with an asymmetry of IOP can be indicative of early damage. This has a special meaning if retinal nerve fiber layer defects can be identified or there is a history of disk hemorrhages in these patients. Localized narrowing of the neuroretinal rim or even rim notches are highly indicative for beginning manifest glaucoma definitely requiring therapy. Circumlinear vessels at the rim margin or bridging of vessels in the cup are also highly suspicious for damage of the disk.

If cupping is considered solely 'glaucoma-like'

cupping is an important differential diagnosis. 'Glaucoma-like' cupping can occur in ischemic optic atrophy, in arteritic optic nerve head lesions, in compressive optic nerve lesions or in congenital optic nerve head anomalies. The size and the configuration of the cup has to be seen in context of other aspects. A generalized increase in the size of the cup can be due to diffuse axonal loss being paralleled by diffuse field loss, occurring predominantly in high IOP's. Rim notches, peripapillary hemorrhages, and parapapillary halos may indicate focal damage to the optic disk, predominantly occurring in normal or moderately elevated IOP's. The information of the disk over time can be essentially increased using computerized biomorphometry with modern imaging equipment like a laser tomographic scanner. This enables to interprete cup and rim size and configuration in relation to the true size of the optic disk.

The information of the visual field

To obtain the best possible information from perimetry, adequate test strategies, well problem-orientated have to be used. The recommendation to use a dynamic test strategy which renders a short duration of the test is fair. A perimetric test analysis in the follow-up can be very helpful in visualizing the area of initial damage in the graphical display of the perimetric examination. Due to the neuronal redundance in the eye it must be questioned, whether very early neuronal damage has already a perimetric equivalent. Most likely discrete optic nerve changes precede the early visual field defect, accepting that subtle diffuse field loss is very difficult to verify. Local field loss is more specific, however, frequently accompanied with diffuse loss. Many other psychophysical and electrophysiological tests claiming to sort out ocular hypertension from early glaucoma like color vision, flicker fusion, motion detection, contrast sensitivity, photostress, recovery time or pattern electroretinogram have not found their way to clinical routine. Many positive and encouraging results have been published with those, however, our expectations with respect to specificity and sensitivity could not be fulfilled.

Conclusion

If the decision to treat can not be made at a given time, careful follow-up will be the basis to revisit the decision when it seems appropriate. Follow-up with respect to IOP means repeated measurements to identify over all trends or changes in the range of fluctuations. Follow-up with respect to the optic nerve should be performed with a modern technique of biomorphometry if possible. Follow-up with respect to visual field testing should consider a dynamic strategy and a trend analysis.
During decision making one should not forget that glaucoma is not the only threat of elevated IOP. We know very well, that the risk of a retinal vein occlusion is probably five times higher in high IOP than in normal. Nevertheless, treatment of all ocular hypertensive patients may be unnecessary as treatment of late stage glaucomas may be ineffective. If the decision is made in favour of treatment one should not forget that the more advanced the glaucomatous damage is, the greater is the required IOP reduction. A therapeutic IOP level reflecting at least 30% reduction from the untreated IOP level is an acceptable guideline.

Start ocular hypotensive therapy:
- at earliest functional or anatomical abnormality
- at IOP levels which make those in long-term inevitable
- modify significance of given IOP level by presence or absence of other risk factors
- at any IOP level if damage is evident
- at any elevated IOP level if there are more than one risk factor
- at IOP's exceeding 25 mm Hg if there is no other risk factor.

Lowering of Intraocular Pressure in the Treatment of Glaucoma

L. Bonomi and M. Marraffa

Department of Neurological and Vision Science, Eye Clinic, University of Verona, 37126 Verona, Italy

Introduction

Elevated intraocular pressure (IOP) is generally considered the most important risk factor for development of glaucoma. Although other factors may be involved, the only method today available for treating glaucoma is lowering IOP.
A great deal of evidence has been gathered about the effectiveness of antiglaucoma therapy in reducing eye pressure, but a direct and indisputable demonstration of optic nerve and/or visual field protection by treatment is still lacking [1]. Because of ethical obstacles unbiased, long-term, controlled clinical trials comparing treated and untreated patients with demonstrated glaucoma damage are not available. A few correctly designed studies comparing treated and untreated ocular hypertensives have been carried out and gave unconclusive results [2-4]. Further experimentation on this subject is in progress, but the results are not yet known [5].
The clinical impression of most ophthalmologists is that in many glaucomatous patients the progression of optic nerve damage is not arrested despite the pressure normalization produced by the treatment [6-8].
The existence of so-called normal pressure glaucoma and of patients with long-term ocular hypertension without glaucomatous damage casts further doubts on the actual role of IOP in the course of the disease. Some authors go so far as to deny that elevated IOP is a causative factor in primary open-angle glaucoma [6, 7].
In recent years, some careful studies carried out on glaucoma patients reported that, in the long-term, further progression of glaucomatous damage actually happens in a number of eyes despite the seeming effectiveness of treatment [8-11]. These studies, however, clearly demonstrate that the functional worsening is strictly correlated with the level of eye pressure attained by the therapy.
On the whole it is apparent that a dependable protection is obtained only with very low levels of IOP and that the variability of this parameter, as expressed by the standard error or the standard deviation, is of importance. Here, we provide a preliminary report on the long-term behaviour of the visual field in patients suffering from POAG, under medical treatment and studied by means of automated perimetry.

Patients and Methods

The study was carried out on 82 patients suffering from POAG under medical treatment at the outpatient glaucoma service of the Eye Clinic of the University of Verona. The demographic data concerning the group are shown in Table1.
Patients included in the study had IOPs controlled only by medical therapy. All of them had some degree of glaucomatous optic atrophy and definite visual field defect, as assessed by threshold automated perimetry (Octopus 2000, program G1).
Exclusion criteria were: other types of glaucoma, previous ocular surgery, concomitant ocular diseases different from glaucoma, neurological diseases potentially damaging visual field, reduced clarity of optical media and poor compliance in taking their medication or attending their outpatient appointments. Patients with far advanced functional loss were not included also.

Table 1. Patient characteristics

	Mean	SD
Age	54.09	14.47
Female	27	
Male	55	
Visual acuity	0.93	0.19
Refraction (SE)	-2.56	- 3.91
Perimetry		
MD	9.16	5.82
CLV	24.95	39.72
SF	2.03	0.66
IOP[a]	19.87	4.62

MD, Mean defect; CLV, Corrected loss variance; SV, Short term fluctuation.
[a]At the beginning of follow-up, most patients were already under treatment.

Patients were followed-up at 3 month intervals or more frequently if needed. At each visit they were examined by one of us (L.B.) by slit-lamp, ophthalmoscopic, tonometric, and visual acuity examination. Mean IOP was calculated as the mean of all tonometric measurements recorded during the follow-up period. The visual field was tested at intervals of 6-8 months by means of Octopus automated perimetry (G1 program). The criterion for visual field deterioration was a loss of mean sensitivity greater than 5 dB, confirmed in two or more consecutive determinations. A change of this extent is usually considered out of the range of long-term fluctuation. To avoid interference from the learning effect the first visual field determination of each patient was discarded.
For each patient only one eye, chosen randomly, was considered for the study. The mean follow-up was 45.27 months ± 4.62 (range 1-8 years).
The data were subjected to survival analysis according to the method of Kaplan-Meier. The possible correlations between visual field worsening and factors like age of the patient, extent of the original defect and variability of the eye pressure (S.D. of the individual tonometric readings) were studied by linear regression.

Results

The time course of the IOP in the entire group is shown in Fig. 1.
The visual field of 55 patients remained stable throughout the study, while a decrease of mean sensitivity of 5 dB or more was observed in 27 patients. However, only one patient suffered a loss of sensitivity greater than 10 dB.
Figure 2 shows the distribution of mean IOP in patients with stable visual field and in those with progression of perimetric damage. It is apparent that all patients with eye pressure below 18 mm Hg remained stable, while all those with mean IOP above 22 mm Hg underwent further damage of their visual field. With mean eye pressure between 18 and 22 mm Hg, nearly 50% of patients suffered a progression of perimetric damage.
A survival distribution for the development of a visual field deterioration at three different levels of mean IOP was computed using the Kaplan-Meier method: the results are shown in

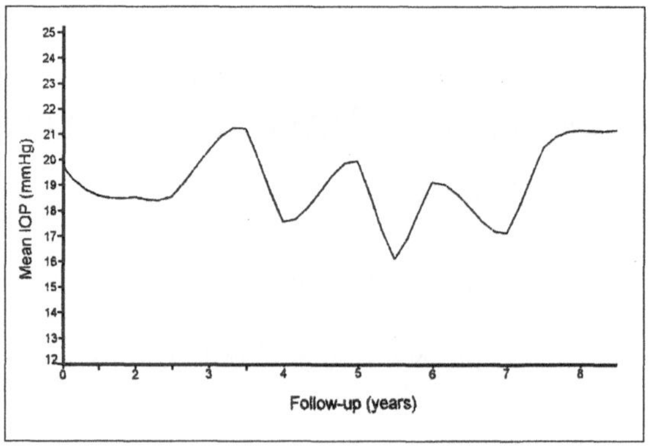

Fig. 1. Time course of mean IOP in the 82 eyes during follow-up

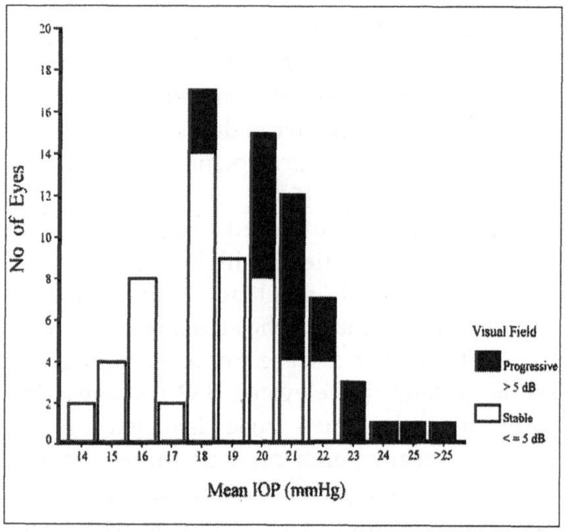

Fig. 2. Distribution of mean IOP in patients with stable visual field and in patients with progression of perimetric damage

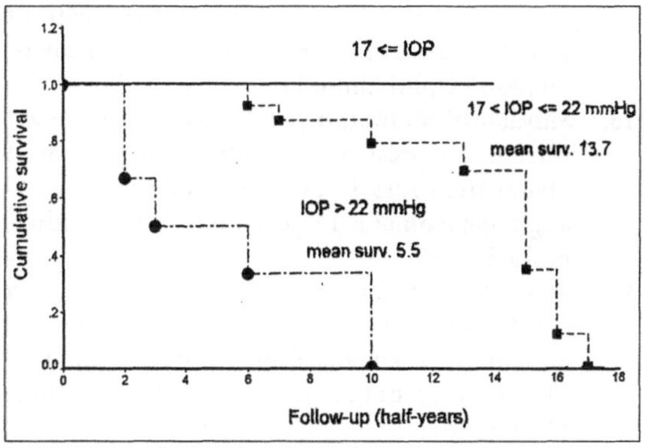

Fig. 3. Survival distribution for the development of a visual field deterioration of 5 or more dB at three different levels of mean IOP

Fig. 3. We can confirm that the eyes with stable eye pressure below 18 mm Hg are not at risk of further visual field deterioration. Above this limit, a definite risk is present, which increases with time and with the level of IOP. Between 18 and 22 mm Hg, mean survival is 81 months, while above 22 mm Hg it is only 33 months.
A significant correlation ($p< 0.01$) was found between visual field worsening and variability of the pressure as expressed by the standard deviation of the tonometric readings recorded in the same patient. The severity of the original defect (MD) was very strictly correlated with the extent of further damage ($p< 0.0009$). No correlation was found with the age of the patient.

Discussion

Our results substantially confirm those obtained by other authors in previous studies of the same design [11-14]. In our series one third of the patients underwent further visual field damage despite a degree of tonometric control that most ophthalmologists might have considered as reasonably good. In fact, only patients with eye pressure stabilized below 18 mm Hg turned out to be fully protected. With higher levels of IOP, the visual field damage progressed in many cases. The probability of worsening was clearly dependent on the height of pressure. For the higher levels (above 22 mm Hg), progression is absolutely certain.
The second most important factor is time. In the present study the mean follow-up of eyes with progressive damage was 66 months, while that of stable eyes was only 35 months. It may be expected that with further follow-up the disease many additional patients will get worse. This is confirmed by the shape of the survival curve: above 17 mm Hg the probability of losing visual field rises with time, finally reaching 100%, the mean survival being 5.5 months above 22 mm Hg and 13.5 months between 18 and 22 mm Hg. Other factors worsening the prognosis are the original severity of the mean perimetric defect (MD) and the variability of eye pressure.
It may be concluded that, in order to secure a reasonably effective protection in the long run to patients suffering open-angle glaucoma, the IOP must be constantly kept below the mandatory limit of 18 mm Hg and large fluctuations of pressure must be avoided. In far advanced cases the safe limit may be even lower [13, 14]. This is not an easy goal. Since the best antiglaucoma drugs induce a decrease of pressure of no more than 20%-30%, in most cases multiple medications are needed or surgical techniques must be resorted to.

References

1. Rossetti L, Marchetti I, Orzalesi N, et al. (1993) Randomized clinical trials on medical treatment of glaucoma. Are they appropiated to guide clinical practice? Arch Ophthalmol 111:96-103
2. Kass MA, Gordon MO, Hoff MR, et al. (1989) Topical timolol administration reduces the incidence of glaucomatous damage in ocular hypertensive individuals. Arch Ophthalmol 107:1590-1598
3. Schulzer M, Drance SM, Douglas GR (1991) A comparison of treated and untreated glaucoma suspects. Ophthalmology 98:301-307
4. Epstein DL, Krug JH, Hertzmark E, et al. (1989) A long-term clinical trial of timolol therapy versus no treatment in the management of glaucoma suspects. Ophthalmology 6:1460-1467
5. Kass MA (1994) The ocular hypertension treatment study. J Glaucoma 3:97-100
6. Quigley HA, Maumenee AE (1979) Long-term follow-up of treated open-angle glaucoma, Am J Ophthalmol 87:519-525
7. Grant WM, Burke JF (1982) Why do some people go blind from glaucoma? Ophthalmology 89:991-998
8. Odberg T (1987) Visual field prognosis in advanced glaucoma. Acta Ophthalmol (Suppl) 65:27-29

9. Bengtsson B (1981) Aspects of the epidemiology of chronic glaucoma. Acta Ophthalmol (Suppl) 146:1-48
10. Krakau (1981) Intraocular pressure elevation cause or effect in chronic glaucoma? Ophthalmologica 182:141-147
11. Mao LK, Stewart WC, Shields MB (1991) Correlation between intraocular pressure control and progressive glaucomatous damage in primary open-angle glaucoma. Am J Ophthalmol 111:51-55
12. O'Brien C, Schwartz B, Takamoto T, Wu DC (1991) Intraocular pressure and the rate of visual field loss in chronic open-angle glaucoma. Am J Ophthalmol 11:491-500
13. Shirakashi M, Iwata K, Abe H, Namba K (1993) Intraocular pressure dependent progression of visual field loss in advanced primary open-angle glaucoma: a 15-year follow up. Ophthalmologica 207:1-5
14. Stewart WC, Chorak RP, Hunt HH, Sethuraman G (1993) Factors associated with visual loss in patients with advanced glaucomatous changes in the optic nerve head. Am J Ophthalmol 116:176-181

The Adverse Effects of Topical Anti-Glaucoma Drugs

P. Demailly

Saint Joseph Hospital Foundation, Institute of Glaucoma, 185 rue Raymond-Lasserand, 75574 Paris, France

Adverse Effects of Cholinergic Eye Drops [4]

The treatment of glaucoma currently includes numerous drugs to reduce intraocular pressure. But, regardless of their effectiveness, these drugs are never innocuous for either the eye or the body as a whole. The frequency and occasional severity of the adverse effects that they cause substantiate an old aphorism: *"glaucoma patients rarely complain about their disease but always about their treatment"*.

The adverse effects of cholinergic eye drops such as pilocarpine are mainly local. Allergic blepharo-conjunctivitis is usually due to the drop's wetting agent rather than the pilocarpine itself.

Induced myosis may lead to reduced vision, especially at night, and more so in patients with early cataract changes. With prolonged myosis, posterior synechiae may form. One should be careful to periodically dilate glaucoma patients treated with myotics. Also, in the presence of a narrow angle, a myotic may actually create a pupillary block.

Accomodative spasm may be induced by action on the ciliary muscles, with headaches, eye pain and a reduction in visual acuity usually found in myopic and young patients. The awareness of floaters may be increased by myotics due to a pinhole effect when there is a posterior vitreous detachment. In addition, myotics may cause posterior vitreous detachment and traction on the retinal periphery due to ciliary spasm. All glaucoma patients should undergo careful examination of the retinal periphery before instillation of myotic treatment, as well as periodically thereafter.

Myotics can also cause iatrogenic cataracts. This is true of anticholinesterase agents. Anterior capsular vacuoles may form which, if seen in time, may be reversible when the eye drops are stopped.

For several reasons, compliance with myotic treatment is far from optimal. This is why a sustained-release system would be advantageous, providing prolonged action lasting at least 12 hours. To date, the best solution is Ocusert, for which the time of action is 6/7 days and the adverse effects are limited, especially with Ocusert 20.

Anticholinesterase agents such as phospholine iodide should not be used in phakic eyes due to the significant risk of posterior synechiae, hindering examination of the disk and retinal periphery. Cardiovascular and gastrointestinal adverse effects may also occur in predisposed patients.

Adverse Effects of Sympathomimetic Eye Drops [5]

These are numerous and often responsible for poor compliance with treatment.

Local Adverse Effects

Mydriasis may be more or less bothersome but, in general, does not last long. Adrenaline should not be prescribed to patients with narrow angles due to the risk of acute angle closure. Gonioscopy should be systematically conducted

as part of the initial assessment.
Conjunctival infection may appear after a white and is due to reflex vasodilation after an initial vasoconstriction. Prostaglandin release may also play a role. Red eyes may represent an aesthetic problem.
Allergic reactions are relatively common and treatment must be discontinued in these cases.
Conjunctival pigmentation due to adrenaline may occur after months or years of treatment. Adrenaline can color soft lenses.
Cystoid macular edema has been reported in aphakic subjects and is generally reversible when the treatment is stopped. Corneal edema has occasionally been observed due to the endothelial toxicity of adrenaline. Blurred and fogged vision is not necessarily due to increased intraocular pressure in these cases.
Finally, there may be a vasoconstrictor effect of adrenaline on the optic nerve head.

Systemic Adverse Effects

One drop of 2% adrenaline may lead to systemic absorption of 2 mg adrenaline. This may induce extrasystoles, tachycardia, arrhythmia, elevated blood pressure and cerebrovascular accidents. Care should thus be taken when using adrenaline in patients with coronary insufficiency or severe arteriosclerosis. Due to the lower concentration of adrenaline in its dipivefrin form, less adverse effects can be expected; however, mydriasis and conjunctival injection may still occur.
With the combination of guanethidine and epinephrine, the reduction in intraocular pressure is improved but, unfortunately, adverse effects are often increased, including ptosis, which makes the use of these drugs less widespread.

Adverse Effects of Topical β-blockers [6-8]

Local Tolerance

Subjective tolerance varies from one β-blocker to another and from one patient to another.
β-blocker eye drops are sometimes responsible for unpleasant sensations : stinging, sensation of a foreign body, pruritis, burning sensations. Carteolol, [3, 15, 18], followed by timolol and levobunolol is better tolerated than befunolol, metripranolol or betaxolol.

Regarding objective tolerance, three phenomena may be observed:

1. A reduction in tear production: In general, this is mild, whatever the β-blocker used, and does not affect the corneal epithelium. It mainly concerns a deterioration in the mucosal layer of the lacrimal film [10]. However, it can exacerbate existing lacrimal dryness related to age, particularly in postmenopausal women or in the event of intake of oral β-blockers and tranquillizers or neuroleptics [3].
2. Corneal hypoesthesia: This is a reflection of a masked membrane-stabilizing activity of β-blockers or a specific β-blocking action on presynaptic nerve transmissions or the β-receptors of the corneal epithelium. It is still very rare with the β-blockers currently in use and has no clinical repercussions, except, of course, in predisposed subjects.
3. Allergic reactions: Immediate or late-onset eye allergies are rare but possible. The preservative seems to be usually, but not always responsible, since allergic reactions to preservative-free single-dose forms can be observed, such as with befunolol.

In summary, the local tolerance of β-blockers is still excellent in comparison with cholinergics or sympathomimetics, for the great majority of glaucoma patients undergoing this treatment.

Topical β-Blockers and Contact Lenses [18]

Hard gas-permeable contact lenses absorb benzalkonium, which can deteriorate the biomaterial and reduce visual acuity. Soft hydrophilic lenses retain any chemical molecule with a molecular weight less than 500 (β-blocker and benzalkonium).
The phenomena of retention and re-release, which have the following consequences should thus be taken into account: (a) in the eye, a greater reduction in intraocular pressure, an exacerbation of local effects, an increase in systemic effects (bradycardia); (b) in the soft lenses, a certain amount of limitation in transparency.

Systemic Adverse Effects

In fact, the adverse effects of topical β-blockers are mainly systemic. Topical β-blockers expose subjects to the same clinical risks as administration by the oral route. The blood concentrations obtained are low but the effects of their active ingredient are promoted by the absence of hepatic passage and conditioned by their pharmacokinetic and pharmacodynamic properties.

Cardiovascular Signs

These are dominated by the negative chronotropic effect and include:

1. Bradycardia: All nonselective topical β-blockers induce sinus bradycardia with no clinical signs. β1-selective betaxolol is the only one which does not significantly modify pulse rate in comparison with a placebo and a more selective β-blocker (timolol), probably as a result of its strong binding to plasma proteins (Fig. 1).
2. Arterial hypotension: This is possible but rare, as is orthostatic arterial hypotension.
3. Serious cardiovascular complications: heart failure and syncopal tendency, which can lead to sudden death, occur only in patients who already present with cardiovascular disease. Elderly subjects with arrhythmia or atrioventricular conduction disorders are particularly vulnerable. The decrease in heart rate can trigger cerebrocirculatory insufficiency or even neurological deficit accidents. These complications generally occur in the first few days following instillation of the β-blocker. Finally, the rebound phenomenon may induce tachycardia and an increase in blood pressure.

Bronchopulmonary Complications

The β2-blocking effect induces bronchospasm. This phenomenon may, at least cause dyspnea on exertion and, at worst, reactivation of previous asthma, exacerbation of pre-existing asthma, or respiratory exacerbation of chronic bronchitis (Fig. 2).
Betaxolol is the only one which, in studies, does not modify respiratory state. In fact, great care should be taken when prescribing it to glaucoma patients with respiratory insufficiency. In the event of the slightest doubt, respiratory function tests should be conducted and the opinion of a pneumologist should be sought.

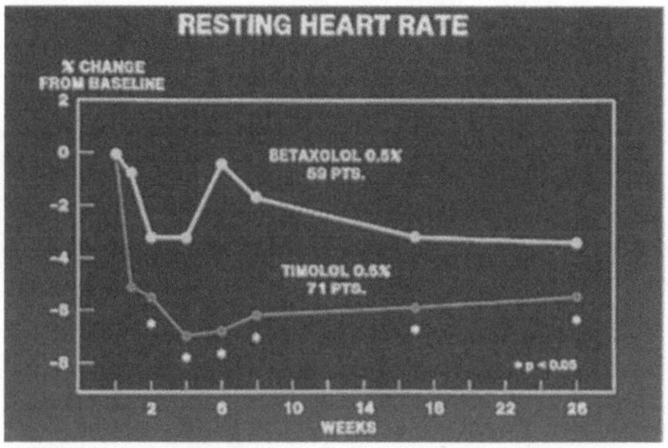

Fig. 1. Resting heart rate curve: comparison between betaxolol and timolol

Neuropsychiatric Signs

Numerous disturbances have been observed, especially in the U.S.: depression, mental confusion, headaches, disorientation, hallucinations, nightmares. The problem is to concretely link these to the β-blocker effect. Two mechanisms may be involved: 1) the active ingredient crossing the hemato-meningeal barrier, in particular with liposoluble β-blockers [18], 2) exacerbation of cerebrocirculatory insufficiency in elderly arteriosclerosis patients.
Cases of sexual dysfunction have been reported, but without irrefutable proof of the role played by the β-blocker.
A few cases of myasthenia have been decompensated with timolol, due to a decrease in

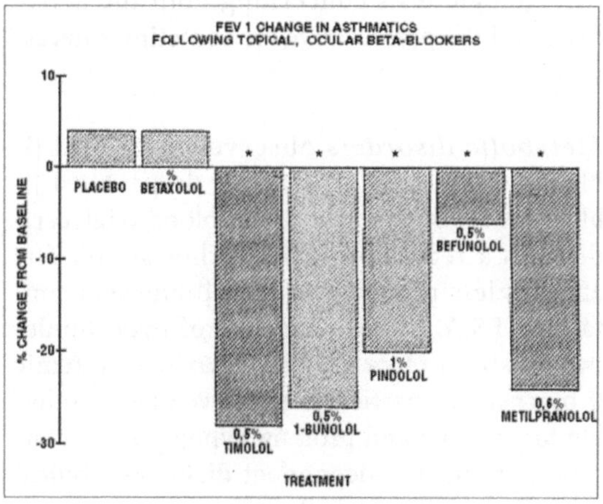

Fig. 2. V.E.M. effects

peripheral neuromuscular transmission or presynaptic block.

Peripheral Vascular Signs

Blocking of the β2-receptors of the vascular walls may exacerbate Raynaud's syndrome or distal arteritis. It may be necessary to conduct a Doppler scan to obtain arterial velocimetric curves. In theory, β-blockers containing I.S.A., betaxolol β1-selective, provide better protection against these signs than non-selective β-blockers, but, once again, there are numerous individual variations.
The effects on vascularization of the optic nerve are still debatable. Some studies demonstrate a vasoconstrictive effect, in particular a reduction in the diameter of retinal arteries and a prolongation in retinal circulatory times. Other studies tend towards correct maintenance of vascularization of the optic nerve, in particular due to an increase in retinal blood flow, or to no further deterioration in (a) glaucoma eyes with statistically normal pressure, (b) telediastolic rate, or (c) the resistance index of the ophthalmic artery and the ciliary arteries on color Doppler imaging [9].
Finally, recent studies have demonstrated a reduction in perimacular leukocyte circulatory velocity linked to the long-term use of topical β-blockers in normal eyes with an increase in macular sensitivity threshold. This phenomenon persists after treatment discontinuation.

Miscellaneous

Cutaneous signs reflect allergic phenomena. Allergologic tests concerning both the active drug and the preservative are sometimes necessary.

Metabolic disorders observed with oral β-blockers rarely occur with eye drops. Most β-blockers induce an increase in blood triglycerides and a reduction in HDL cholesterol. The effect is less pronounced with β-blockers containing I.S.A. [7, 15]. One case of hyperlipidemia has been reported with betaxolol. Systemic β-blockers, in particular selective ones, are liable to promote and prolong hypoglycemic conditions in insulin-dependent diabetics. Topical β-blockers may mask the adrenergic warning signs of hypoglycemia (sweating, tachycardia).

Topical β-blockers have not been studied in pregnancy, but the fact that they cross the placental barrier exposes the fetus to cardiovascular effects. During breast-feeding, β-blocker levels in breast milk are significantly higher than in blood plasma. Repercussions are thus possible in the infant (bradycardia, asthma, apnea).

Drug Interactions

The combination of oral and topical ß-blockers generally increases efficacy with respect to intraocular pressure but it may also increase the adverse effects.
In combination with calcium inhibitors, there is a potentiation of the depressive effects with a risk of syncopal accidents or heart failure in predisposed subjects. This phenomenon is essentially observed with verapamil. Apart from this drug, all other anti-calcium drugs can be used with topical β-blockers.
The digitalic drugs, quinidine and amiodarone accentuate the negative chronotropic and dromotropic effects of topical β-blockers; it is thus necessary to monitor the heart rate of treated patients.
Regarding general anesthesia there is a particular problem with the combination of oral β-blockers and volatile halogenic anesthetics, with the risk of myocardial depression, a reduction in cardiac output and slowed conduction. The anaesthetist must thus be warned of treatment with topical β-blockers, but the latter must not be discontinued.

Conclusion

The good local tolerance of β-blockers has led to millions of glaucoma patients receiving this treatment throughout the world. But, these drugs can have adverse effects due to their systemic passage. It is thus necessary to comply with the contraindications. Absolute contraindications are asthma and stage II and III atrioventricular block. Relative contraindications include heart failure, chronic bronchopneumopathy, Raynaud's syndrome and severe obstructive arterial disease, sinus bradycardia, and certain cases of severe myasthenia.
In the event of the slightest doubt, the ophthalmologist and general practitioner must consult closely before instigating such treatment and

then conduct long-term monitoring.
Insertion of a pace-maker may be necessary.
Systemic passage can be reduced by naso-lacrimal occlusion for 5 min [17, 18]. This occlusion also enables reduction of the concentration of the β-blocker for the same efficacy on intraocular pressure. As the adverse effects are dose-dependent, sustained-release timolol essentially yelds a reduction in the dose for the same efficacy [17].
Finally, the greater vulnerability of elderly patients to the systemic effects of β-blockers should be pointed out [12, 15]. These patients often present with latent obstruction of the respiratory tract, which although not detected is likely to be exacerbated under the effects of long-term treatment with topical β-blockers. It would thus be logical to conduct respiratory function tests in these patients before any treatment.

Adverse Effects of Apraclonidine in Long-Term Treatment

The adverse effects of long-term treatment with apraclonidine are not negligible (39% of cases) and the drug must be discontinued in 23% of cases [2]. The two most common adverse effects are: (1) a reduction in visual acuity attributed to a decrease in posterior ciliary artery flow on colour-Doppler imaging; and (2) intense allergic conjunctivitis with chemosis. Other rarer effects have been reported and include blurred vision, discomfort, conjunctival hyperhemia, sensation of foreign body, dry mouth, and systemic effects such as nausea.

Side-Effects of Topical Carbonic Anhydrase Inhibitors [14]

Carbonic anhydrase-inhibitors are well tolerated, especially dorzolamide. Mild stinging and burning upon instillation can occur but resolve within minutes. A bitter taste following ocular instillation has been noted in some patients [11, 16].

Adverse Effects of Topical Prostaglandins

Adverse effects are minimal with Latanoprost [1]; there may be a slight increase in conjunctival injection.
With PGF2α-IE [13], there may be foreign body sensation, irritation, conjunctival hyperemia.
Iris pigmentation has been observed in glaucoma patients.

Adverse Effects on Conjunctiva [19, 20]

Adverse effects on conjunctiva after long-term treatment of antiglaucoma drugs are now well documented. The role of the drop's wetting agent, mainly benzalkonium, is mainly responsible but sympathomimetics and myotics may also work adversely.
Long-term treatment (more than 1 year) indirectly causes an alteration of lacrimal film and directly causes alterations of epithelial cells, inflammation and fibrosis. These conjunctival disorders can increase the risk of failure in filtering surgery with the development of fibroblasts proliferation and cystic bleb.

Conclusion

Medical anti-glaucomatous treatment compliance is mainly dependant on its tolerability, which is nevertheless variable from one human being to another. Systemic effects are the most redoubtable and force the ophthalmologist to strictly respect contraindications of the products. The most recently marketed drugs, such as topical carbonic anhydrase inhibitors or prostaglandin analogs, are devoid of such disadvantages. Their long-term efficacy as monotherapies remains to be evaluated.

References

1. Alm A, Widengärd I, Kjellgren D, Söderström M, Friström B, Heijl A, Stjerschantz J (1995) Latanoprost administered once daily cause a maintained reduction of intraocular pressure in glaucoma patients treated concomitantly with timolol. Br J Ophthal-mol 79:12-16
2. Araujo S, Bond J, Wilson R, Moster M, Courtland M, Schmidt Jr, Spaeth G (1995) Long term effect of apraclonidine. Brit J Ophthalmol, 79:12, 1098-1101
3. Cohen J (1995) Topical β-blocker therapy in the

aging female patient with glaucoma. Adv Therapy 12:121-128
4. Demailly P (1989) Traitement actuel du glaucome primitif à angle ouvert, Masson Editeurs. Rapport Soc Franç Ophtalmol 103-111
5. Demailly P (1989) Traitement actuel du glaucome primitif à angle ouvert, Masson Editeurs. Rapport Soc Franç Ophtalmol 111-122
6. Demailly P (1989) Traitement actuel du glaucome primitif à angle ouvert, Masson Editeurs. Rapport Soc Franç Ophtalmol 123-207
7. Freedman S, Freedman N, Shields B, Lobaugh B, Samsa G, Keates E, Ollie A (1993) Effects of ocular carteolol and timolol on plasma high density lipoprotein cholesterol level. Amer J Ophthalmol 116:600-611
8. Frishman W, Fuksbrumer M, Tannenbaum M (1994) Topical ophthalmic β-adrenergic blockade for the treatment of glaucoma and ocular hypertension. J Clin Pharmacol 34:795-803
9. Harris A, Spaeth G, Sergott RC, Katz LJ, Cantor L, Martin BJ (1995) Retrobulbar arterial hemodynamic effects of betaxolol and timolol in normal-tension glaucoma. Amer J Ophthtalmol 120:168-175
10. Herreras J, Pastor C, Calonge M, Asensio N (1992) Ocular surface alteration after long-term treatment with an antiglaucomatous drug. Ophthalmol 99:1082-1088
11. Lippa EA, Schuman JS, Higgingbotham EJ, et al. (1991) MK507 vs Sezolamide: comparative efficacy of two topically active carbonic anhydrase inhibitors. Ophthalmology 98:308
12. O'Donoghue E (1995) β-blockers and elderby with glaucoma: are we adding insult to injury? Brit J Ophthalmol STET 79:794-796
13. Lee PY, Shao H, Camras C, Podos S, (1991) Additivity of prostaglandin F2-α (1-Isopropyl ester to timolol in glaucoma patients. Ophthalmology 98:1079-1082
14. Serle JB, Podos S (1995) Topical carbonic anhydrase inhibitors in the treatment of glaucoma, Ophthalmol Clin North America 8:315-325
15. Stewart W (1994) Carteolol, an ophthalmic β-adrenergic blocker with intrinsec sympathomimetic activity. J Glaucoma 3:339-345
16. Wilkerson M, Cyrlin M, Lippa EA, et al. (1993) Four-week safety and efficacy study of dorzolamide, a novel active topical carbonic anhydrase inhibitor. Arch Ophthalmol 111:1343
17. Zimmerman T (1994) Safety of β-blockers in clinical practice. J Ophthalmol 10:56-59
18. Zimmerman T (1993) Topical ophthalmic β-blockers: a comparative review. J Ocular Pharmacol 9:373-384
19. Baudouin C, Garcher C, Houat N, Bron A, Gastaud P (1994) Expression of inflammatory membrane marker by conjunctival cells in chronically treated glaucoma patients. Ophthalmology 101:454-460
20. Broadway DC, Grierson I, O'Brien C, Hitchings R (1994) Adverse effects of topical antiglaucoma medications. The outcome of filtration surgery. Arch Ophthalmol 112:1446-1454

The Role of Visual Field Examination During Treatment of Glaucoma

M. Zingirian

Ophthalmological Eye Clinic, University of Genoa, S. Martino Hospital, 16132 Genoa, Italy

Introduction

The role of perimetry is different according to the stage of glaucoma. In the very early stage of the disease, when the glaucomatous damage has not yet been definitely established and the proper therapy is still questionable, perimetry has a diagnostic role and can tell us whether a visual field defect exists or not. In apparent glaucoma, perimetry has two different roles: (1) the assessment and (2) the follow-up of visual field damage. In this case perimetry provides information about the type and severity of damage and its variations over time.

Computerized perimetry provides this information using a typical numerical language consisting of maps, indices and plots. The maps are graphic charts in which light sensitivity, measured in a determined pattern of field locations, is reported numerically (decibels, dBs) or in grey scale symbols, according to strictly topographic criteria (Fig. 1).

Perimetric indices are simple numbers obtained by processing the measured values of sensitivity in order to improve interpretation of the defect features [1]. The main indices are: (1) the mean defect (MD), which represents the severity of the global damage in dBs; (2) the short-term fluctuation (SF), which indicates that thresholds are unstable and visual field, even if normal, is going to deteriorate when its value exceeds the normal limit of 2 dBs; (3) the corrected loss variance (CLV of the Octopus system) and the corrected pattern standard deviation (CPSD of the Humphrey system), which are both indices of inhomogeneous or localized damage. Since standard deviation is the square root of variance ($SD = \sqrt{V}$), the range of inhomogeneity is above 4 dBs for CLV and above 2 dBs for CPSD ($2 = \sqrt{4}$). Finally the plots are linear representations obtained by sorting the deviation from normal sensitivity values in an arithmetic progression from the best to the worst one. They indicate how wide and homogeneous the distribution is (Fig. 2).

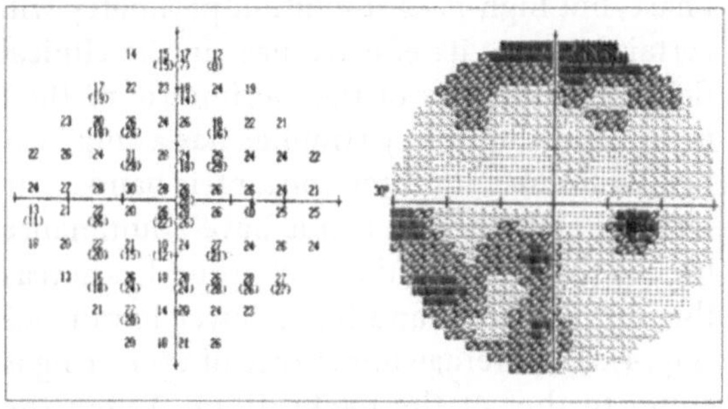

Fig. 1. Numerical and grey scale maps

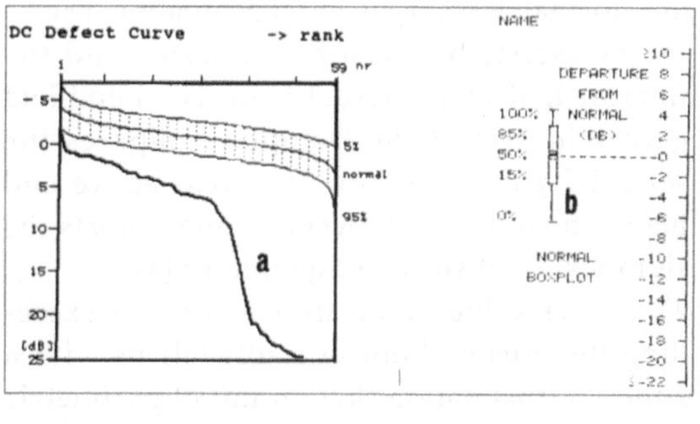

Fig. 2a, b. Two types of plots: **a** Cumulative defect curve (Octopus); **b** box-plot (Humphrey). Both represent the deviation from normal sensitivity of every point of a visual field, sorted in an arithmetic progression from the best to the worst value, thus indicating how wide and homogeneous the distribution is

Diagnostic Role

Perimetry fulfils its diagnostic role by answering our first question: “Does a visual field defect exist?” The answer is given in the following ways.

1) Mapping: it is easy to recognize a defect in a perimetric map, if it is pronounced: the sensitivity values are remarkably reduced (Fig. 3a) and the the darkest areas on the gray scale map are where the defect has its maximum density.

It is much more difficult to detect the defect when it is very slight, but the computer offers substantial help in this case by providing the so-called “differential maps” (Fig. 3b). These maps report the differences between the values measured and those of a normal population, available in the computers database for every point tested. This allows us both to recognize the locations where the sensitivity differs from the expected values and to read the relevant variations in dBs.

The Humphrey field analyzer gives additional information by means of a third type of map, which indicates how common or rare are the single variations in the normal population and therefore if they represent true, significant defects or not [2, 3]. Probability map classifies the statistical significance of the defects in four percentage levels (Fig. 3c).

Sometimes all the threshold values of a map are normal, but a typical glaucomatous asymmetry exsists between the superior and the inferior half of the visual field. The hemifield glaucoma test of the Octopus compares the sensitivity of corresponding areas above and below the horizontal meridian and reports the significance of such an asymmetry [4].

2) Indices values: a mean defect (MD) exceeding the normal limit of 2 dBs tels us with a good approximation that an initial perimetric defect exists. When CLV (or CPSD) and SF are also increased, this means that the defect has a typical glaucomatous character and is destined to deteriorate.

3) Through new devices. Today new perimetric systems are available to carry out *high-pass resolution perimetry* or *ring perimetry* [5] and *blue-yellow perimetry* [6]. Thus, early glaucomatous defects of visual field can be discovered before they become evident using the conventional computerized perimetry.

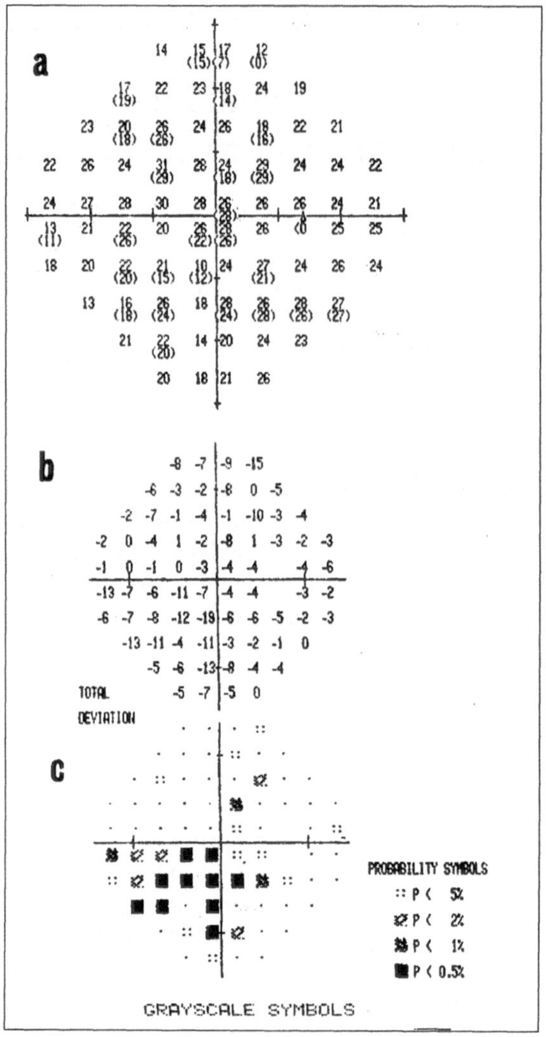

Fig. 3a-c. **a** Numerical map; **b** differential map; **c** probability map

Both techniques are still in a experimental phase, but high-pass resolution perimetry will certainly prove its effectiveness in the clinical field. The rationale of this perimetric method is the following: every stimulus has a ring-shaped structure with three concentric bands. The internal and external bands have a luminance higher than that of the background, whereas the intermediate band has a lower luminance (Fig. 4). The average luminance of every ring is equal to that of the background. When the resolution power of an eye does not distinguish between the three bands because the ring is too small or ocular function has deteriorated, the eye perceives neither the ring-shape nor the presence of the stimulus, because the reso-

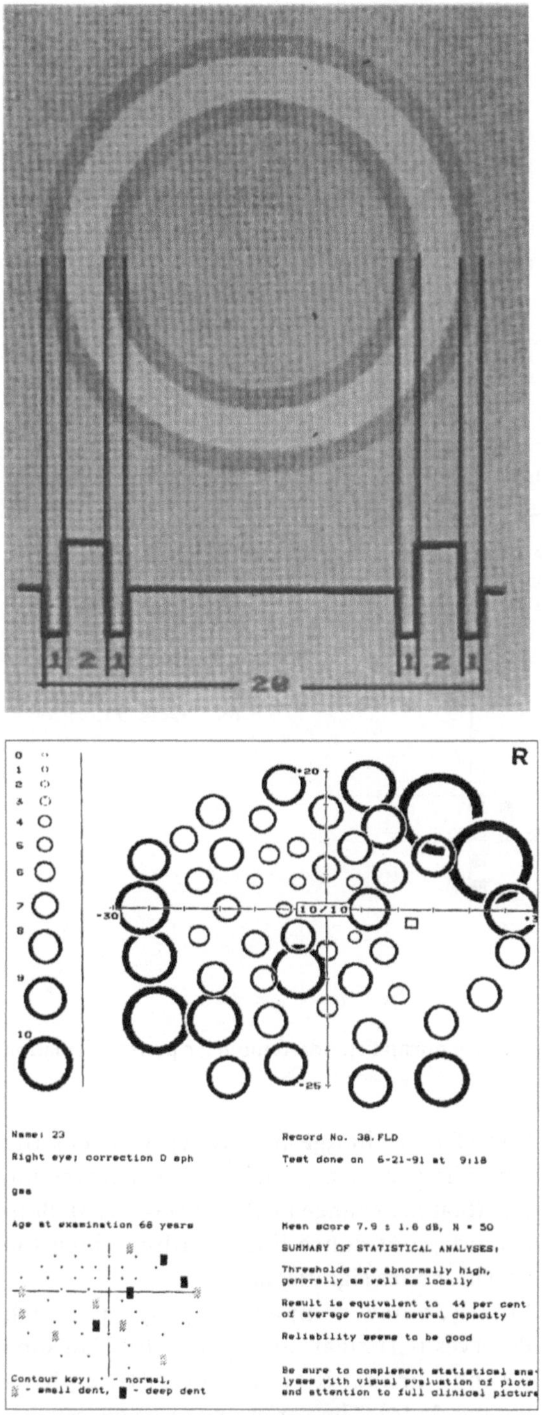

Fig. 4. High-pass resolution perimetry; *up*: the ring-shaped stimulus; *down*: an example of a ring perimetry map

lution and the perception thresholds coincide for this type of structured stimulus.

The capacity to perceive structured stimuli is assumed to be linked to the functional integrity of receptive fields of the retinal ganglion cells, where the initial glaucoma damage takes place. This explains the great importance of a method that detects glaucomatous defects at a very early stage.

Assessment Role

Now we would like to consider how computerized perimetry fulfills its assessment role, in order to answer our question: "How severe is the visual field loss?" For this purpose the numerical and grey scale maps provide data suitable for showing how wide is the deviation of the sensitivity from the normal average in every point tested. However, the most exact information is provided by the MD, since it is the perimetric index which quantifies the global loss in dBs, thus allowing a precise functional assessment of the glaucomatous eye.

A second question that computerized perimetry answers in relationship to its assessment role is: "Is the defect diffuse or localized?" The importance of this question is explained by the fact that diffuse defects are commonly related to preretinal factors, most frequently to a cataract, whereas localized defects are mostly typical of glaucoma. The Humphrey perimeter allows us to distinguish between diffuse and localized defects by comparing the sensitivity values of a visual field with both the normal standard and the patients individual models [3]. This provides a *total deviation map* (in which the diffuse and localized damage are added toghether) and a *pattern deviation map* (where only the localized damage are present) (Fig. 5).

For the same purpose, the Octopus perimeter plots 59 threshold values determined by the G1 program on a diagram, thus forming a curve (cumulative defect curve or Bebié curve) (Fig. 2a) in which the diffuse and the localized components of the defect are easy to recognize [7].

Follow-Up Role

Finally we must consider the follow-up role of perimetry, from which we expect an answer to our question: "Has the perimetric defect changed with respect to previous examinations?"

The importance of this information is of fundamental value for the ophthalmologist, who must establish whether the patient's glaucoma

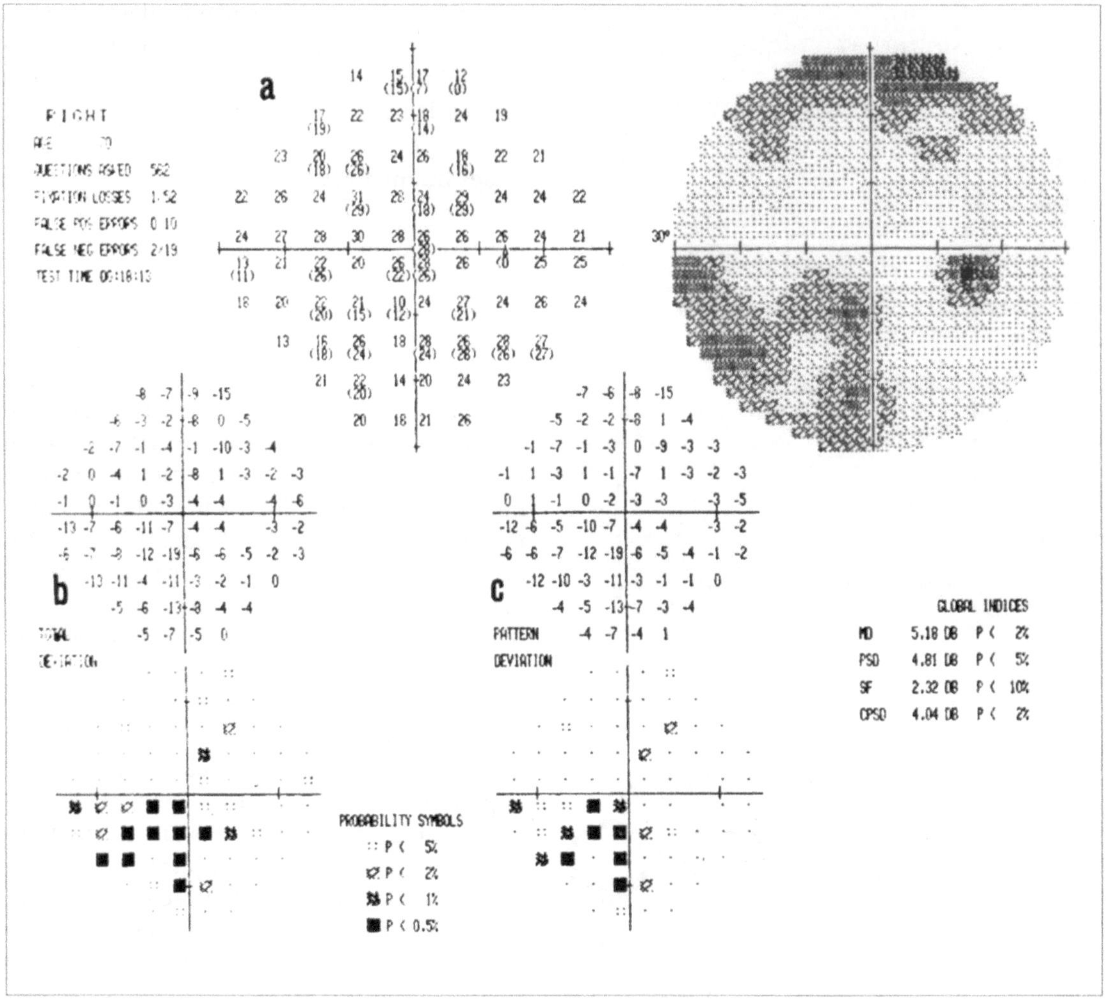

Fig. 5 a-c. a numerical map; **b** total deviation map, related to the normal standard model; **c** pattern deviation map, related to the individual model

is stable or requires new therapeutic approaches. The comparison between the last and the previous examinations can be performed by direct observation of a series of successive visual fields of the same eye or by means of statistical analysis.

In direct observation, the ophthalmologist can easily observe in the series of fields whether the defects have become progressively denser or have enlarged over time, whether the MD and other indices have worsened, or, whether, by contrast, the maps and indices have remained stable (Fig. 6).

In a statistical comparison, the computer compares the variations in MD in a series of successive visual fields of the same eye with those of a normal population. The Octopus system [8] performs this comparison using Student's *t* test (Delta change program), whereas the Humphrey system [3] uses a linear regression test (Statpac-change analysis) (Figs. 7, 8). Both provide confidence limits within which the variations are significant.

Finally, a new comparison program which deserves particular attention is the Glaucoma Change Probability Analysis (Humphrey Statpac 2) [4]. The variations of single sensitivity values in a series of fields, related to a previous visual field of reference, are compared with those of a population with stable glaucoma (Figs. 9, 10). The significance of this comparison is statistically evaluated. This program offers additional help to the ophthalmologist, in making a decision about maintaining or changing the patient's therapy.

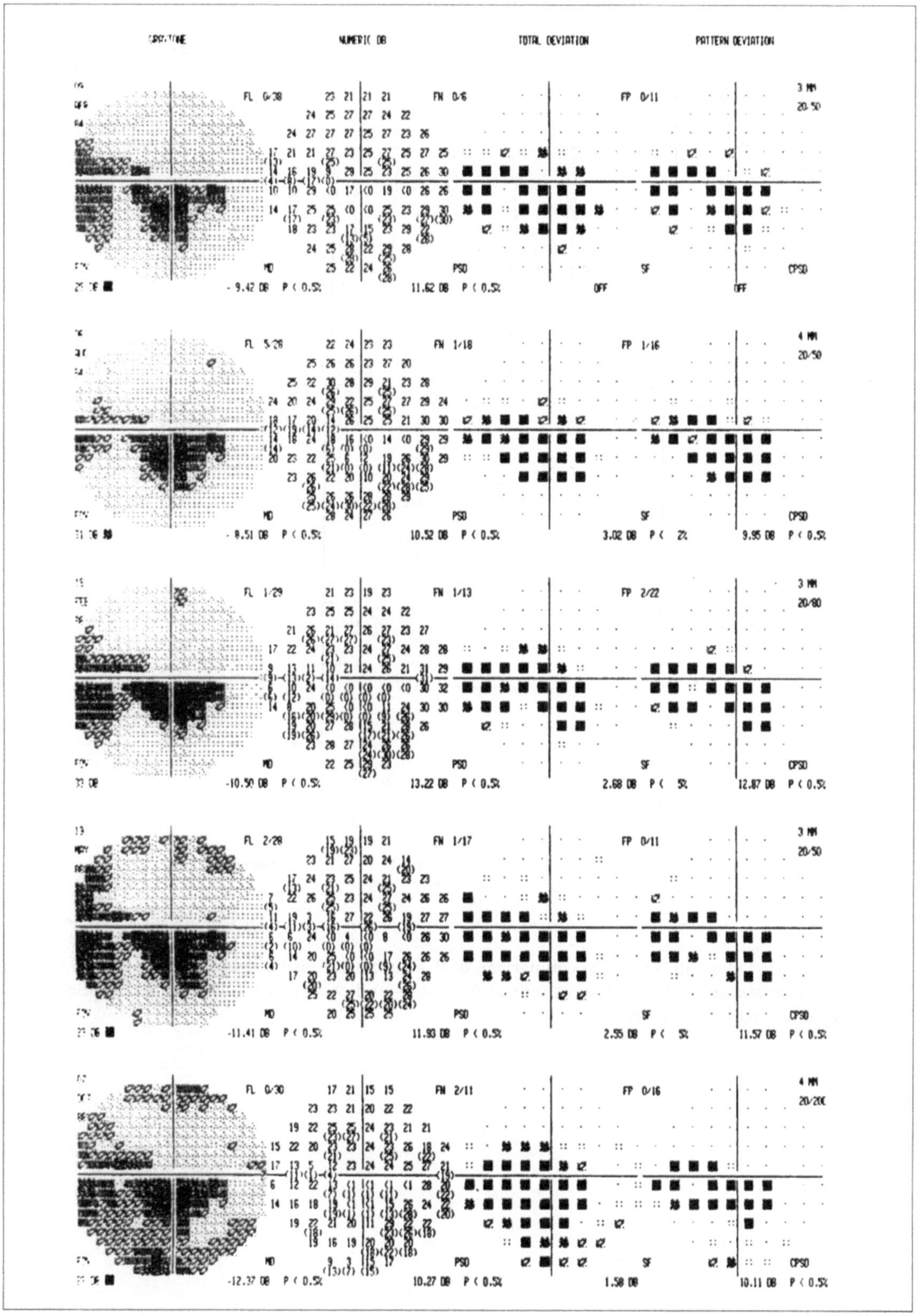

Fig. 6. Perimetric follow-up. Five successive visual fields of the same patient are printed so as to be directly evaluated by the ophthalmologist together with the relevant total deviation and pattern deviation maps (Statpac overview printout)

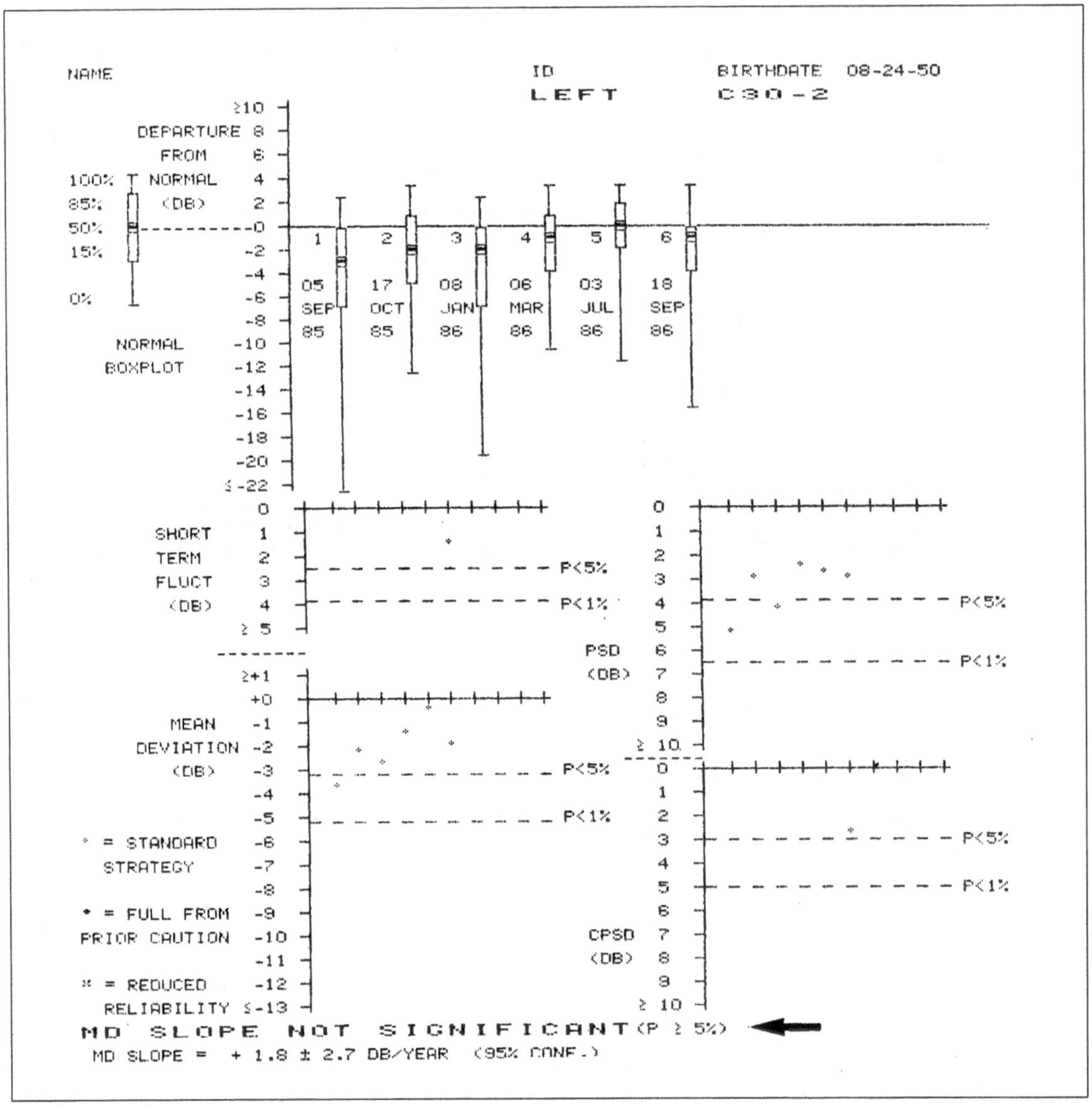

Fig. 7. Perimetric follow-up. Statistical comparison of five successive visual fields (Statpac change analysis printout). The mean defect (*MD*) slope is indicated as not significant (*arrow*), with respect to the normal data, using linear regression analysis

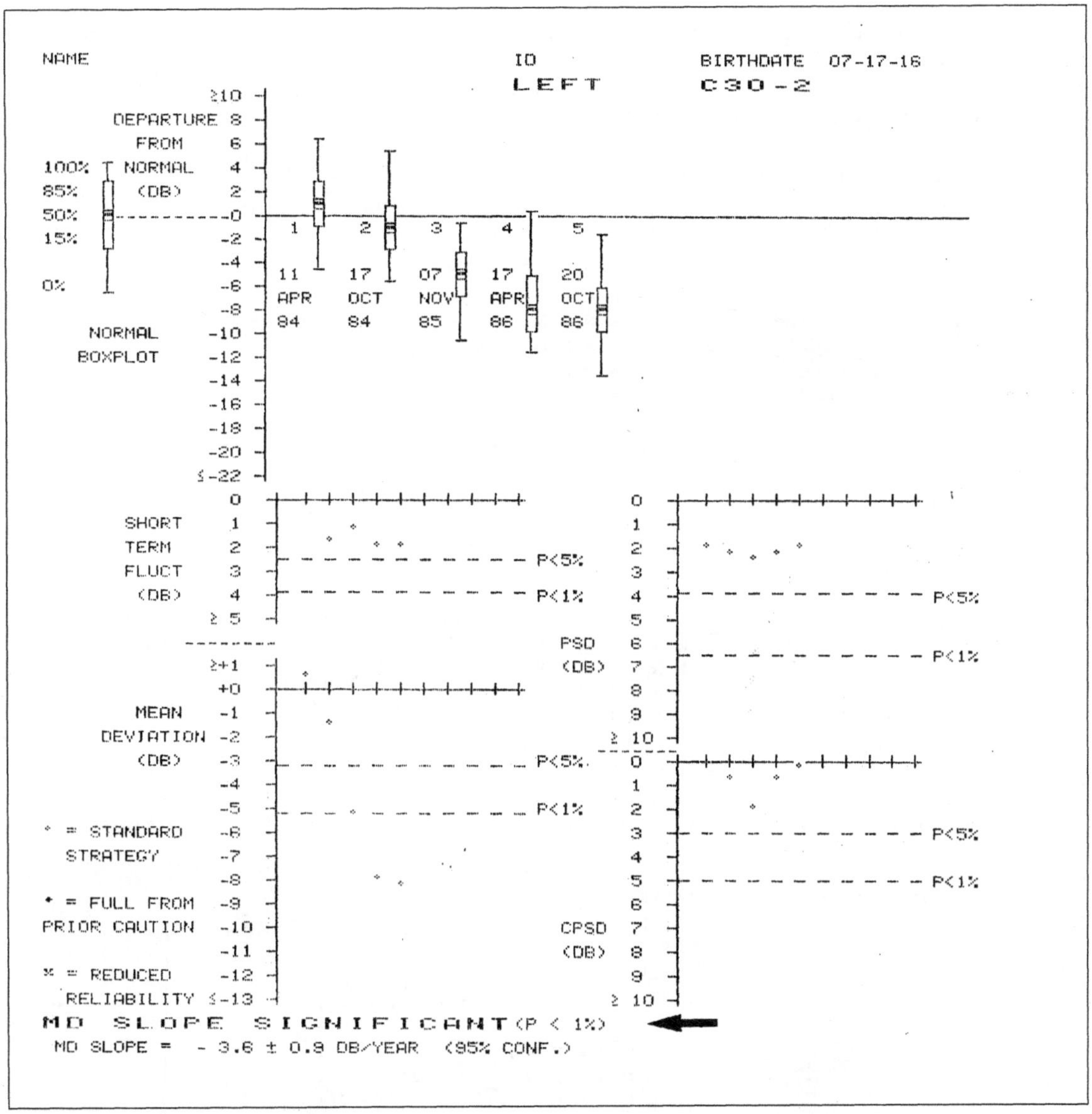

Fig. 8. Perimetric follow-up. Statistical comparison of four successive visual fields (Statpac change analysis printout). The mean defect (*MD*) slope is indicated as significant (*arrow*) with respect to the normal data, using linear regression analysis

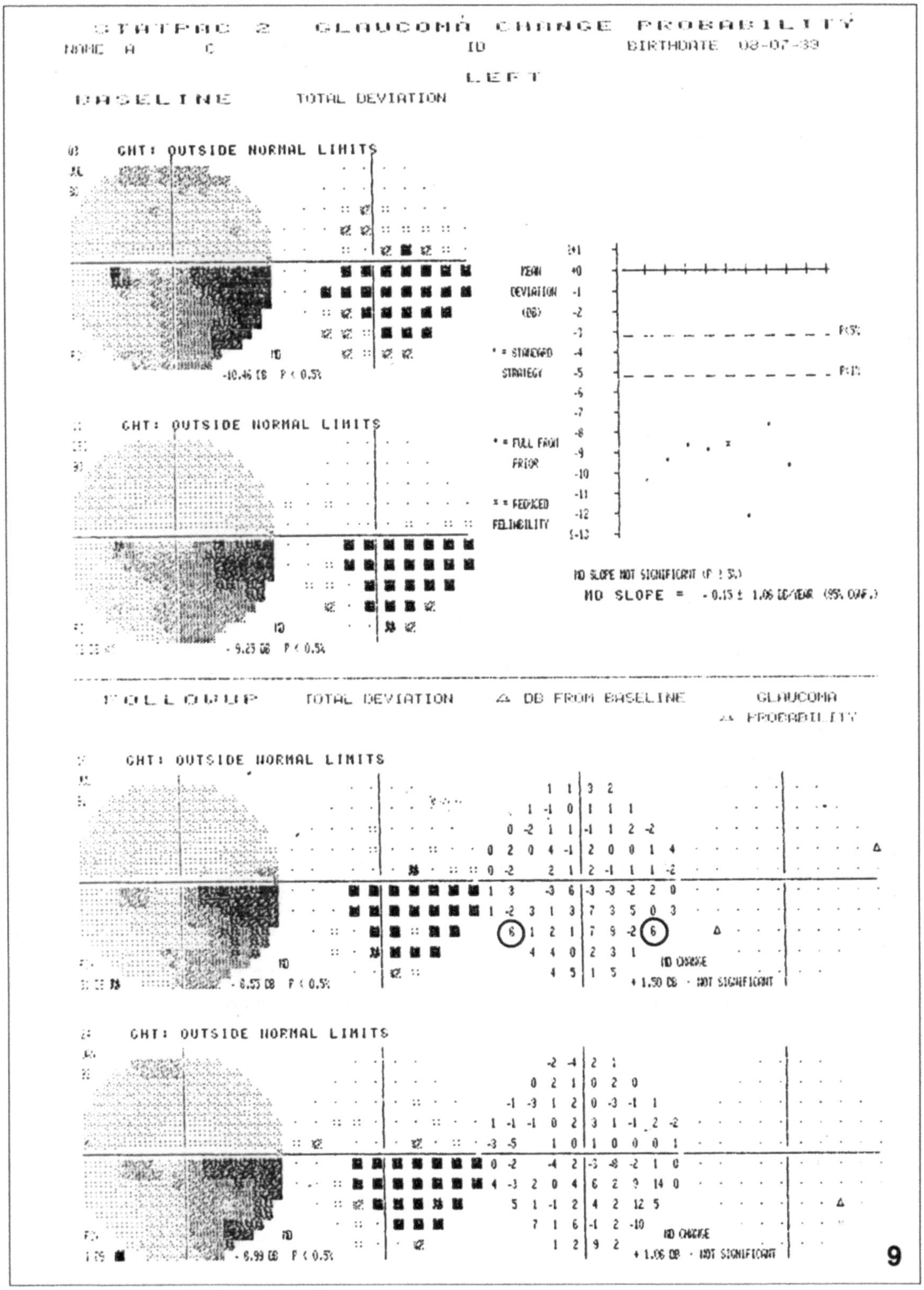

Figs. 9, 10. Perimetric follow-up. Statistical comparison of eight successive visual fields (Statpac 2 Glaucoma Change probability Analysis). The variations of single sensitivity values in every field, related to a previous field of reference (*baseline*), are compared with those of a population with stable glaucoma. The statistical significance is indicated

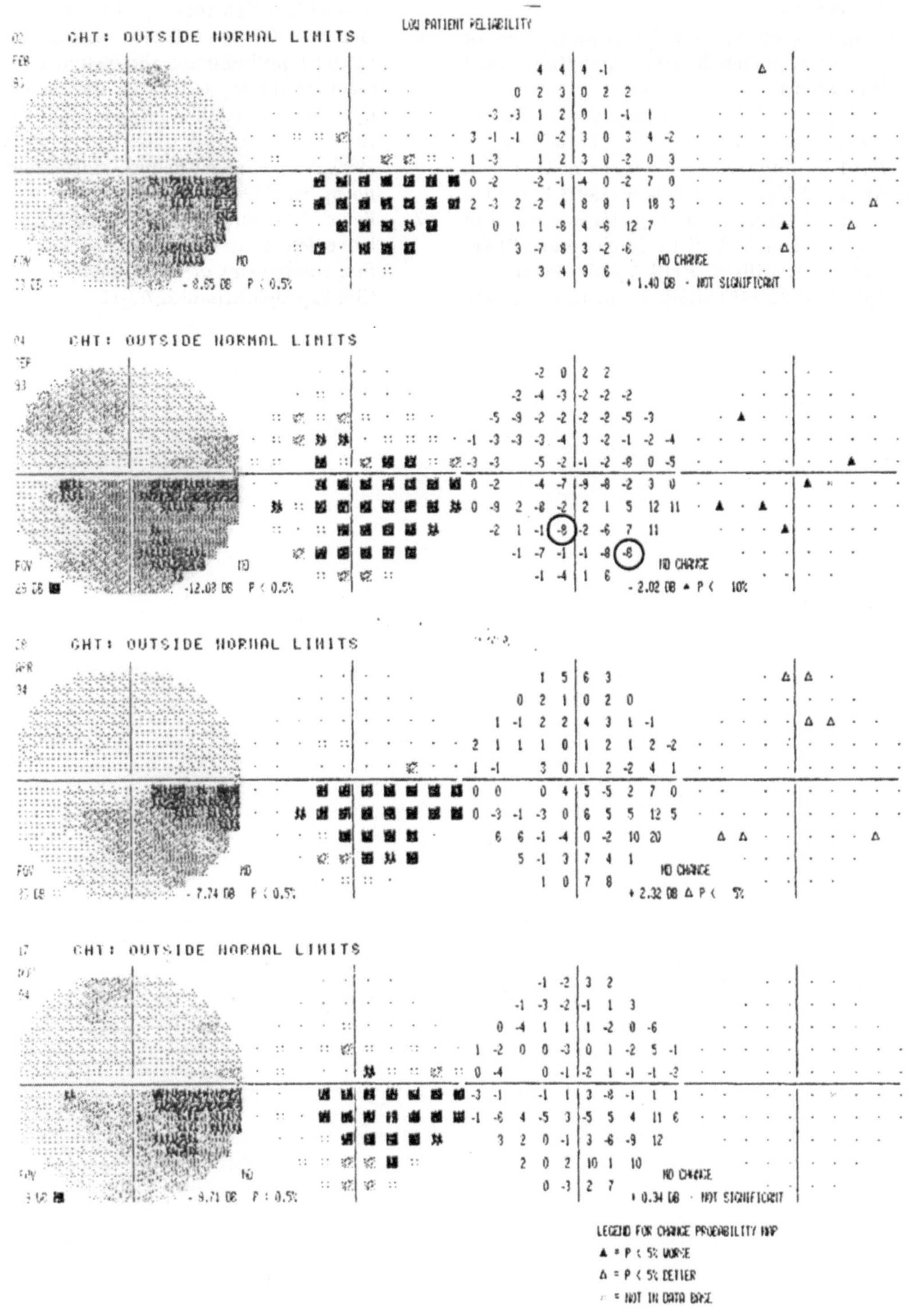
LOW PATIENT RELIABILITY
GHT: OUTSIDE NORMAL LIMITS
NO CHANGE
+ 1.40 DB - NOT SIGNIFICANT
GHT: OUTSIDE NORMAL LIMITS
NO CHANGE
- 2.02 DB ▲ P < 10%
GHT: OUTSIDE NORMAL LIMITS
NO CHANGE
+ 2.32 DB Δ P < 5%
GHT: OUTSIDE NORMAL LIMITS
NO CHANGE
+ 0.34 DB - NOT SIGNIFICANT
LEGEND FOR CHANGE PROBABILITY MAP
▲ = P < 5% WORSE
Δ = P < 5% BETTER
= NOT IN DATA BASE

10

References

1. Flammer J (1986) The concept of visual field indices.Graefe's Arch Clin Exp Ophthalmol 224:389-392
2. Heijl A, Asman P (1989) A clinical study of perimetric probability maps. Arch Ophthalmol 107:199-203
3. Allergan H (1987) Statpac User's Guide. Humphrey Instruments Inc., San Leandro, CA
4. Heijl A, Lindgren G, Lindgren A, Olsson J, Asman P, Myers S, Patella S (1991) Extended empirical statistical package for evaluation of single and multiple fields in glaucoma: STATPAC 2. In: Mills R, Heijl A (eds) Perimetry update 1990/1991. Kugler Ghedini, Amsterdam-Milano, pp 303-315
5. Frisén L (1993) Resolution theory and high-pass resolution perimetry (HRP). In: Mills R (ed)Perimetry update 1992/1993. Kugler, Amsterdam-New York, pp 419-427
6. Hart WM, Gordon MO, Silverman SE, Kass MA (1991) Equilluminant blue-yellow color contrast perimetry (CCP) in high risk ocular hypertension (OHT) and glaucoma (POAG). In: Mills R, Heijl A (eds) Perimetry update 1990/1991. Kugler Ghedini, Amsterdam-Milano, pp 325-329
7. Bebie H, Flammer J, Bebie T (1989) The cumulative defect curve: separation of local and diffuse components of visual field. Graefe's Arch Clin Exp Ophthalmol 227:9-12

Discussion

Question: L. Quaranta

To Prof. Zingirian. Your school suggested a bracketing index. What is the clinical meaning of this index ? What is the clinical value of the Brusini stadiation modified by Zingirian?

Answer: Zingirian

These are specific questions. The bracketing index is an index that we obtained in the development of a new system of automated perimetry. The purpose was to point out all the information on the sensibility for a specific point in the visual field to be seen by the patient. The Brusini stadiation is useful to establish how advanced the glaucomatous damage is. It is based on the correlation of the mean defect with the index of variance. So we know how much the visual field defect progresses and also if it is localized or diffuse.

Question:

To Dr. Weinreb. In your conclusion you said that for the diagnosis and treatment of glaucoma we should focus, in 1996, on the optic nerve and not on ocular hypertension. I understand that for diagnosis, but what do you do for treatment?

Answer: Weinreb

The question relates to the slide where I indicated that we should be focusing on the optic nerve and not on intraocular pressure. I don't mean to underestimate the importance of intraocular pressure. After all in 1996 the only treatment we have for glaucoma is to lower intraocular pressure. Nevertheless, it's clear to all of us that glaucoma is not solely a disease of intraocular pressure.
I think it's important to focus on the optic nerve and particularly when we plenty utilize some of the new structural tests such as the one shown by Prof. Krieglstein. Some of the new functional tests such as swap that I talked about. We keep in mind that we are treating a glaucomatous optic neuropathy and not solely a disease of intraocular pressure.

Question: Demailly

I have two questions: first, what's the relationship between the swap research and the development of cataract? Second, are the early deficits recorded with swap reversible with treatment?

Answer: Weinreb

These are both excellent questions relating to the relationship between SWAP visual fields and cataract. This is a very important issue, because as one ages one develops a cataract. When we initially began to do these tests 12 years ago, we developed a method for measuring the density of the cataract and we would correct our visual fields according to the density of the lens. Subsequently, we developed a statistical method based on the age of the patients so that we no longer need to go through a procedure to measure the lens density. This correction factor is now implemented in software for color perimetry using the Humphrey visual field analyzer. So, to summarize, it is necessary to take into account the presence of the cataract and statistical means in software available with the visual field instrument that has been used. The second question is also quite interesting and relates to the reversibility of short weavening visual field defects. In my lecture I mentioned that the swap visual field defects appear to be more sensitive than standard white on white defects. In other words, we may be packing up glaucoma, and we think we are packing up glaucoma at an earlier stage than possible with standard white on white perimetry. So one may question: Where packing it up earlier is possible through other treatments which means lowering intraocular pressure, is it possible that some or all of these defects might not be reversible? There is no definitive answer to this question, Prof. Demailly.

Question:

To Dr. Weinreb. What is the method you utilize to evaluate the cataract density and if visual field defects detected by SWAP have the same topography of those detectable by b/w perimetry.

Answer: Weinreb

The first question relates to how lens density is measured, but I remind you again that this is no longer necessary when performing swap in clinical practice. The three methods that we used to validate the statistical method for correcting lens density included first of all the use of a lens opacitymeter, second the use of the digitized camera, and third a psychophysical test of lens density that we developed. Again this is not necessary in clinical practice. The second question relates to the correlation between visual field defects obtained with short weaving testing and with standard achromatic perimetry. There is an excellent correlation; the most common scenario is a patient who is an ocular hypertensive patient who has standard white on white visual field and a defect in swap. The patient is followed for several years and then subsequently develops glaucoma characterized by a visual field defect in swap, in standard white on white perimetry which was originally normal. Most often, the location of the defect is the same location as was earlier present with SWAP, the size of the defect very often is similar to the size of that defect as well. This is not always the case, but one of the very exciting things for us about swap that we noticed using the longitudinal tests was that swap predicted not only the presence of visual field defect but also its location.

Question: Maraini

I think I have two questions for you: which is your definition of progression, provided that progression is eventually confirmed in consecutive visits? The second question is: did you observe regression in your swap technique?

Answer: Weinreb

For confirmation in any of the studies that we do we insist not only on confirmation in consecutive visits but we require confirmation onto subsequent visual fields obtained within a time period that ranges between two weeks and four weeks depending on the study. Again we do observe regression in hypertensive patients who have swap defects, who are treated, but it is something that was ongoing and that we were evaluating in longitudinal clinical trials. This is a very interesting question, certainly one that gets at the fundamental issues of glaucoma and glaucoma therapy.

Question: Traverso

I have a question for Dr. Krieglstein, Dr. Demailly and Dr. Weinreb. The only outcome we are interested in is the patients' quality of life, which obviously seems to be related to visual field defects evolution and to how we are able to lower IOP enough to stop the progression of damage at least in the majority of patients.

So, it seems that a key factor is to find in each individual the appropriate target pressure. Do you think it is realistic at this point, and at this stage of our knowledge, to try and find in each patient the appropriate target pressure just looking for a reversal of either visual field or disc defects, so that we can lower their pressure until we observe such a phenomenon and then accept that as individual target pressure? Do you think this is a realistical thing to look for?

Answer: Krieglstein

Probably it would be a very nice perspective if you had means to identify the pressure required, if you would have dignostic means identifying the pressure required to prevent incidence of field loss or to prevent progression.

The rule is to get pressure as low as possible when the decision to treat is made, depending on the pressure level at which the early abnormalities, morphological and functional, occurred. But it's very difficult to sign it individually.

Answer: Demailly

In my opinion, the best therapeutic control of IOP is a control which in a stated lapse of time doesn't modify the visual field. There are no magic values of IOP.

Answer: Weinreb

I think the question of reversibility is very interesting and important, and certainly one we don't know much about.

When one considers reversibility of a structure, one needs to be very careful; for example yesterday Dr. Quigley mentioned that he has not seen or he has very rarely seen a nerve fiber layer defect that reverses, so once you have that type of structural damage perhaps you don't have reversibility. I think we need to know a lot more about how the disc and the visual field or any other functional test respond to lowering intraocular pressure.
In the future, I think it is certainly reasonable to speculate on this, because at the moment there is not any scientific evidence supporting it, and perhaps we might findi a point for treatment that relates to some type of reversal or change in a structural or functional parameter.

Answer: Bonomi

We don't know the critical pressure. We theoretically know that with "low" values of intraocular pressure values the optic nerve is reasonably safe. On the other hand, there is a wide band of intraocular pressure values in which the patient may be safe or not. It would be very useful to know which patients at 20 mmHg will worsen and which will not. However, at present we cannot establish it, so we have to try to decrease the intraocular pressure below "security limits ". That is very hard because obtaining 16 mmHg in a glaucomatous patient is not easy. In addition, we don't know if there are any peaks of increased intraocular pressure, for example at hours in which the patient isn't followed by us. So, I suggest to follow these patients rather frequently with a threshold perimetry. I don't see other way; if, in 2-3 following visits, this method confirms also a small worsening, our therapy is not sufficient.

Question: Bisantis

I wanted to ask the first three speakers about diagnostic and therapeutic monitoring, what importance has today the relationship between tonometric curve and blood pressure monitoring during 24 hours.

Answer: Krieglstein

I don't think, frankly speaking, that the correlation of systemic blood pressure and intraocular pressure has a diagnostic meaning, however we see very rarely nowadays that topic nerve circulation can suffer from both extremes of abnormal blood pressure. If you are on a low side, you get a perfusional loss and you get a normal tension glaucoma, if you are on a high side if you have systemic hypertension you may get an ischemic optic neuropathy. An abnormal blood pressure either on the low or the high side is an additional risk factor, additional to the elevated intraocular pressure.

Question: Maccaluso

My question is to Dr. Weinreb. Of course, SWAP perimetry is looking at a different pathway than luminance perimetry, but how selective is this? Of course, it's looking at something different because it is clear that the stimulus is different and you get different visual fields appearance from what you get with white on white visual field; but with the projection perimeter you get anyway a luminance difference between target and background, that is, since you are projecting the target onto a background its luminance will be higher. How selective can the stimulus be if there is a luminance difference and this is not seen by the short wave insensitive system but rather through a very low contrast by the magnocellular?

Answer: Weinreb

We are not sure that swap is detecting visual field defects at an earlier stage than standard achromatic perimetry. Yesterday we heard about the magnocellular and parvocellular pathways. The magnocellular pathway of course shows a haze of the cells that have the larger axons, appear to get damaged earlier. As Dr. Quigley noticed yesterday, both parvocellular and magnocellular ganglion cells appeared to be damaged in glaucoma. The speculation is that by isolating parvocellular cells with the swap mechanism what we are doing is stressing the system. We are detecting damage in a system where some cells perhaps have been lost, and by isolating that we are able to detect the drop out of cells better than if we are looking both at the magnocellular and the parvocellular systems.

Agonist Adrenergic Drugs

A.L. Robin*

Lake Falls Prof. Bldg., 6155 Falls Rd., Baltimore, MD 21209-2226, USA

What I'd like to do in the next twenty minutes is give you an overall perspective of the history of the alpha agonists as we use them in glaucoma, what their short cause and long run cause and future potentiality are. Put this all in perspective in a fond way if you had to take one lesson from what I am going to say, is that there is a role that relatively safe medications and most of the side effects perhaps are dose related. The first developed alpha agonist is clonidine. Clonidine is predominantly an alpha 2 agonist at higher concentrations it also has alpha 1 effects. These alpha 1 effects include conjunctival vasoconstriction, elevation of interpalpebral fissure, mydriasis and decreased oxygen tension in the conjunctival vessels. It was first developed as a nasal decongestant because of the alpha 1 effects and in the first preclinical studies it was realised that many of the normal subjects who were developed using this nasal spray began fating from systemic hypotension. In the sixties it was then realized that topical clonidine also lowered intraocular pressure, the initial one-dose studies above eight and quarter per cent clonidine was very impressive and showed that it was more effective than vehicle slightly less effective than pilocarpine but much better tolerated. Regrettably all good things come to an end. Studies in the early eighties compared clonidine to a placebo and apraclonidine and placebo to pilocarpine and found that clonidine in both eight and quarter per cent concentration worked very well, but markedly lowered blood pressure in over 50% of individuals. There is greater than 30 mm Hg drop in systolic blood pressure and 30% had a greater than 20 mm Hg drop in diastolic blood pressure. These studies and others quickly diminished the enthusiams that many researchers had for this topical agent. Then came apraclonidine. How is apraclonidine different from clonidine, looking at the chemical structure, is on the see four position of the benzene ring there is now a minor group which is substituted. This, however, greatly changes the chemical activity of this medication so that it is much less likely to penetrate the central nervous system and changes its ability to penetrate the blood aqueous barrier. Because of this, the safety of apraclonidine has greatly increased. In multiple studies with apraclonidine and also brimonidine we have seen no effects, absolutely no effects on systemic blood pressure or heart rate. We have looked at exercises or used tachycardia and seen none with either one of upper set of apraclonidine. The only safety issues that we have seen have been the slight rises, which is statistically significant but clinically insignificant, in conjunctival blenching and lid retraction. There has been no data to date to support any long term effect or deleterious effect on the posterior segment circulation, I want to repeat it, no evidence at all to show that with apraclonidine there is any deleterious effect on the posterior segment circulation. In addition I would like to add that apraclonidine from a systemic point of view is probably one of the safest drug that we have seen and there has really been no effects on cardiovascular parameters, no effect on lipid parameters, no effect on CNS parameters, no

*From recording of the presentation.

depression we have not yet seen with this. Its initial use is mentioned with acute and prevention of intraocular pressure spikes associated with both argon laser trabeculoplasty, iridotomy and capsulotomy. Using 360 degrees argon laser trabeculoplasty all over two third of 26 treated eyes are randomized with apraclonidine, timolol, pilocarpine, acetazolamide and dipivefrin. Apraclonidine was the only medication to have a mean IOP lowering effect. There is only 1% of eyes that had an IOP raise over 5 mm of mercury of a base line where there was no significant difference between pilocarpine, dipivefrin, timolol, acetazolamide in that they all had initial IOP increase. This was a 360 degrees treatment and now we found that there is no reason to treat 360 degrees for most individuals. Additionally, as we mentioned, we compared it to timolol for the treatment of the IOP rise after iridotomy which has a high rate of IOP rise. Here too there is an initial IOP decrease with apraclonidine compared to the initial IOP increase with timolol. The other real damage goes back to the vasoconstriction where we see much less iris bleeding both in subhuman primates studies and in human studies although this has not been a major problem. There is nothing worse than having this little vessel break iridotomy. One of the things that apraclonidine does do, that beta blockers don't do is that apraclonidine does decrease aqueous flow during sleep. There are some suggestions that it works similar to timolol in aqueous flow suppression. There are many suggestions that it may increase uveo-scleral outflow but I am very dubious of this as I am of recent report that brimodine increases uveo-scleral flow, as a single therapeutic agent. It does work very well in those eyes with early glaucoma where a beta blocker alone is not a sufficient therapy. There is also a group of eyes who were very familiar with multiple medications and really cannot have surgery because of physical elements or refused to have surgery despite our best judgement. It's interesting to look at the history of this kind of individuals. In a masked cross-over study only 38% of eyes had at least 4 mm IOP lowering when timolol was added, and 18% of eyes had a masked 4 mm IOP lowering when placebo was added. In essence timolol didn't really do that well but did twice as well than placebo. You see very similar results here with apraclonidine. This was a multi-centered study, placebo-controlled masked study where apraclonidine was added to individuals who underwait to the operating room to see if surgery could be avoided. I am not saying that it is the right thing to do as a new algorithm of therapy of glaucoma, but that was for half the study was designed, it was a very heterogeneous group of individuals, all of them had advanced glaucoma. Interestingly enough it is that apraclonidine did twice as well as placebo and decreased as after surgical intervention. The patients who benefited most were those with open angle glaucoma and those who are not onto aqueous suppressance but have only one aqueous suppressant. Most patients did have open angle glaucoma so we are not sure how well they would work in other forms of secondary glaucoma. The placebo effect is a real effect and is something we have to deal with especially in that very heterogeneous group of patients but it did better in another group of patients what timolol did a decade and a half ago. The main limiting side effect wich is bothersome is red allergic response.

We don't know what kind of allergic response it is and we are going to speak about allergy in a few minutes but it is not a typical type one or type two or type four allergy; we are not really sure of what it is and there are probably multiple different allergic responses involved. A nice thing about that is that apraclonidine either works or doesn't or has allergic response or not, they engender things such as depression associated with beta blockers or the potential for having brown eyes associated with latanoprost or retina detachment with pilocarpine. This is a self-limited complication. Let's go over to other alpha agonists as I conclude, let me talk both about clonidine and brimonidine. Clonidine if you look at the major side effects associated with alpha agonists, tachyphylaxis should be really a decreased tolerance for the drug. Initial IOP lowering is not as good as later IOP lowering. Allergy, systemic hypotension and CNS effects such as headache, depression are probably all dose related. What one wants is a concentration of the drugs that lower the intraocular pressure adequately but also minimize the side effects; so you have lower concentration to give less side effects but higher concentration to get adequate IOP lowering. One of the things we have seen with clonidine is that clonidine in low doses, 0.063%, appears to have very good IOP lowering but had minimum effect on diastolic blood pressure and systemic blood pressure; so it could be that the problem with clonidine in the eighties was a too higher dose.

About brimonidine, the only comparison I had in my hand was from a dose response study above 0.5% iopidine and 0.2% brimonidine to compare the IOP lowering with iopidine and brimonidine. Iopidine is working slightly better but I am not sure it really would be a clinically significant difference. In addition, there appears not to be a clinically significant difference in the rate of allergy with about 15% for apraclonidine and, as I heard last night, 9.6% for brimonidine. The allergy with brimonidine is the type of allergy which seems to be different. It seems that you really are not hidrolizing the quinone to become a stable hapten which may react as an allergy as we see with propine or with apraclonidine or iopidine. Brimonidine doesn't appear to have the same allergic pathway for oxidation. Whether or not this is really the pathway it is unclear. Apraclonidine does work as brimonidine in preventing IOP spikes after lasers. But the true role is probably better than that, than the topical carbonic anhydrase inhibitors. My fear with them is that those medications dwell in your systemic circulation; their half- life I think it is approximately 140 days. It's gary for me to think of what kind of complications we may have. Here there is really not much of a complication except for the allergy and in the lack of tolerance. I think for the formulation on delivery system that is imperative for the work on allergy. I think that the drug is now promising and will be more promising in the future.

Prostaglandins in the Treatment of Increased Intraocular Pressure

A. Alm

Department of Ophthalmology, University Hospital, 701 85 Uppsala, Sweden

Effects of Natural Prostaglandins

Early studies in experimental animals demonstrated that low doses of naturally occurring prostaglandins caused a pronounced reduction of the intraocular pressure (IOP) in rabbits, cats, and monkeys [1]. However, these studies also showed that there were marked species differences with respect to the IOP response, the resistance of the blood-aqueous barrier, and the dose needed to obtain an ocular hypotension. Thus prostaglandin $F_{2\alpha}$ ($PGF_{2\alpha}$) reduced IOP in rabbits at a low dose, but the effect was rapidly lost due to tolerance development and the blood-aqueous barrier was disrupted [2]. Higher doses of $PGF_{2\alpha}$ will reduce IOP effectively in cats and monkeys with no or little effect on the blood-aqueous barrier [3-4] and the main mechanism of action seems to be increased by uveoscleral outflow [5-7].

Applied as eye drops the tromethamine salt of $PGF_{2\alpha}$ is a potent ocular hypotensive drug also in the human eye, but it causes unacceptable ocular side effects in the form of conjunctival hyperemia and ocular irritation [8-9]. The isopropylester ($PGF_{2\alpha}$-IE) is much more lipid soluble and the dose could be reduced to about 1% of the effective dose for the tromethamine salt without loss of effect on IOP in normal [10-11] and glaucomatous eyes [12-13]. Still there was no acceptable separation of effect and side effects and an attempt to use a diester of $PGF_{2\alpha}$ also failed to reduce the ocular side effects sufficiently for clinical use [14]. Studies on aqueous humor dynamics showed that $PGF_{2\alpha}$-IE has no effect on aqueous flow [10-11] and that the effect on IOP is additive to that of timolol [15-16].

Phenylsubstituted Analogues

In order to avoid, or at least considerably reduce, the ocular side effects a large number of $PGF_{2\alpha}$ analogues were synthezised and evaluated [17-19]. One of them, a phenyl-substituted analogue, code name PhXA34, retained the ocular hypotensive effect of $PGF_{2\alpha}$-IE despite a marked reduction of conjunctival hyperemia and ocular irritation [20-22]. In all later studies the *R*-epimer latanoprost (code name PhXA41 13,14-dihydro-17-phenyl-18,19,20-trinor-$PGF_{2\alpha}$-IE) which is more pharmacologically active, was used. None of the epimers had any effect on aqueous flow [20, 23]. In monkeys increased uveoscleral outflow is responsible for the reduction in IOP [24] and indirect measurements suggest that this is the case also in human eyes [25].

Latanoprost is a more selective *FP-receptor* agonist than $PGF_{2\alpha}$ which may explain its lack of vasoactivity. Topical application has no effect on intraocular blood flow [24].

Dose and Dose Regimen

A dose-response relationship was found when three different concentrations (0.0035%-0.035%) of PhXA34 were tested in a single dose study in normal eyes [20]. In patients with ocular hypertension, 0.0115% PhXA34 produced an almost maximal IOP reduction but very little conjunctival hyperemia [21]. Two single dose-response studies have been reported for latanoprost, which should be about twice as potent as PhXA34. In one study, latanoprost caused a dose-dependent reduction of IOP from 4 h to 24 h post-dose with 0.003%, 0.005%, and 0.01% latanoprost applied to healthy volunteers [26]. In the other study, 0.005% and 0.01% latanoprost, applied as a single dose to 35 patients with ocular hypertension or glaucoma, caused a significant reduction of IOP from 4 h to 24 h post-dose without any difference between the two concentrations [27]. From these studies it was concluded that a concentration of latanoprost of about 0.005% was optimal.

The effect on IOP of repeated administrations of placebo or one of three different concentrations of latanoprost, 0.0035%, 0.006%, or 0.0115%, was determined in patients with increased IOP [28]. The eye drops were administered twice daily to 60 patients in a three-center study. The effect was evaluated by comparing the mean diurnal IOP at baseline (that is the mean of IOP measurements at 8 a.m., noon, and 4 p.m.) and after 2 and 28 days of treatment. Mean pre-treatment IOP ranged between 22.5 mm Hg and 24.4 mm Hg for the four treatment groups. All three doses reduced IOP significantly better than placebo but the difference between the three doses was small. There was a clear-cut short-term escape during the first 2 weeks of treatment. Thus on day 2 the reductions of the IOP were 32%, 33% and 38% for the three concentrations of latanoprost, and 19%, 20%, and 22% on day 28. The most pronounced effect on IOP was seen at 8 a.m., that is 12 h post-dose. The highest concentration, 0.0115%, was considered supramaximal.

Subsequent studies have demonstrated that the dose regimen with one eye drop twice daily is too much and that a better effect on IOP is obtained with once daily applications. This was studied in 50 patients with ocular hypertension who were treated for 2 weeks: 10 patients with placebo, 20 with 0.006% latanoprost twice daily and 20 with the same dose applied only in the evening [29]. On the second day of treatment mean diurnal IOP was reduced, from an untreated level of about 25 mm Hg, by 4%, 30%, and 36%, respectively, with placebo, once and twice daily latanoprost. After 2 weeks of treatment the efficacy was reversed for the two groups treated with latanoprost. Once daily caused a 36% reduction compared to 28% with twice daily. Thus there was a striking difference between the two dose regimens. Given once daily, the effect is slightly improved from day 2 to day 14, while the reverse was seen with twice daily applications. In another study patients with glaucoma with an IOP of at least 22 mg Hg despite 0.5% timolol twice daily were included [30]. This was a parallel group study, in which 0.006% latanoprost was added to timolol to one eye twice daily in 25 patients and once daily (in the evening) to 25 patients for 3 months. Throughout the study latanoprost once daily reduced IOP more efficiently than latanoprost twice daily at all time points. The difference in mean diurnal IOP on the last examination was significantly lower in the once daily group than in the twice daily group, 15.7 mm Hg and 18.0 mm Hg, respectively, although they started at almost identical IOP levels, 24.8 mm Hg and 24.9 mm Hg. From these two studies it seems clear that once daily application of latanoprost is at least as good as, and probably better than, twice daily application. The reason for this is not clear but the first study, in which twice daily was initially more effective, suggests some receptor adaptation. It is known that down-regulation of FP-receptors occurs [31]. Thus latanoprost applied once daily reduces IOP for 24 h since latanoprost, unlike β-adrenergic receptor blockers [32], is effective also during the night [33].

Additivity

As latanoprost acts by increasing uveoscleral outflow one would expect that the effect on IOP would be additive to that of an aqueous flow reducer, such as a β-adrenergic receptor blocker. An additive effect of latanoprost to that of timolol has also been observed in patients with elevated IOP [30-34] and the effect of adding latanoprost once daily to patients on timolol caused a further reduction of the mean diurnal IOP from 24.8 mm Hg to 15.7 mm Hg after 3 months of treatment, indicating that the two drugs are fully additive [30].

Somewhat more surprising is the observation that latanoprost also caused an added reduction of IOP by about 15% when added to pilocarpine [35], since pilocalpine contracts the ciliary muscle and inhibits the effect of prostaglandins in monkeys [5]. The difference between the clinical study and the study in monkeys is probably due to age and/or dose. One should expect a less intense contraction of the ciliary muscle in elderly glaucoma patients than in young animals used in laboratory experiments, and the dose of pilocarpine used in monkeys was twice the maximal dose in terms of accommodation in order to ensure maximal contraction of the ciliary muscle. In the clinical study a 2% solution of pilocarpine was used three times daily, which may be a submaximal dose for contraction of the ciliary muscle in the elderly human eye.

Long-term Studies

Three 6-month masked trials comparing latanoprost to timolol have recently been reported, one from the Scandinavian countries [36], one from the USA [37] and one from the UK [38]. These are all basic studies for evaluation of the efficacy as well as the safety of latanoprost. All three studies included patients with open angle glaucoma or ocular hypertension. They were treated for 6 months with either timolol 0.5% twice daily or latanoprost 0.005% once daily in a randomized, double-masked, parallel group study. The three studies included a total of 829 patients, 460 on latanoprost and 369 on timolol. There were minor differences in the three studies. In the US study patients previously treated with β-adrenergic receptor blockers were allowed to be included after wash-out of the timolol effect for 3 weeks.

In the other two studies patients previously treated with β-adrenergic receptor blockers were excluded.

In the UK and the US study latanoprost was applied in the evening, in the Scandinavian study a cross-over design was used with application either in the evening or the morning with a switch after 3 months. In all three studies the efficacy of the two drugs was based on difference in mean diurnal IOP after 6 months of treatment (Table 1).

Table 1. Untreated mean diurnal IOP and reduction in mm Hg after 6 months of treatment with 0.005% latanoprost once daily (Lat) or 0.5% timolol twice daily (Tim) in three phase III clinical trials [From 36-38].

	US		UK		Scand	
	Lat	Tim	Lat	Tim	Lat	Tim
Initial IOP (mm Hg)	24.4	24.1	25.2	25.4	25.1	24.6
Reduction, 6 months (mm Hg)	6.8	5.2	8.5	8.3	8.2	6.7

Mean diurnal IOP is defined as the mean of three IOP measurements, at 8 a.m., noon and 4 p.m.

In the three studies latanoprost reduced mean diurnal IOP significantly, with between 28% and 34% from the untreated level of 24.4-25.2 mm Hg, and timolol with between 22% and 33%, from the untreated level of 24.1-25.4 mm Hg. Latanoprost was equally effective in all three studies while timolol was significantly less effective than latanoprost in the US and the Scandinavian studies. The different outcomes in the three studies may well be due to chance variation, but a meta-analysis of the three studies showed that timolol was more efficient in males than in females and the UK study contained 65% males compared to 43% and 44% in the US and Scandinavian studies, respectively.

Treatment with oral β-adrenergic receptor blockers was permitted in the inclusion criteria. That may theoretically reduce the effect of timolol but is unlikely to influence the results in these studies. Only 4%-6% of patients randomized to timolol were on oral β-adrenergic receptor blockers.

The Scandinavian study provided added information on the best time of application of latanoprost, morning or evening. Evening administration of latanoprost was statistically superior to morning administration. The most likely explanation is that: (1) IOP measurements at 8 a.m., noon, and 4 p.m. provide IOP values 4, 8 and 24 h post-dose for morning applications and 12, 16, and 20 h post-dose for evening applications and (2) a late and prolonged maximum for the effect on IOP favors evening application when IOP was measured during daytime.

Patients completing the phase III studies were asked to continue in an open label follow-up with 0.005% latanoprost once daily, choosing between morning or evening administration [39]. By May 1, 1994 there were 198 patients who had been treated with latanoprost for 1 year and an analysis of the effect on IOP showed an insignificant increase in IOP, from 17.2 to 17.4 mm Hg, between 6 and 12 months. This difference is not larger than what can be expected if some patients switch from evening to morning administration. The results thus indicate that there is little loss of efficacy during 1 year's treatment.

Ocular Safety

Most of the information on ocular safety can be found in the three phase III studies [36-38] and the interim follow-up of 1 year of treatment [39]. The following presentation is based on a combined analysis of the three studies.

Conjunctival hyperemia was reported as an adverse event in 4.6% of patients treated with latanoprost and 1.4% of patients treated with timolol, and it was noted in the case report form as an ocular sign in 4.6% and 3.0% respectively [36-38]. In the continuation of the phase III studies [39], hyperemia was reported as an adverse event in seven of 198 patients (3.4%). In four of these patients [2%], hyperemia was reported more than once, indicating that conjunctival hyperemia may be a clinical problem in about 2% of patients treated with latanoprost.

Ocular irritation or discomfort was reported as an adverse event or noted in the case report forms 266 times for 460 patients treated with latanoprost and 208 times for 369 patients treated with timolol [36-38]. Thus the frequency of ocular discomfort is the same for latanoprost as for timolol. The high number of reports for the two drugs probably reflects the level of ocular discomfort induced by any eye drop.

A slight flare was reported in two of 460 patients on latanoprost and two of 369 patients on timolol. Thus the long-term studies confirm previous short-term studies with noninvasive determination of the aqueous protein concentration, indicating that latanoprost has no significant effect on the blood-aqueous barrier [23-27].

Corneal punctate erosions were observed in 9.4% of patients on latanoprost and 8.7% on timolol. Most of these punctate epithelial erosions were mild sporadic events, but some were reported as adverse events, 15 (3.3%) on latanoprost and five (1.4%) on timolol. Latanoprost, as well as the vehicle used as placebo, contains twice the amount of the preservative benzalkonium chloride as timolol, which may explain the small difference between the two treatments. One of 460 patients treated with latanoprost was withdrawn from the study because of corneal erosions.

The only clinically significant ocular side effect that has emerged in these studies is an increase of the amount of pigment in the iris. Among 460 patients enrolled in the 6 month study with latanoprost, increased pigmentation of the iris was observed or suspected in 31 patients (6.7%) [36-38]. The majority of these cases have been mild and only detected by careful comparison between pre- and post-treatment iris photographs. With increased treatment time the number has increased, and of 214 patients (198 treated for 1 year and 16 withdrawn earlier due to increased pigmentation of the iris) there were a total of 29 cases (13.6%) [39]. The change in iris pigmentation has occurred only in eyes with an iris color that is already partly brown (naevi and freckles not included). An example of a blue-brown eye with increased pigmentation is shown in Fig. 1. Thus no definite change in iris color has been observed in pure blue, grey, green, or brown irides during treatment for up to a year. The highest frequency is seen in green-brown irides (56.4%) and yellow-brown irides (37.5%) after 1 year's treatment, while in blue-brown irides the figure is 18.4% (Table 2).

All patients that have developed increased pigmentation of the iris have been withdrawn from the studies.

During a maximum follow-up time of 2 years, the developed change in iris pigmentation has been stable without any sign of reversibility or further increase.

Table 2. Frequency of increased iris pigmentation during treatment for 1 year

Iris color	Number of eyes	Pigmented (%)	
Blue/grey	103	0	(0.0)
Blue/grey-brown	38	7	(18.4)
Green	1	0	(0.0)
Green-brown	39	22	(56.4)
Brown	25	0	(0.0)
Yellow/brown -brown	8	3	(37.5)
Total	214	32	(15.0)

Clinical studies can only give limited information on iris pigmentation. Slit lamp examinations and iris photographs have not revealed any changes apart from an increased amount of brown pigment, usually within an area spreading peripherally from a concentric brown area around the pupil (Fig. 1).

Naevi and freckles have not changed color or size. Apart from the change in color, the iris looks normal and no pigment has been seen on the corneal endothelium. Two iridectomy specimens from an iris with increased pigmentation have been evaluated electron microscopically and judged to be normal (Grierson, personal comm.). In monkeys it is clear that the change in color is due to an increased amount of melanin in the stromal melanocytes of the iris without any structural or cellular changes involved [40]. Neither latanoprost nor naturally occurring prostaglandins induce cell division in melanocytes in vivo [40]. Thus it seems likely that the change in iris pigmentation has only cosmetic consequences. The possibility of a late loss of pigment and induction of a pigmentary glaucoma also seems unlikely. The melanin content of the stromal melanocytes is only a few percent of the total amount of iridial melanin and the iridial melanocytes are continent and do not lose melanin [41]. This is supported by the fact that follow-up of eyes with increased iris pigmentation for more than 2 years has not indicated any loss of pigment or late complication due to the increased iris pigmentation.

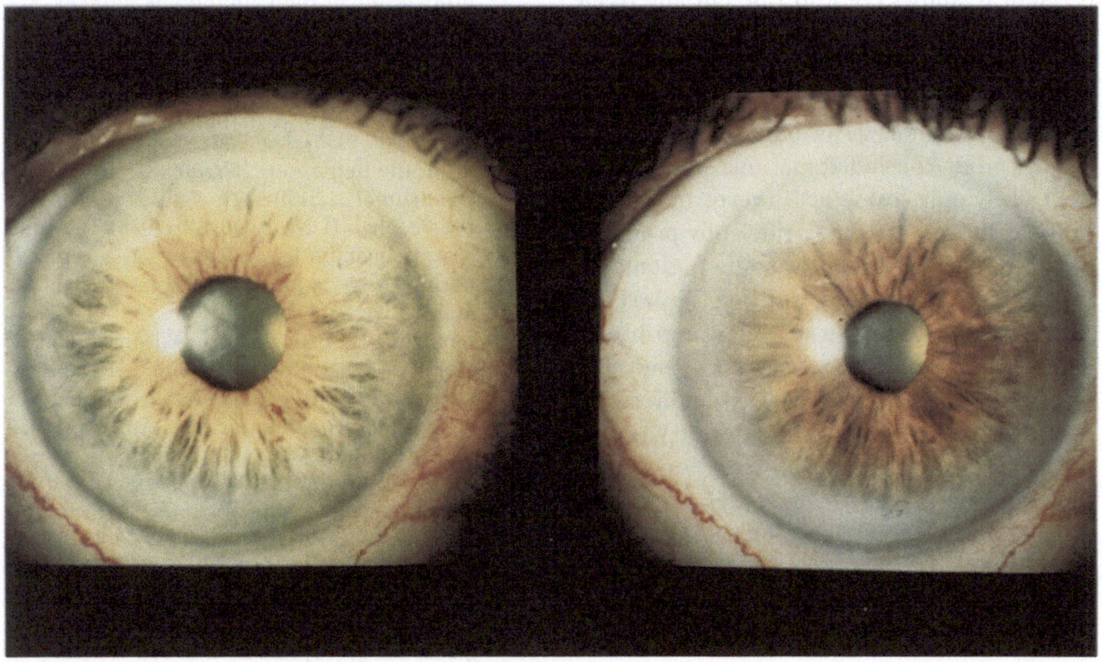

Fig. 1. The left eye of one patient treated with latanoprost (*left*) before and (*right*) after 6 months of treatment. The iris is classified as blue-brown with a brown zone surrounding the pupil before treatment

Systemic Safety

The low systemic dose of latanoprost when applied as one or two 0.005% eye drops once daily suggests that drug-related systemic side effects are unlikely. Most reports of systemic symptoms or signs concerned transient events despite continued treatment, and there was no pattern suggesting a particular systemic effect of latanoprost in the phase III studies.

Conclusions

Latanoprost is a potentially very useful drug for the treatment of glaucoma. In terms of eye pressure reduction there is no doubt that latanoprost offers considerable advantages. It is a very potent drug, more potent than the β-adrenergic receptor blocker timolol, and it has a unique mechanism of action which permits added IOP reduction in combination with other drugs. The only clinically significant ocular side effect observed is an increased iris pigmentation seen in 15% of eyes treated for 1 year. The clinical studies have not revealed any harmful effect of the increased pigmentation despite follow-up for more than 2 years and preclinical studies seem to rule out any tissue change apart from an increased melanin content in already existing stromal melanocytes. Thus since neither mitosis nor structural changes of the melanocytes or other cells are involved, it can be concluded that this side effect is most likely only cosmetic. However, the change in iris color may become sufficiently pronounced to be unacceptable for some patients. In mixed blue and brown, and particularly in mixed green and brown or yellow and brown iridises, the probability of an increased pigmentation with time is quite large and it seems advisable to use latanoprost with restriction in such eyes until information from longer follow-up of already pigmented iridises is available. With this reservation it seems reasonable to conclude that latanoprost will become a useful addition to present glaucoma treatment.

References

1. Bito LZ, Camras C, Gum GG, Resul B (1989) The ocular hypotensive effects and side effects of prostaglandins on the eyes of experimental animals. In: Bito LZ, Stjernschantz J (eds) The ocular effects of prostaglandins. Liss, New York, pp 349-368
2. Camras CB, Bito LZ, Eakins KE (1977) Reduction of intraocular pressure by prostaglandins applied topically to the eyes of conscious rabbits. Invest Ophthalmol Vis Sci 16: 1125-1134
3. Lee P, Podos SM, Severin C (1984) Effect of prostaglandin $F_{2\alpha}$ on aqueous humor dynamics of rabbit, cat, and monkey. Invest Ophthalmol Vis Sci 25:1087-1093
4. Camras CB, Bhuyan KC, Podos SM, Bhuyan DK, Master RWP (1987) Multiple dosing of prostaglandin $F_{2\alpha}$ or epinephrine on cynomolgus monkey eyes. II. Slit-lamp biomicroscopy, aqueous humor analysis, and fluorescein angiography. Invest Ophthalmol Vis Sci 28:921-926
5. Crawford K, Kaufman PL (1987) Pilocarpine antagonizes prostaglandin $F_{2\alpha}$-induced ocular hypotension in monkeys. Evidence for enhancement of uveoscleral outflow by prostaglandin $F_{2\alpha}$. Arch Ophthalmol 105:1112-1116
6. Nilsson SFE, Samuelsson M, Bill A, Stjernschantz J (1989) Increased uveoscleral outflow as a possible mechanism of ocular hypotension caused by prostaglandin $F_{2\alpha}$-1-isopropylester in the cynomolgus monkey. Exp Eye Res 48:707-716
7. Gabelt BT, Kaufman PL (1989) Prostaglandin $F_{2\alpha}$ increases uveoscleral outflow in the cynomolgus monkey. Exp Eye Res 49:389-402
8. Giuffre G (1985) The effects of prostaglandin $F_{2\alpha}$ in the human eye. Graefe's Arch Clin Exp Ophthalmol 222:139-141
9. Lee PY, Shao H, Xu L, Qu CK (1988) The effect of prostaglandin $F_{2\alpha}$ on intraocular pressure in normotensive human subjects. Invest Ophthalmol Vis Sci 29:1474-1477
10. Kerstetter JR, Brubaker RF, Wilson SE, Kullerstrand LJ (1988) Prostaglandin $F_{2\alpha}$- 1-isopropylester lowers intraocular pressure without decreasing aqueous humor flow. Am J Ophthalmol 105:30-34
11. Villumsen J, Alm A (1989) Prostaglandin $F_{2\alpha}$-isopropylester eye drops: effects in normal human eyes. Br J Ophthalmol 73:419-426
12. Villumsen J, Alm A, Soderstrom M (1989) Prostaglandin $F_{2\alpha}$-isopropylester eye drops: effect on intraocular pressure in open-angle glaucoma. Br J Ophthalmol 73:975-979
13. Camras CB, Siebold EC, Lustgarten JS, Serle JB, Frisch SC, Podos SM, Bito LZ (1989) Maintained reduction of intraocular pressure by pro-

staglandin $F_{2\alpha}$-1-isopropylester applied in multiple doses in ocular hypertensive and glaucoma patients. Ophthalmology 96:1329-1337
14. Villumsen J, Alm A (1990) The effect of adding prostaglandin $F_{2\alpha}$-isopropylester to timolol in patients with open angle glaucoma. Arch Ophthalmol 108:1102-1105
15. Villumsen J, Alm A (1990) Ocular effects of two different prostaglandin $F_{2\alpha}$ esters. A double masked cross-over study on normotensive eyes. Acta Ophthalmol 68:341-343
16. Lee P, Shao H, Camras CB, Podos SM (1991) Additivity of prostaglandin $F_{2\alpha}$-1-isopropylester to timolol in glaucoma patients. Ophthalmology 98:1079-1082
17. Stjernschantz J, Resul B (1992) Phenyl substituted prostaglandin analogs for glaucoma treatment. Drugs Future 17:691-704
18. Resul B, Stjernschantz J (1993) Structure-activity relationships of prostaglandin analogues as ocular hypotensive agents. Curr Opin Ther Pat 3:781-795
19. Resul B, Stjernschantz J, No K,Liljebris C, Selén G, Astin M, Karlsson M, Bito LZ (1993) Phenyl substituted prostaglandins potent and selective antiglaucoma agents. J Med Chem 36:243-248
20. Alm A, Villumsen J (1991) PhXA34, a new potent ocular hypotensive drug: A study on dose-response relationship and on aqueous humor dynamics in healthy volunteers. Arch Ophthalmol 109:1564-1568
21. Villumsen J, Alm A (1992) PhXA34-a prostaglandin $F_{2\alpha}$ analogue. Effect on intraocular pressure in patients with ocular hypertension. Br J Ophthalmol 76:214-217
22. Camras CB, Schumer RA, Marsk A, Lustgarten JS, Serle JB, Stjernschantz J, Bito LZ, Podos SM (1992) Intraocular pressure reduction with PhXA34, a new prostaglandin analogue, in patients with ocular hypertension. Arch Ophthalmol 110:1733 1738
23. Ziai N, Dolan JW, Kacere RD, Brubaker RF (1993) The effects on aqueous dynamics of PhXA41, a new prostaglandin $F_{2\alpha}$ analogue, after topical application in normal and ocular hypertensive human eyes. Arch Ophthalmol 111:1351-1358
24. Selen G, Karlsson M, Astin M, Stjernschantz J, Resul B (1991) Effects of PhXA34 and PhD 100A, two phenyl substituted prostaglandin esters, on aqueous humor dynamics and microcirculation in the monkey eye. Invest Ophthalmol Vis Sci 32 (ARVO suppl): 869 (Abstr)
25. Toris CB, Camras CB, Yablonski ME (1993) Effects of PhXA41, a new prostaglandin $F_{2\alpha}$ analog, on aqueous humor dynamics in human eyes. Ophthalmology 100:1297-1304
26. Hotehama Y, Mishima HK, Kitazawa Y, Masuda K (1993) Ocular hypotensive effect of PhXA41 in patients with ocular hypertension or primary open-angle glaucoma. Jpn J Ophthalmol 37:270-274
27. Hotehama Y, Mishima HK (1993) Clinical efficacy of PhXA34 and PhXA41, two novel prostaglandin $F_{2\alpha}$-isopropyl ester analogues for glaucoma treatment. Jpn J Ophthalmol 37:259-269
28. Alm A, Villumsen J, Törnquist P, Mandahl A, Airaksinen J, Tuulonen A, Marsk A, Resul B (1993) Intraocular pressure-reducing effect of PhXA41 in patients with increased eye pressure: A one-month study. Ophthalmology 100: 1312-1317
29. Nagasubramanian S, Sheth GP, Hitchings RA, Stjernschantz J (1993) Intraocular pressure-reducing effect of PhXA41 in ocular hypertension: Comparison of dose regimens. Ophthalmology 100:1305-1311
30. Alm A, Widengard I, Kjellgren D, Söderström M, Friström B, Heijl A, Stjernschantz J (1995) Latanoprost administered once daily caused a maintained reduction of intraocular pressure in glaucoma patients treated concomitantly with timolol. Br J Ophthalmol 79:12-16
31. Deaciuc IV, Spitzer JA (1991) Down-regulation of prostaglandin $F_{2\alpha}$ receptors in rat liver during chronic endotoxemia. Prostaglandins Leukot Essent Fatty Acids 42:191-195
32. Topper JE, Brubaker RF (1985) Effects of timolol, epinephrine, and acetazolamide on aqueous flow during sleep. Invest Ophthalmol Vis Sci 26:1315-1319
33. Racz P, Ruzsonyi MR, Nagy ZT, Bito LZ (1993) Maintained intraocular pressure reduction with once-a-day application of a new prostaglandin $F_{2\alpha}$ analogue (PhXA41): An in-hospital, placebo-controlled study. Arch Ophthalmol 111:657-661
34. Rulo AH, Greve EL, Hoyng PF (1994) Additive effect of latanoprost, a prostaglandin $F_{2\alpha}$ analogue, and timolol in patients with elevated intraocular pressure. Br J Ophthalmol 78:899-902
35. Friström B, Nilsson SEG (1993) Interaction of PhXA41, a new prostaglandin analogue, with pilocarpine: A study on patients with elevated intraocular pressure. Arch Ophthalmol 111: 662-665
36. Alm A, Stjernschantz J and the Scandinavian Latanoprost Study Group (1995) Effects on intraocular pressure and side effects of 0.005% latanoprost once daily, evening or morning. A comparison with timolol. Ophthalmology 102:1743-1762
37. Camras CB, the rest of the USA Latanoprost Study Group (1996) Comparison of latanoprost and timolol in patients with ocular hypertension and glaucoma – six-month, masked USA multicenter trial. Ophthalmology 103:138-147
38. Watson P Stjernschantz J, the Latanoprost

Study Group in United Kingdom (1996): A six month randomized, double-masked study comparing latanoprost to timolol in open angle glaucoma or ocular hypertension. Ophthalmology 103:126-137
39. Camras CB, Alm A, Watson P (1995) Glaucoma treatment for 1 year with latanoprost, a prostaglandin analog, in the USA, Scandinavia and UK. American Academy of Ophthalmology, Annual Meeting, Atlanta, p 89 (Abstr)
40. Selén G, Stjernschantz J, Resul B, Bito LZ (1996) Prostaglandin-induced increase in iris pigmentation. Survey Ophthalmol (in press)
41. Prota G (1992) Melanins and Melanogenesis. Academic, San Diego

Development of a Topically Active Carbonic Anhydrase Inhibitor

I. Adamsons

Merck Research Laboratories, 10 Sentry Parkway BL 1-3, Blue Bell, PA 19422, USA

There are several classes of drugs that are used to treat open-angle glaucoma and ocular hypertension. Among these classes are carbonic anhydrase inhibitors (CAIs) which, up until 1995, were available only as oral agents. Inhibition of carbonic anhydrase in the ciliary processes of the eye by CAIs decreases aqueous humor secretion by slowing the formation of bicarbonate ions. This results in a reduction in sodium and fluid transport into the posterior chamber and consequently in a reduction in intraocular pressure (IOP) [1]. Oral CAIs are very effective in lowering IOP but are poorly tolerated; up to 50% of patients experience side effects such as anorexia, nausea, vomiting, diarrhea, fatigue and weight loss, numbness and tingling [2].

The first oral CAI synthesized was acetazolamide, which was found to have an ocular hypotensive effect in 1954. The poor tolerability of oral agents quickly led to research efforts into the development of a topically active agent which would be better tolerated. Merck Research Laboratories initiated its own research program in this area in 1978. Over 1200 compounds were synthesized and tested, and in 1995 dorzolamide hydrochloride (Trusopt) became the first topically active CAI to be made commercially available. The development of dorzolamide required such an extended period of time because of the complexity of the challenges involved. First, it was necessary that the drug inhibit the appropriate isoenzyme of carbonic anhydrase: there are at least seven different carbonic anhydrase isoenzymes [3] and it is carbonic anhydrase isoenzyme II that is involved in aqueous humor production [4]. Second, it was necessary that the drug be a potent inhibitor of carbonic anhydrase: in order to obtain a reduction of IOP, the blockade of carbonic anhydrase in the ciliary process must be higher than 99% [5]. In vitro experiments showed that dorzolamide was a potent inhibitor of human erythrocyte carbonic anhydrase II: its IC_{50} is 0.16 nM compared to 3.37 nM for acetazolamide [6]. Next, the drug had to possess adequate aqueous-lipid solubility to allow for good ocular penetration. This was achieved with dorzolamide by adding a basic secondary amine group to the compound's ring structure [6]. Thus, dorzalamide is amphoteric, that is, it contains both an acidic sulfonamide group and a basic secondary amine group and, as shown in preclinical studies with pigmented rabbits, is a good ocular penetrator [6]. Finally, the drug had to be largely free from the extraocular side effects generally associated with oral CAIs.

Clinical evaluation began after extensive preclinical research on dorzolamide had been completed. The goals of the early (Phase II) clinical studies included establishing the dosing regimen of Trusopt, evaluating its pharmacokinetics, and assessing the additivity of Trusopt to timolol.

In order to establish the dosing regimen of Trusopt, two issues had to be addressed. The first was determining the optimal concentration of the drug, and the second was determining the optimal frequency of drug administration. Among the studies conducted to address these issues was the following 12-day study [7]: Seventy-four patients with either ocular hypertension or open-angle glaucoma were enrolled and randomized into one of four study groups. Three groups received dorzolamide at either 0.7%, 1.4%, or 2.0% concentration. The fourth group of patients received placebo. Patients were instructed to take their masked study medication twice a day for the first 5 days of the study, and three times a day for the final week of the study. Diurnal curves were performed at baseline (Day 0) and on Days 5 and 12. A diurnal curve was defined as an IOP measurement every 2 h beginning at Hour 0 (immediately before their morning dose of study medication) through Hour 12.

The groups of patients receiving 0.7% and 1.4% dorzolamide did not experience as large a decrease in IOP as the group of patients receiving 2% dorzolamide. Therefore, this presentation will be limited to the data obtained from the patients receiving 2.0% dorzolamide and from those receiving placebo.

After 5 days of b.i.d. dosing, 2.0% dorzolamide (Trusopt) lowered IOP over a range that varied from 13% at morning trough (immediately before the morning dose of study medication) to 21% at morning peak (2 h after dosing). This effect on IOP was statistically greater than that of placebo administered twice a day for 5 days. After 1 week of t.i.d. dosing, the magnitude of the IOP lowering effect ranged from 18% at morning trough to 22% at morning peak. This effect on IOP was statistically greater than that of placebo administered three times a day for a week. Furthermore, compared to twice a day dosing, three times a day dosing resulted in more consistent IOP lowering throughout the day.

Thus, it was concluded that the 2.0% concentration was more effective than the 0.7% or the 1.4% concentration, and that three times a day dosing was more effective for monotherapy than twice a day dosing.

With the optimal dosing schedule determined, it was possible to evaluate the pharmacokinetics of Trusopt with the following 20-week study [5]. Study medication was administered orally in order to minimize the variability in drug absorption that is associated with ocular administration. Because the effect on IOP of orally administered dorzolamide is inconsequential, healthy volunteers rather than glaucoma patients were enrolled. Dorzolamide 2.0 mg b.i.d. taken orally was determined to provide the same maximum systemic exposure as one drop of 2.0% dorzolamide t.i.d. OU. Thirteen study volunteers were randomized in a 2:1 ratio to receive either masked dorzolamide or masked placebo. These individuals were evaluated at baseline, every week for 12 weeks, and then every other week for the final 8 weeks of the study. Whole blood, plasma, and urine samples were obtained to measure levels of drug, drug metabolite, carbonic anhydrase-II (CA-II) activity, total carbonic anhydrase (CA) activity, and numerous elecrolytes.

Dorzolamide is hepatically metabolized to a single metabolite (N-desethyl dorzolamide) and both dorzolamide and its metabolite are renally excreted. Dorzolamide binds preferentially to CA-II, which is found on the red blood cell membranes. In the presence of dorzolamide, the metabolite binds primarily to carbonic anhydrase-I (CA-I) which is also found on the red blood cell membranes. When all the red blood cell binding sites are saturated, dorzolamide and metabolite are found free in the plasma. Study results showed that steady state levels of dorzolamide were achieved in the red blood cells after 4 weeks of dosing and after 13 weeks for the metabolite. And at no point in this 20-week study were plasma levels of either dorzolamide or its metabolite detected. This implies that, even at steady state, all of the red blood cell CA-II and CA-I sites were not saturated.

The critical question was how much systemic carbonic anhydrase activity remained after steady state was reached? Study results showed that, at steady state, CA-II inhibition was 94%-96%, and that total CA inhibition was 81%-88%. While these levels of systemic inhibition may appear high, they are in fact too low to result in the systemic side effects associated with oral CAIs. The renal side effects of carbonic anhydrase inhibition occur in the presence of greater than 99% inhibition of CA-II. The respiratory side effects of carbonic anhydrase inhibition occur in the presence of at least 96% inhibition of total CA. Thus, these study results imply that Trusopt would be devoid of these systemic side effects which are associated with oral CAIs. Additionally, no systemic biochemical changes of the plasma or urine were detected.

The short term additivity of Trusopt to timolol was assessed in the following 8 day study [8]. Patients with either ocular hypertension or open-angle glaucoma were eligible to participate if their IOP was ≥ 22 mm Hg O.U. 2-4 h after receiving 0.5% timolol O.U. Thirty-two patients were randomized to receive either 0.5% timolol b.i.d. and masked Trusopt b.i.d. or 0.5% timolol b.i.d. and masked placebo b.i.d. Since diurnal variability in IOP is reduced in patients receiving timolol, Trusopt was evaluated in a b.i.d. dosing regimen for adjunctive therapy. Diurnal curves were performed on day 1 and on day 8. A diurnal curve was defined as an IOP measurement every 2 h beginning at Hour 0 (immediately before their morning dose of study medication) through Hour 12. After 8 days of adjunctive therapy to timolol, Trusopt b.i.d. lowered IOP over a range that varied from 13.2% at morning trough to 21.0% at morning peak. This effect on IOP was statistically greater than that of placebo administered as adjunctive therapy to timolol for 8 days. These results showed that Trusopt b.i.d. further lowers IOP in patients who are concurrently receiving 0.5% timolol.

The conclusions from these key Phase II studies were as follows. Optimal IOP lowering activity was obtained with the 2.0% concentration of dorzolamide. Three times a day dosing was more effective for monotherapy than twice a day dosing. At steady state, systemic inhibition of CA-II was 94%-96% and systemic inhibition of total CA was 81%-88%; these levels of inhibition are below those required for the renal and respiratory, respectively, side effects of carbonic anhydrase inhibition. No clinically significant systemic biochemical changes were found. Trusopt administered b.i.d. was an effective short-term adjunctive therapy to timolol.

With this information the Phase III program of long-term, large clinical studies was undertaken. Its goals were to establish the efficacy of Trusopt both as monotherapy and as add-on therapy, and to establish the safety profile of Trusopt.

The efficacy of Trusopt versus ocular β-blocker monotherapy was evaluated in a 12-month, double-masked, randomized trial conducted in 523 patients with either open-angle glaucoma or ocular hypertension [9]. Patients were randomized in a 3:1:1 ratio to receive either Trusopt t.i.d., or 0.5% timolol b.i.d., or 0.5% betaxolol b.i.d. IOP was measured at Hour 2 (peak drug effect), at Hour 5, and at Hour 8. The Hour 8 measurement was taken immediately before the afternoon dose of masked study medication and is the afternoon trough measurement. The mean reduction in IOP from baseline at morning peak and afternoon trough at the and of the study was 6.2 and 4.3 mm Hg with Trusopt, 5.7 and 4.0 mm Hg with betaxolol, and 7.1 and 5.4 mm Hg with timolol. Thus, after 12 months of therapy, the IOP-lowering effect of Trusopt was equivalent to that of betaxolol, whereas timolol was somewhat more effective than either Trusopt or betaxolol.

The efficacy of Trusopt as add-on therapy to timolol was evaluated in a 6-month, double-masked, randomized trial conducted on 261 patients with either open-angle glaucoma or ocular hypertension [8]. After a 2-week placebo-controlled, double-masked period patients were randomized to receive either Trusopt b.i.d., 0.7% dorzolamide b.i.d., or 2.0% pilocarpine q.i.d. in addition to 0.5% timolol b.i.d. for 6 months. IOP was measured at Hour 0 (morning trough), Hour 2 (peak drug effect), and at Hour 4. The IOP lowering effect of 0.7% dorzolamide was not consistently as great as that of 2.0% dorzolamide (Trusopt), once again confirming the drug concentration that was selected. The mean reduction in IOP from baseline (on timolol) to morning peak and trough at the end of the study was 2.8 and 3.6 mm Hg with Trusopt, and 2.8 and 2.8 mm Hg with pilocarpine. Thus, as adjunctive therapy to 0.5% timolol, Trusopt b.i.d. and 2.0% pilocarpine q.i.d. produced similar lowering of IOP for up to 6 months.

The safety profile of Trusopt was also carefully evaluated in the 1108 patients who received Trusopt while enrolled in one of the Phase III studies [6]. The incidence in these patients of the side effects typically associated with oral CAIs was of particular interest. Headache was the most frequent of these side effects with an incidence of 5%. Other side effects typical of oral CAIs which occured with a frequency of 1% or greater were dizziness (2%), paresthesias (2%), fatigue (1%), and rash (1%). Trusopt was generally well-tolerated. Approximately 5% of patients discontinued therapy with Trusopt because of a drug-related adverse experience of any sort. Overall, approximately 3% of the patients discontinued because of an ophthalmic adverse event, most commonly conjunctivitis and lid reactions, which generally resolved on discontinuation of drug therapy. The most frequently reported symptoms were transient bitter taste (26.0%), ocular burning (11.6%), and ocular stinging (11.6%).

Other ocular symptoms that were commonly reported were ocular itching, tearing, and blurred vision. In most cases, the majority of ocular symptoms were characterized as mild in intensity.

The role of Trusopt in the treatment of glaucoma is twofold. It is indicated in the treatment of open-angle glaucoma, pseudoexfoliative glaucoma, and ocular hypertension as adjunctive therapy when IOP is not adequately controlled with β-blockers alone. It is also indicated for use as monotherapy in the treatment of the above conditions when β-blockers are inappropriate. When Trusopt is used as adjunctive therapy the recommended dosage is one drop in the affected eye(s) twice daily. The recommended dosage of Trusopt used as monotherapy is one drop in the effected eye(s) three times daily. When more than one topical ophthalmic drug is being used, the drugs should be administered at least 10 min apart. When Trusopt is being substituted for another topical glaucoma therapy, the other agent should be discontinued at the and of one day and Trusopt begun at the start of the next day.

Trusopt represents an important new addition to the armamentarium available for the treatment of glaucoma. Twice daily Trusopt offers an equally effective and more convenient alternative to four times daily pilocarpine for adjunctive therapy in patients inadequately controlled on timolol alone. Monotherapy with three times a day Trusopt provides meaningful IOP lowering in patients in whom the use of topical β-blockers is inappropriate. Topical administration of Trusopt results in lower systemic carbonic anhydrase inhibition than occurs with the use of oral CAIs: carbonic anhydrase inhibition in red blood cells after orally administered therapeutic doses of dorzolamide was found to be below the levels which produce the renal and respiratory side effects of carbonic anhydrase inhibition. Finally, in clinical trials, Trusopt was generally well tolerated. The adverse events typically associated with oral CAIs occured at low frequencies, and the ocular symptoms and adverse clinical reactions that did occur were generally characterized as mild to moderate.

References

1. Maren THI (1974) HCO_3 - formation in aqueous humor: mechanism and relation to the treatment of glaucoma. Invest Ophthalmol 13(7):479-484
2. Lichter PR et al (1978) Patient tolerance to carbonic anhydrase inhibitors. Am J Ophthalmol 85:495-502
3. Tashian RE (1989) The carbonic anhydrases: widening perspectives on their evolution, expression and function. Bio Essays 10(6): 186-192
4. Wistrand et al (1986) Carbonic anhydrase isoenzymes CAI and CAII in the human eye. Invest Ophthalmol Vis Sci 27:419-428
5. Merck Sharp & Dohme, data on file.
6. Sugrue MF et al (1990) A comparison of L-671, 152 and MK-927, two topically effective ocular hypotensive carbonic anhydrase inhibitors, in experimental animals. Curr. Eye Res. 9(6):607-615
7. Lippa EA et al (1992) Dose response and duration of action of dorzolamide, a topical carbonic anhydrase inhibitor. Arch Ophthalmol 110:495-499
8. Strahlman ER et al (in press) The use of dorzolamide and pilocarpine as adjunctive therapy to timolol in patients with elevated intraocular pressure. Ophthalmology
9. Strahlman ER et al (1995) A double-masked, randomized 1-year study comparing dorzolamide (Trusopt), timolol, and betaxolol. Arch Ophthalmol 113:1009-1016

Recovery of Glaucomatous Damage Following Treatment of Glaucoma

B. Schwartz

20 Park Plaza, Suite 535, Boston, MA 02116, USA

Introduction

Primary open-angle glaucoma has been described as a progressive optic neuropathy [1]. Lowering the ocular pressure has at best been shown to slow down the rate of progression of the optic neuropathy as evidenced primarily by visual field loss [2-4]. In some instances, even with filtering surgery, visual field progression has been noted to continue in spite of normal ocular pressures [5]. In several series of cases, treatment -both medical and surgical- to lower ocular pressure has resulted in reversibility of visual field loss [6-12] or optic disc cupping, particularly in juvenile glaucoma [13-18]. The purpose of this report is to summarize the results of a therapeutic trial of ocular hypertension which resulted in reversibility of glaucomatous damage, particularly optic disc cupping, pallor, retinal nerve fiber layer thickness, and retinal vessel width. The detailed aspects of this trial have been reported previously [19-22].

Methods

The effect of timolol drops vs placebo drops was evaluated in a double-masked, randomized therapeutic trial in ocular hypertensives, that is, patients who had elevated ocular pressure consistently greater or equal to 21 mm Hg without evidence of field loss, as determined by the Goldmann perimeter both by kinetic and static means.

The objective end points of the trial were measurements of optic disc cupping, pallor, retinal nerve fiber layer thickness, and retinal vessel width. Subjects were examined every 3 months for approximately 2 years of follow-up. At each examination visual acuity, ocular pressures and optic disc photographs with the Zeiss and Donaldson simultaneous stereo fundus camera [23] were obtained. Visual fields were determined with the Goldmann perimeter by kinetic and static means every 6 months.

Measurements of optic disc cupping including cup volume, cup area, cup depth and cros-sectional area of the cup at 0.2 and 0.5 depths (volume profile) were obtained from simultaneous stereo photographs using stereophotogrammetry [24, 25]. Optic disc pallor was measured from single photographs by computerized image analysis, which determined the area of pallor expressed as a percentage of area of disc [26]. Retinal nerve fiber layer thickness was measured from simultaneous stereophotographs, using stereophotogrammetry [27]. Retinal vessel width was measured by using computerized image analysis [21].

Measurements from the optic disc photographs were made masked as to type of therapy, timolol or placebo, and the clinical status of the subjects. All measurements were made at least in duplicate from independent photographs. For optic disc cup volume, the percent coefficient of variation (standard deviation/mean x 100) excluding cup volumes less than 8% was 9.7% ± 7.1% (454) (mean ± standard deviation) (number of measurements), for optic disc pallor it was 3.0% ± 2.4% (826), for retinal nerve fiber layer thickness it was 3.54% ± 2.55% (413), and for retinal vessel width for the average of the superior temporal artery, inferior temporal artery, superior temporal vein and inferior temporal vein, it was 3.63% ± 3.17% (497).

A total of 37 ocular hypertensive subjects underwent the clinical trial, 20 were randomly assigned to placebo one drop in both eyes twice a day and 17 were randomly assigned to 0.5% timolol one drop in both eyes twice a day (Table 1).

For statistical analyses univariate and multivariate evaluations are done [28-31] and two-tailed tests were used with $p < 0.05$ chosen as significant.

Results

Fourteen subjects were discontinued during the study, six on placebo drops and eight on timolol drops. The subjects were discontinued for various reasons: six for noncompliance or unavailability for follow-up (three placebo, three timolol), and the others for various vascular complications such as a branch vein occlusion and disc hemorrhage in the placebo group and in the timolol group, red eyes and bradycardia. Figure 1 shows the change of mean ocular

Table 1. Subject characteristics at baseline

Characteristics	Placebo (n = 20)	Timolol (n = 17)
Age (years)[a]	60.0 ± 2.9	60.3 ± 3.7
Sex (male/female)	10/10	9/8
Race (white/black)	20/0	14/3
Iris color (light/dark)	7/13	5/12
Visual acuity [a,b]		
OD	0.9 ± 0.06	0.96 ± 0.07
OS	0.94 ± 0.07	0.95 ± 0.07
Refractive error (diopters-spherical equivalent)[a]	-0.51 ± 0.60	-0.12 ± 0.43

From [19].
[a]Mean ± standard error.
[b]Visual acuity determined as ratio, e.g., 20/20 = 1, 20/30 = 0.67.

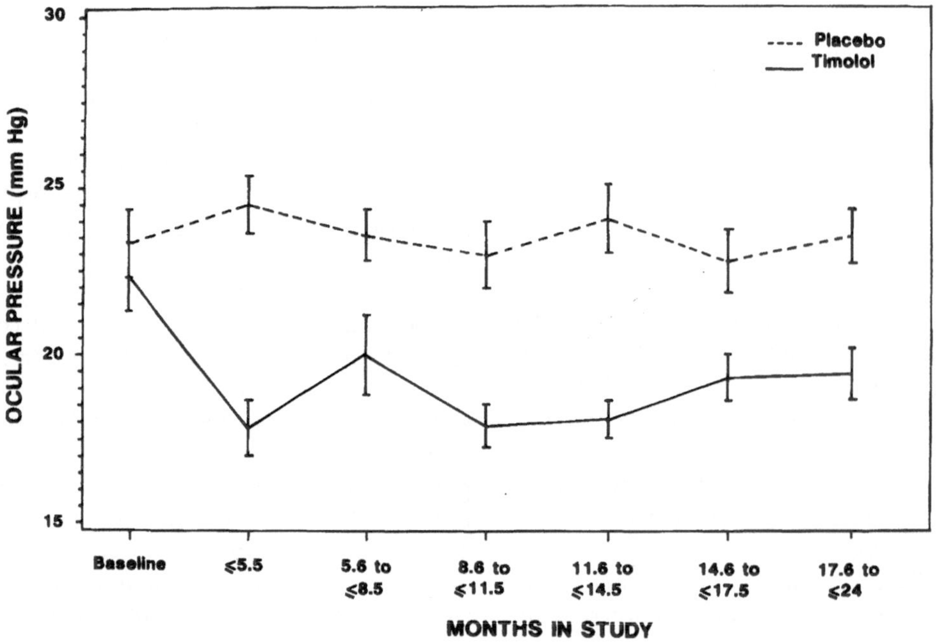

Fig. 1. Change of mean ocular pressure for left eye over time for placebo and timolol groups. *Vertical bars* indicate the standard error of the mean (From [19])

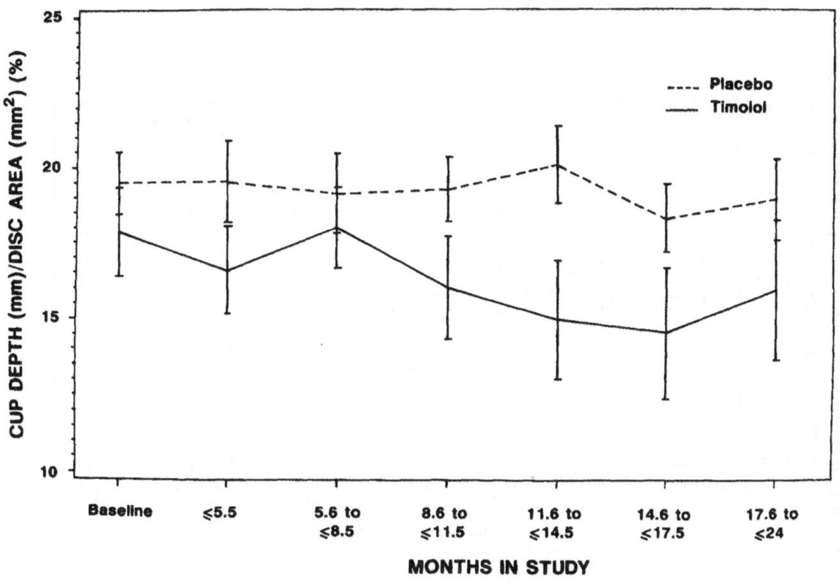

Fig. 2. Change of mean optic disc cup depth for total disc for left eye over time for placebo and timolol groups. *Vertical bars* indicate the standard error of the mean (From [19])

pressure for the left eye over time for the placebo and timolol groups.

There were highly significant differences between the two groups, which persisted throughout the study.

Univariate Analysis

Optic Disc Cupping and Pallor

Figure 2 shows the changes in cup depth for the total disc for the left eye over time for the placebo and the timolol groups. The placebo group remained fairly constant throughout the period of the trial however the timolol group showed a decrease in cup depth, which is particularly significant for the temporal aspect of the cup [$p = 0.04$]. Similar to cup depth, the other parameters of the cup showed a significant decrease in their measurements during the study, greater for timolol than placebo, particularly cup area, cup volume, the cup area at 0.5 depth and the area of pallor in various quadrants of the disc.

Table 2. Retinal nerve fiber layer thickness for total disc comparison of placebo and timolol groups for change from baseline (period minus baseline)

Period	Placebo	Timolol	*t*	*p*
0-9 months				
OD	- 0.010 ± 0.010 (20)	0.016 ± 0.0006 (17)	- 2.277	0.030
OS	- 0.021 ± 0.006 (20)	0.018 ± 0.012 (17)	- 2.850	0.009
>9-15 months				
OD	- 0.028 + 0.011 (19)	0.032 ± 0.012 (12)	- 3.515	0.002
OS	- 0.019 ± 0.008 (19)	0.029 ± 0.016 (12)	- 2.886	0.007
>15-24 months				
OD	- 0.013 ± 0.010 (16)	0.030 ± 0.011 (10)	- 2.809	0.010
OS	- 0.030 ± 0.008 (16)	0.015 ± 0.018 (17)	- 2.313	0.038

From [20].
t test; mean ± SE; number of eyes is shown in parentheses.
OD, right eye; OS, left eye

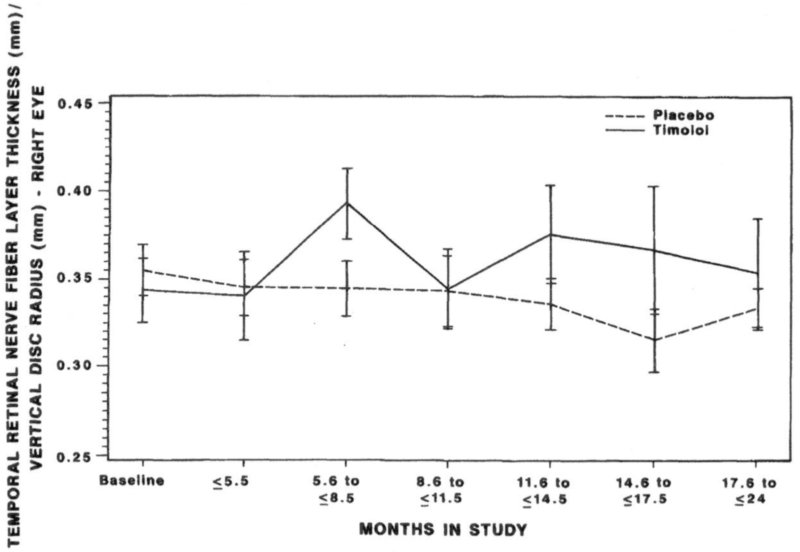

Fig. 3. Mean values of retinal nerve fiber layer thickness for the temporal quadrant for the right eye for the placebo and timolol groups over time. *Vertical bars* indicate the standard error of the mean. (From [20])

Retinal Nerve Fiber Layer Thickness

A similar trend was noted for retinal nerve fiber layer thickness. Figure 3 shows the mean values of retinal nerve fiber layer thickness for the temporal quadrant for the right eye, for the placebo and timolol groups over time. There is a continuous decrease of the placebo group compared to the increase of the timolol treated group, which particularly becomes significant at about 8 months. Table 2 compares the retinal nerve fiber layer thickness for the total disc for change from baseline. Comparison of the placebo and the timolol groups shows the placebo group decreasing, while the timolol group shows an increase with a significant difference for all three periods of the study and for both eyes.

Retinal Vessel Width

Figure 4 shows the plot of mean values of retinal vessel width for the inferior temporal artery for the left eye for the placebo and timolol groups over time. The placebo group showed mostly a significant decrease over time, while the timolol group appeared to show an increase over time, as indicated by the slopes of retinal vessel width for the placebo and the timolol groups for the retinal arteries and veins (Tables 3, 4). The slopes of the placebo group both for right and left eyes are negative and mostly show a significant decrease over time, while some of the slopes of the timolol group for right and left eyes are positive in sign, or relatively less negative than the slopes of the placebo group.

Changes in retinal vessel width from baseline were more evident for the retinal veins than for the retinal arteries. Table 5 shows the comparison of placebo and timolol groups for the change from baseline for the superior temporal vein with a number of significant differences noted for the various periods of time, both for the right and left eyes. The placebo group showed a mean decrease in retinal vessel width from baseline, while the timolol group showed a relative mean increase compared to the placebo group.

An evaluation of the extent of the changes that occurred in the optic disc, retinal nerve fiber layer thickness and retinal vessel width during the therapeutic trial is shown in Table 6. The maximum percent increases of various parameters ranged from 8.6% to 20.4%.

Multivariate Analyses

Multivariate analyses were done to evaluate the changes in the end point of the optic disc measurements for cupping and pallor, retinal nerve fiber layer thickness and retinal vessel width, in

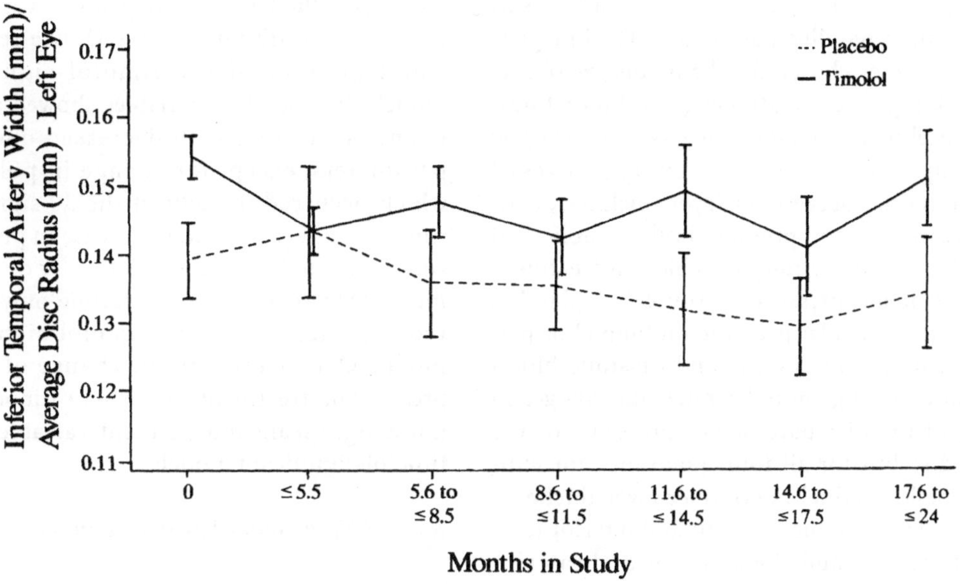

Fig. 4. Mean values of retinal vessel width for inferior temporal artery for the left eye for the placebo and timolol groups over time. *Vertical bars* indicate the standard error of the mean. (From [22])

Table 3. Slopes of retinal vessel width with time for the placebo group

	Placebo OD Slope	*p*	OS Slope	*p*
Artery				
Superior temporal	- 0.662 ± 0.207 (20)	0.0047	- 0.751 ± 0.361(20)	0.0508
Inferior temporal	- 0.609 ± 0.217 (20)	0.0111	- 0.602 ± 0.283 (20)	0.0468
Vein				
Superior temporal	- 0.789 ± 0.203 (20)	0.0010	- 0.461 ± 0.381 (20)	0.2413
Inferior temporal	- 0.898 ± 0.350 (20)	0.0188	- 1.273 ± 0.635(20)	0.0592

From [22].
p value for significant differences of slope from zero; mean ± SE x 10^{-3}; number of eyes is shown in parentheses.
OD, right eye; OS, left eye.

Table 4. Slopes of retinal vessel width with time for the timolol group

	Timolol OD Slope	*p*	OS Slope	*p*
Artery				
Superior temporal	+0.452 ± 0.573 (17)	0.4410	+0.000327 ± 0.269 (17)	0.9990
Inferior temporal	-0.128 ± 0.333 (17)	0.7041	-0.361 ± 0.248 (17)	0.1643
Vein				
Superior temporal	-0.174 ± 0.489 (17)	0.7260	+0.315 ± 0.451 (17)	0.4942
Inferior temporal	-0.446 ± 0.557 (17)	0.4351	-0.203 ± 0.491 (17)	0.6846

From [22].
p value for significant differences of slope from zero; mean ± SE x 10^{-3}; number of eyes is shown in parentheses.
OD, right eye; OS, left eye.

relation to the characteristics of the subjects as well as their baseline parameters. The independent variables chosen for the models were age, iris color, gender, treatment (placebo or timolol), baseline parameters, such as baseline optic disc cup volume, area of pallor, retinal vessel width, retinal nerve fiber layer thickness, ocular pressure, blood pressure both diastolic and systolic, and pulse rate; variables on treatment such as ocular pressure on timolol or placebo, or change of ocular pressure on timolol or placebo, changes in systolic and diastolic blood pressures, change in pulse rate; and changes in some of the disc parameters, not only for the total disc but for all four quadrants, for cupping, pallor, retinal nerve fiber layer thickness and the width of the superior and inferior temporal arteries and the superior and inferior temporal retinal veins.

Optic Disc Cupping and Pallor

For cupping and pallor, of the 60 possible models for the total disc and the four quadrants for cup volume, area, depth, cup area at 0.2 and 0.5 depth levels (volume profile), and area of pallor for the right and the left eyes, 30 models were obtained with timolol as a significant independent variable. The models indicated that a decrease in the optic disc parameters of cupping and pallor was associated with timolol therapy. The baseline optic disc cup parameter was another significant independent variable so that the larger the baseline cup parameter, the larger the dependent variable of the measured disc parameter. Only a relatively small number of the timolol-significant models' independent variables showed a significant association with decreased optic disc parameters, except for change in pulse rate which occurred in eight of the 30 significant timolol models. A greater decrease in pulse rate was associated with a smaller optic disc parameter. Ocular pressure at baseline only occurred significantly in one timolol-significant model. Ocular pressure or change of ocular pressure on treatment (placebo or timolol) was not a significant independent variable in the timolol-significant models.

Retinal Nerve Fiber Layer Thickness

Of the possible ten models for both eyes for the total disc and the four quadrants, eight showed timolol as the significant independent variable associated with an increase in retinal nerve fiber layer thickness during the trial. Baseline retinal nerve fiber layer thickness was also a significant independent variable, so that the larger the baseline retinal nerve fiber layer thickness, the larger the retinal nerve fiber layer thickness during the trial. Similar to the multivariate analyses of the optic disc cupping and pallor, ocular pressure at baseline only occurred in a very small number of timolol -significant models but ocular pressure or change of ocular pressure on treatment did not occur as a significant independent variable.

Table 5. Superior temporal retinal vein retinal vessel width (mm)/average disc radius (mm): comparison of placebo and timolol groups for change from baseline (period minus baseline)

Period	Placebo	Timolol	*t*	*p*
0-9 months				
OD	-11.3 ± 4.31 (19)	+7.33 ± 4.70(17)	-2.92	0.006
OS	-10.0 ± 6.32 (18)	+7.44 ± 5.01 (17)	-2.17	0.038
>9-15 months				
OD	-15.2 ± 4.41 (19)	-1.62 ± 4.63 (12)	-2.13	0.043
OS	-12.8 ± 5.96 (18)	-2.90 ± 4.80 (12)	-1.29	0.207
>15-24 months				
OD	-16.3 ± 4.78 (17)	-1.22 ± 6.16 (10)	-1.93	0.069
OS	-2.06 ± 5.32 (17)	+5.60 ± 7.88 (10)	-2.75	0.014

From [22].
t test; mean ± SE x 10^{-3}; number of eyes is shown in parentheses.
OD, right eye; OS, left eye

Table 6. Maximum percent change with timolol[a]

Depth of cup	-20.4%
Pallor	-8.6%
Retinal nerve fiber layer thickness	+14.3%
Retinal vessel width	+12.3%

[a] $\frac{\text{Max timolol-baseline}}{\text{Max timolol+baseline/2}} - \frac{\text{Max placebo-baseline x 100}}{\text{Max placebo + baseline/2}}$

Change in cup volume did not occur as a significant independent variable in any of the timolol-significant models, indicating that the increase in retinal nerve fiber layer thickness was not associated with any change in cup volume.

Retinal Vessel Width

Of the total number of eight models for the retinal vessel width of the superior and inferior temporal arteries and veins in both eyes, timolol occurred as a significant variable in five of these models indicating that a larger retinal vessel width was associated with timolol treatment. Again, similar to the models developed with optic disc cupping and pallor and retinal nerve fiber layer thickness, baseline ocular pressure as well as ocular pressure on treatment occurred significantly in only a very small number of models. As with the other analyses, baseline retinal vessel width occurred as a significant independent variable in all eight models with the larger the baseline retinal vessel width, the larger the retinal vessel width during the trial.

Discussion

This therapeutic trial of timolol vs placebo in ocular hypertensives has demonstrated that a decrease in optic disc cupping and area of pallor occurred, as well as an increase in retinal nerve fiber layer thickness, and retinal vessel width which was significantly associated with timolol therapy. These observations suggest reversibility of parameters of the glaucomatous optic neuropathy with timolol therapy. Ocular pressure on treatment or change of ocular pressure on treatment did not occur as a major significant independent variable, indicating that the effect of timolol was independent of its effect of lowering ocular pressure. However the decrease in the optic disc parameters, retinal nerve fiber layer thickness and retinal vessel width with timolol therapy was associated with the baseline values, so that the larger the baseline values, the less the decrease. This suggests that the decrease or the reversibility is related to the amount of glaucomatous damage, or the stage of the disease. The effect of timolol in reversing these parameters occurred in most of the subjects but not all.

Reversibility or improvement of the visual field in glaucoma has been described in other reports, generally associated with a decrease in ocular pressure, usually by surgery [6, 7, 32] and more recently with betaxolol [33, 34]. As far as we are aware, this is the first study that demonstrates reversibility of optic disc parameters, retinal nerve fiber layer thickness and retinal vessel width in a therapeutic trial with a double-masked randomized design in the early stage of the disease. Visual field reversibility described in the literature has to be viewed with caution, since it is well known that visual fields vary in nature and to demonstrate a worsening of the visual field in normal pressure glaucoma at least four, probably six, visual fields would be required [35]. Therefore, to demonstrate worsening of the visual field, one would also have to have a significant number of visual fields or show this on a regression analysis which involves a relatively large sample of visual fields [4]. Optic disc reversibility has also been documented by photographs or actual measurements [36], in specific cases, and but not in a group of subjects as in a therapeutic trial.

Studies of glaucomatous patients, particularly those under therapy, have indicated a definitive progression of the disease. Two studies indicate that at least two thirds showed progression over 5 years as measured by visual field loss involving qualitative evaluation of the visual fields [2, 3].

However, a study with a shorter period of follow-up, namely 3-4 years, using linear regression techniques for the analysis of change in the visual fields, has shown that only one third of the patients progressed with treatment [4]. However the patients in these studies had more advanced disease and therefore cannot be compared to the present study, which studied ocular hypertensives.

This study has demonstrated, by objective methods and the use of objective end points, reversibility of glaucomatous damage with medical therapy. It would be important to pursue other studies, using other ß-blockers or other medications, to determine if this effect is also present, regardless of the change of ocular pressure with these medications. Of particular importance would be to define the effect in relation to the stage of disease.

Acknowledgements. This study of the therapeutic trial comparing placebo to timolol was supported by a grant from Merck & Co. Inc., Medical and Scientific Affairs, Human Health Division, Clinical Development, West Point, Pennsylvania. The author, Bernard Schwartz, has applied for a patent on the use of timolol for maintaining or decreasing optic disc cupping and pallor and for maintaining or increasing retinal nerve fiber layer thickness.

References

1. Hoskins HD Jr, Kass MA (1989) Diagnosis and therapy of the glaucomas. 6th ed CV Mosby, St. Louis, p 277
2. Hart WM Jr, Becker B (1982) The onset and evolution of glaucomatous visual field defects. Ophthalmology 89:268-279
3. Mikelberg FS, Schulzer M, Drance SM, Lau W (1986) The rate of progression of scotomas in glaucoma. Am J Ophthalmol 101:1-6
4. O'Brien SC, Schwartz B, Takamoto T, Wu DC (1991) Intraocular pressure and the rate of visual field loss in chronic open-angle glaucoma. Am J Ophthalmol 111:491-500
5. Werner EB, Drance SM, Schulzer M (1977) Trabeculectomy and the progression of glaucomatous visual field loss. Arch Ophthalmol 95:1374-1377
6. Drance SM, Bryett J, Schulzer M (1977) The effects of surgical pressure reduction on the glaucomatous field. Doc Ophthalmol Proc Ser 14:153-157
7. Greve EL, Dake CL, Verduin WM (1977) Pre- and post-operative results of static perimetry in patients with glaucoma simplex. Doc Ophthalmol 42:335-351
8. Heilmann K (1978) Progression and regression of visual field defects. In: Heilmann K, Richardson KT (eds) Glaucoma; conceptions of a disease: pathogenesis, diagnosis, therapy. WB Saunders, Philadelphia, pp 168-175
9. Armaly MF (1979) Reversibility of glaucomatous defects of the visual field. Doc Ophthalmol Proc Ser 19:177-185
10. Greve EL, Furuno F, Verduin WM (1979) The clinical significance of reversibility of glaucomatous visual field defects. Doc Ophthalmol Proc Ser 19:197-203
11. Iwata K (1979) Reversible cupping and reversible field defect in glaucoma. Doc Ophthalmol Proc Ser 19: 233-239
12. Phelps CD (1979) Visual field defects in open-angle glaucoma: progression and regression. Doc Ophthalmol Proc Ser 19:187-196
13. Neumann E, Hyams SW (1973) Intermittent glaucomatous excavation. Arch Ophthalmol 90:64-66
14. Spaeth GL, Fernandes E, Hitchings RA (1980) The pathogenesis of transient or permanent improvement in the appearance of the optic disc following glaucoma surgery. Doc Ophthalmol Proc Ser 22: 111-126.
15. Pederson JE, Herschler J (1982) Reversal of glaucomatous cupping in adults. Arch Ophthalmol 100:426-431
16. Quigley HA (1982) Childhood glaucoma; results with trabeculotomy and study of reversible cupping. Ophthalmology 89:219-226
17. Katz LJ, Speath GL, Cantor LB, Poryzees EM, Steinmann WC (1989) Reversible optic disk cupping and visual field improvement in adults with glaucoma. Am J Ophthalmol 107:485-492
18. Shin DH, Bielik M, Hong YJ, Briggs KS, Shi DX (1989) Reversal of glaucomatous optic disc cupping in adult patients. Arch Ophthalmol 115:1599-1603
19. Schwartz B, Lavin P, Takamoto T, Araujo DF, Smits G (1995) Decrease of optic disc cupping and pallor of ocular hypertensives with timolol therapy. Acta Ophthalmol Scand 73 (Suppl 215):5-21
20. Schwartz B, Takamoto T, Lavin P, Smits G (1995) Increase of retinal nerve fiber layer thickness in ocular hypertensives with timolol therapy. Acta Ophthalmol Scand 73 (Suppl 215):22-32
21. Wu DC, Schwartz B, Schwoerer J, Banwatt R (1995) Retinal blood vessel width measured on color fundus photographs by image analysis. Acta Ophthalmol Scand 73 (Suppl 215):33-40
22. Schwartz B, Takamoto T, Lavin P (1995) Increase of retinal vessel width in ocular hypertensives with timolol therapy. Acta Ophthalmol Scand 73 (Suppl 215):41-53
23. Donaldson DD, Prescott R, Kennedy S (1980) Simultaneous stereoscopic fundus camera incorporating a single optical axis. Invest Ophthalmol Vis Sci 19:289-297
24. Takamoto T, Schwartz B (1985) Reproducibility of photogrammetric optic disc cup measurements. Invest Ophthalmol Vis Sci 26:814-817
25. Takamoto T, Schwartz B (1984) Stereo measurement of the optic disc cup shape: volume profile method. In: American Society of Photo-

grammetry. Technical Papers of the 50th Annual Meeting. Falls Church, VA: The Society, pp 352-358
26. Nagin P, Schwartz B, Nanba K (1985) The reproducibility of computerized boundary analysis for measuring optic disc pallor in the normal optic disc. Ophthalmology 92:243-251
27. Takamoto T, Schwartz B (1989) Photogrammetric measurement of nerve fiber layer thickness. Ophthalmology 96:1315-1319
28. Murphy EA (1982) Biostatistics in Medicine. Johns Hopkins University Press, Baltimore
29. Mehta CR, Patel NR, Tsiatis AA (1984) Exact significance testing to establish treatment equivalence for ordered categorical data. Biometrics 40: 819-825
30. Ware JH (1985) Linear models for the analysis of longitudinal studies. Am Statist 39:95-101
31. Kim J-O, Mueller CW (1978) Factor analysis: statistical methods and practical issues. Sage, Beverly Hills, CA, pp 14-36
32. Spaeth GL (1985) The effect of change in intraocular pressure on the natural history of glaucoma: lowering intraocular pressure in glaucoma can result in improvement of visual fields. Trans Ophthalmol Soc UK 104:256-264
33. Kaiser HJ, Flammer J, Stümpfig D, Hendrickson P (1994) Long-term visual field follow-up of glaucoma patients treated with beta-blockers. Surv Ophthalmol 38:S156-S160
34. Collignon-Brach J (1994) Long-term effect of topical beta-blockers on intraocular pressure and visual field sensitivity in ocular hypertension and chronic open-angle glaucoma. Surv Ophthalmol 38:S149-S155
35. Schulzer M (1994) Errors in the diagnosis of visual field progression in normal-tension glaucoma. Ophthalmology 101:1589-1595
36. Schwartz B, Takamoto T, Nagin P (1985) Measurements of reversibility of optic disc cupping and pallor in ocular hypertension and glaucoma. Ophthalmology 92: 1396-1407

Discussion

Question: Rolando

I have two questions for Dr. Schwartz. The first concerns nerve fiber layer thickness. Why did you choose the temporal side of the nerve fiber thickness to make your measurement if most actions are in the inferior and posterior bowls? And the second quéstion is, what does it mean clinically the thickening of nerve fibers?

Answer: Schwartz

We measured all the areas of the nerve fiber layer and all parameters of the disc. What I showed is an example of the changes we observed, so we didn't particularly select the temporal side. In glaucoma some axons are dead and not functioning, but there are axons in which the axonplasma transport has been slowed down and perhaps this will lead to recovery.

Question: Quaranta

I wanted to ask Dr. Schwartz if the photographs for evaluation of vessels were taken connected with an electrocardiograph to establish if a photo was taken during the diastolic or the systolic phase. In fact, this is a fundamental parameter to evaluate retinal vessel.

Answer: Schwartz

We did a study on this a number of years ago, and we showed that our measurement may have a little difference in relation to reproducibility of our method.

Question: David

I have a question for Dr. Robin concerning the rate of allergy that you presented, based on the 12-week data. There was 15% of allergy with Apraclonidine and 10% with Brimonidine. Just looking at literature we see that some of the numbers vary, and from recently presented data on several hundred patients the UK were up to 48% using Apraclonidine and 10% with Brimonidine. Do you think that there is a time related connection and that as time goes on more allergies can be expected?

Answer: Robin

You raised a very interesting point. Let me first say, as I tried to do in my presentation, that data on allergy that occurred are very confusing. The determination of allergy ranges from a red eye to a marked blepharoconjuntivitis and I believe it's hard for investigators to make all these as one entity and to spread them into different entities. Let's look at Alvarado's data first. He put a 1% solution and he didn't distinguish between various forms of allergy. If you look at his data, he had approximately 50% of allergy and still it was not clear what allergy we defined. If you look at all the other studies going up to one year, the rate of allergy ranges somewhere between 10 and 25% with Apraclonidine. In my personal experience, having patients being treated up to 6 years, the rate of allergy is approximately 17%. Most of the allergies we have seen with Apraclonidine occurred early, that is approximately 40 days. Once you have reached approximately 2 or 3 months, it is unusual to see an allergy develop. While I am on the podium, I'd like to stress a point made by Dr. Alm regarding the prostaglandines, and by Ingrid regarding the dorzolamide, that these are both new drugs and new formulations of drugs. I still remember and most of you remember that Timolol was first introduced as a panacea. It was a medication that had no side effects, and we have all since learned that it is not the case. Allergologists use this medication with caution because a true side effect profile is not known.

Question: Gay

I have a question for Dr. Adamson or maybe a statement. What you presented, for me, is that Timolol and Trusopt have a negative effect, that's what you said, but I think it's a little misleading because what appears from the data is that Trusopt works when Timolol doesn't work. So in order to know what is the real additive effect of the two drugs, one should determine what each drug does by itself and then what they do together.

Answer: Adamson

I want to try to get the question clear. I presented one patient not adequately controlled on Timolol, so I am really showing additivity. We didn't take people who, let's say, had pressure of 16 on Timolol and put them aided by Trusopt to see if they got additional benefits, but we took people certainly not adequately controlled on Timolol. A good number of them go to additional pillar effect on Trusopt in addition to Timolol. I hope I answered to some degree to your question.

Question: James

I have two questions for Dr. Robin. The first question has to do with the loss of visual acuity associated with Apraclonidine treatment mentioned by Dr. Demailly this morning. Do you have any information about the severity and frequency of that side effect? The second question has to do with the mechanism of action for Apraclonidine. You mentioned that you were dubious about the outflow pathway as a subcomponent of mechanism of action. Do you think a vasoconstriction is a component of a mechanism of action?

Answer: Robin

Before I go on, I'd like to congratulate for your excellent work. You did a very enlightening and excellent work that really should go noticed by this audience. Let me answer your second question regarding the mechanism of action of Apraclonidine or of other agonists in general.

Posterior uveo-scleral outflow is a possible alternative for Apraclonidine and Brimonidine. The technique used has a lot of limitations and I am dubious on the results of these studies. The type of work that really should be done is microsphere in primates or subhuman primates and that has not been done to the best of my knowledge. It could be that uveo-scleral outflow has a portion in some work, but maybe not. Regarding the question of vasoconstriction, it's interesting to see that some of the effects we see initially with alpha-agonists, that is eyelid retraction and conjunctival blenching, disappear with time. A chronic use of alpha agonists is not associated with eyelid elevation or mydriasis, so I wonder whether the effects can still continue. There is no relationship between the discontinuation of this side effects and the IOP lowering effects. I don't know any substantiated case of visual loss with Apraclonidine. That does not mean that it is a perfect drug, but it has different ranges of side effects.

Question: Lamberti

Several studies show that the hypertensive effect of the drug is related to the baseline IOP value.
Is it true?

Answer: Alm

If we look at the data we will find that with Latanoprost, as you do with most drugs, we have a better pressure reduction the higher the pressure is in absolute terms. But if there is a significant difference between Latanoprost and any other drugs, there is no study to show that. So I think it is something we have to find out in the future.

Question: Secchi

A question to Dr. Robin. How do we know that what you call allergic conjunctivitis is really an allergic conjunctivitis, since it could well be due to, for instance, some non specific release of chemical mediators which have nothing to do with allergy?

Answer: Robin

The question is an excellent question and let me repeat it. It is: How do we know that we have to do with a real allergy? The answer is that we really don't. I think that is a term that I and others have coined and it's probably a mistake. It's probably a toxic reaction that involves, for a large part, one of the things we are presently trying to work on. We are trying to get what is causing this type of reaction. There are a lot of theories if you look at type I, type II, type III allergies. It doesn't fit any of these, so most likely it's a multifactorial problem and the toxicant may be a significant factor, but I don't know if it is or not.

Question: Virno

I wish to ask Dr. Robin how these alfa-agonists lower intraocular pressure. We have demonstrated that these substances, both apraclonide and clonidine, inhibit opening of the blood-ophthalmic barrier after paracentesis and "osmotic stress" through a vasoconstrictor action. On the other hand, when we put these drugs on the conjunctiva we see the disappearance of conjunctival capillaries so that when these drugs reach the ciliary body vessels, which are responsible of humor aqueous production, they can induce a reduction of the humor aqueous production by vasoconstriction.

Answer: Robin

If I understand the question correctly, it is that by your research you have shown that there is perhaps a vasoconstriction to the ciliary body that may decrease aqueous humor production. I cannot dispute this, I am not familiar with your work. We don't see further vasoconstriction of the ciliary or the conjunctival vessel or the interior segment vessel, and I wonder if the mechanism of action chronically has really to do with vasoconstriction. I don't know the answer, I am sorry.

Question: Virno

A question to Prof. Alm. The literature says us that there is antagonism of the substances that contract ciliary muscle towards the uveoscleral outflow. If Latanoprost acts increasing the uveoscleral outflow, is there antagonism for pilocarpine, that contracts ciliary muscle, towards the ocular hypotensive effect of Latanoprost?

Answer: Alm

There has been an early study on monkeys showing that one could prevent the effect of prostaglandines by pre-treatment with pilocarpine, so in monkey it was possible to do that. We have few short-term studies where Latanoprost was combined with 2% of pilocarpine given 3 times a day, and the two drugs combined were a little better than other drugs. 2% pilocarpine 3 times a day is a much lower dose than was used in monkeys, and when you reach the age of glaucoma your ciliary muscle is not contracting as actively as it would do in young monkeys.

Question: Virno

So, is there antagonism or sinergism?

Answer: Alm

A guess is that the effect you get from Latanoprost if you pre-treated with pilocarpine, probably is a little bit less than you would have expected otherwise, but that is a pure guess and not easy to show, but if you have them together they are a little bit more effective than if you take either Latanoprost or pilocarpine. But I don't think that terms other than guess would be correct.

Question:

I'd just like a comment about the three drugs which suppress aqueous production. We have three drugs which now suppress aqueous production, and I believe sooner or later we are going to use all three of them together on the same eye. The question is for any of the speakers: do we have any long-term experience or any experience with using all the three drugs which suppress the ciliary body producing the aqueous humor?

Answer: Robin

It may be that the aqueous suppression chronically would have caused cornea and epithelium to be damaged because drug is absorbed and maintened in the cornea; there is probably some damage to the lens because of decreased aqueous flow rates. We have not seen that, we have not a control group to compare to.

Question: Tico

My question is how much are we going to be able to suppress aqueous more than you can do with two aqueous suppressors. Again may be that we should really be working about changing apoptosis which should be worded as calcium channels and gated calcium channels excitatory aminoacids, NMDA pathways; those are really the right ways of looking at glaucoma research. I hope that when Prof. Bucci holds his meeting again in the next decade we are really talking not about intraocular pressure but about protecting axons.

Answer: Adamsons

The best long term data we have is a work where we used aqueous suppressant on patients who are on Timolol and Dorzolomide. We had a 1 year study and a 2 year study, the two year study has just begun. Patients could have been on combination therapy for basically two years minus 15 days or one year minus 15 days. There were previous controls on both medications and it seemed that there haven't been additional problems.

Answer: Alm

Latanoprost doesn't reduce flow. I still would like to make one comment on the question itself, an important one. The question is: Do they, all the three drugs together, really give a very good additivity? I know that there was one study when Apraclonidine and Timolol were added and flow was measured in acute study and single drop study in normal eyes; they had no additive effects in that study. I don't think you get large addition on aqueous flow.

UP-DATING ON HYPOTENSIVE AND NON HYPOTENSIVE GLAUCOMA THERAPY

Dopaminergic Drugs and Ocular Pressure

M. Virno, J. Pecori Giraldi, L. Taverniti, L. Pannarale, and F. De Gregorio

Department of Ocular Physiopharmacology, Eye Clinic, University "La Sapienza", Viale Policlinico 153, 00161 Rome, Italy

Introduction

The identification of novel mechanism of modulating intraocular pressure (IOP) is essential to the development of new antiglaucoma drugs. While the ocular pharmacological effects of β-blockers have been widely studied, the potential for influencing IOP through other adrenergic receptors has not yet been investigated. In the case of dopamine receptors, progress has been limited by the complex pharmacology of dopamine, the lack of appropriate selective dopamine receptors agonists and antagonists, and the different activities of these agents regarding IOP.

The great majority of studies into the role of dopamine (DA) in the eye have examined its function as a neurotransmitter in the retina, whereas its effects on the anterior segment are poorly described. Moreover, the data concerning the activity of dopaminergic drugs on IOP in animal experiences proved to be contradictory, since these drugs were shown to be able either to increase or to decrease IOP or to induce a biphasic response, according to species, type of formulation or concentration. Furthermore, dopamine, in addition to activating D1 and D2 receptors, has a high affinity for α-adrenergic receptors [1-11].

Investigations in animals [1] showed that dopamine itself decreases IOP with a significant controlateral effect, causes vasodilatation without mydriasis and lowers aqueous humor formation.

Our studies on dopaminergic drugs started in 1986 and involved a new dopaminergic agonist, ibopamine (3,4-diisobutyril ester of *N*-methyldopamine: epinine) [12]. Ibopamine proved to have a stimulatory effect on dopaminergic, β-adrenergic and, to a lesser extent, α-adrenergic receptors when administered topically [13]. In comparison with dopamine, epinine has more pronounced effects on D1, D2 and β2-receptors and on prejunctional α2-receptors.

Ibopamine is extensively and rapidly absorbed and is immediately hydrolyzed to epinine by the plasma esterases [14-16]. Studies on rabbits have shown that ibopamine evokes mydriasis when instilled in the conjunctival sac [17]. The drug is well tolerated when given by ocular route, as is shown by biomicroscopic examinations of the anterior segment of the eye [12]. Ibopamine produces a dose-dependent mydriasis with very interesting characteristics: rapid onset, marked pupil dilatation and rapid return to normal pupillary diameter, and no cycloplegic effect (Fig. 1). The mydriatic effect is correlated with the concentration of epinine in the aqueous humor [18].

Moreover, following instillation of a 2% solution, ibopamine has the peculiar pharmacological property of inducing a transient ocular hypertensive effect (120/180 min) only in eyes having intraocular hydrodynamic disorders [19, 20]. No IOP rise has ever been observed in normal eyes [21] (Fig. 2), results which were recently confirmed by other autors [22-27]. The hypertensive effect of ibopamine was shown to be unrelated to the mydriasis induced, since pre-treatment with the α-blocker thymoxamine inhibited the mydriatic activity, but did not significantly affect the hypertensive response [20] (Fig. 3).

The ocular hypertensive effect is due to a D1-dopaminergic effect, since instillation of a

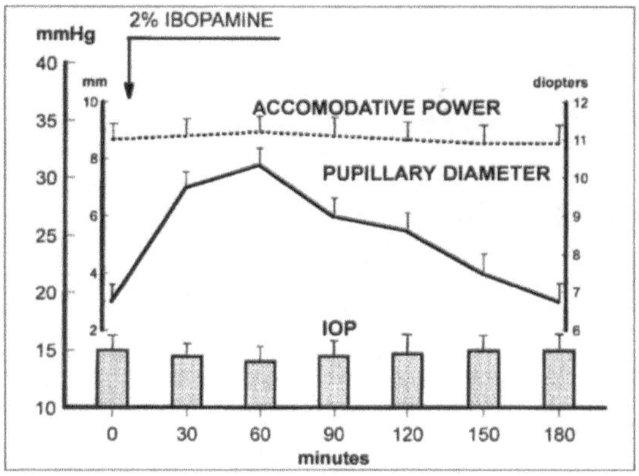

Fig. 1. After topical application, ibopamine is rapidly hydrolyzed to free *N*-methyl-dopamine (a dopamine analogue). It causes a maximal mydriasis of brief duration with no cycloplegic effect

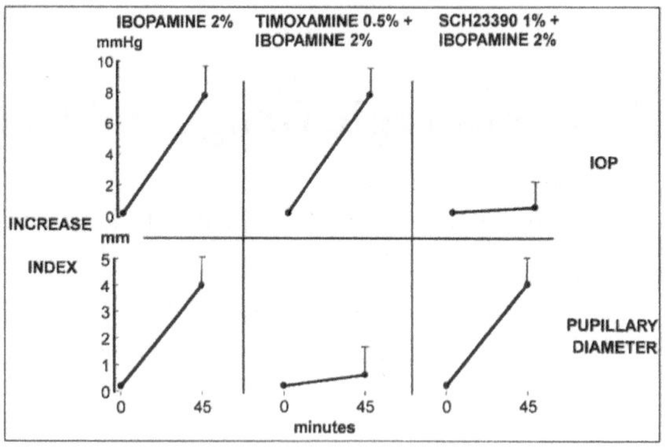

Fig. 3. The effect of ibopamine on IOP is unrelated to the induced mydriasis, since pre-treatment with the α-blocker thymoxamine inhibits the mydriatic activity but does not significantly affect the hypertensive response. By contrast, the IOP increase, but not mydriasis, is antagonized by topical pre-treatment with selective D1 receptor blockers (SCH23390)

selective D1 agonist (1% 3B90 and 1% fenoldopam) caused a behavior similar to that in response to ibopamine. Conversely, the selective D1 antagonist SCH23390 was shown to be able to antagonize the hypertensive effect of ibopamine (Fig. 3). Topical antihypertensive drugs (DPE, β-blockers, α-blockers, clonidine) were unable to significantly inhibit this action, whilst pilocarpine and oral glycerol showed a partial inhibitory effect [28-36].

Fluorophotometric studies have demonstrated an increase in aqueous humor production following instillation of 2% ibopamine both in healthy and glaucomatous eyes. Therefore, since the transient ocular hypertension induced by ibopamine is typical of eyes with ocular hydrodynamic disorders, it would indicate a disparity between inflow and outflow of aqueous humor [37-39] (Fig. 4).

Here, we summarize our studies on dopaminergic drugs and point out their possible clinical applications.

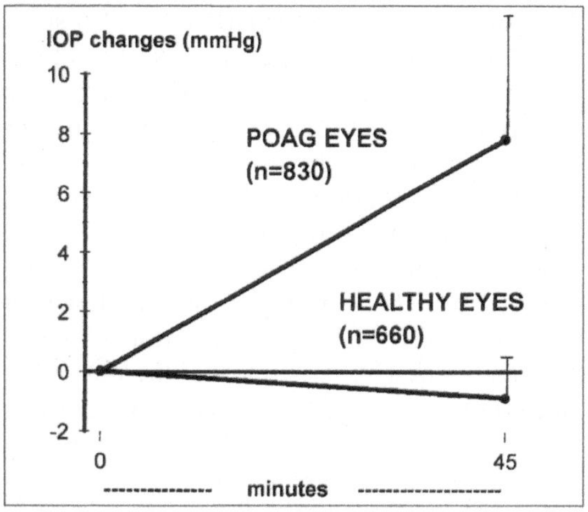

Fig. 2. Effect of 2% ibopamine eyedrops on IOP (45 min after instillation). Ibopamine induces a transient ocular hypertensive effect in 92% of patients with primary open-angle glaucoma. No IOP increase has ever been observed in healthy eyes

Material and Methods

Our series consisted of 25 eyes from 18 healthy subjects (age 45-72 years) and 20 eyes suffering from primary open-angle glaucoma from 10

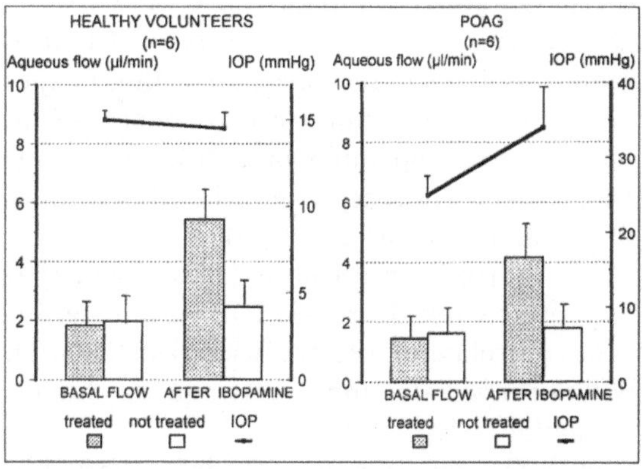

Fig. 4. The hypertensive response to 2% ibopamine instillation is attributable to an increase in aqueous humor production, as demonstrated by fluorophotometry. In eyes with altered outflow structures, the increased production of aqueous humor would involve a transient IOP increase

patients (age 43-72 years).
The experimental procedures were:

1. Applanation tonometry following topical anesthesia by 0.4% oxybuprocaine.
2. Measurement of pupillary diameter by Haag-Streit slit lamp.
3. Topical administration of the drug tested either by instillation of two drops at an interval of 5 min or by an ocular bath lasting 2 min, a method adopted in order to prolong contact of the drug with the eye.
4. Repetition of applanation tonometry and pupillary diameter measurement 45 min after administration.

Pre-treatment with dopaminergic antagonist was performed 20 min prior to instillation of the dopaminergic agonist.
The dopaminergic drugs used were: 2% dopamine, 0.25% *L*-DOPA, 1% fenoldopam, 1% 3B90, 0.8% bromocryptine and 2% ibopamine.
Clinical trials with the different dopaminergic drugs were performed in the 25 healthy eyes and in the 20 POAG eyes under the same experimental conditions at 15–20 day intervals.

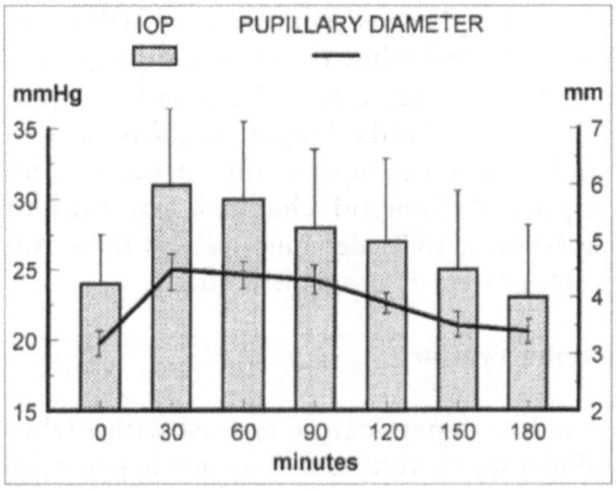

Fig. 5. The ocular hypertensive effect of ibopamine is attributable to a dopaminergic activity (actually ibopamine is the prodrug of N-methyl-dopamine, an analogue of dopamine as far as chemical structure is concerned), since it is comparable to that obtained in the very same patients following an ocular bath with 2% dopamine; such method of administration was adopted in order to prolong the substance's contact with the eye because of its poor intraocular penetration

Results and Discussion

Dopamine

Following an ocular bath of 2% dopamine, no IOP changes were ever observed in the 25 healthy eyes, whereas a mean increase of 9.1 ± 2.55 (SD) mm Hg was obtained 45 min after administration in the 20 POAG eyes (Fig. 5) [16-19]. A slight mydriatic activity was noted in both groups of eyes.
The hypertensive effect of dopamine could not be inhibited by pre-treatment with 1% haloperidol (nonselective dopaminergic antagonist) or with 1% sulpiride (D2 selective dopaminergic antagonist).
The only substance which antagonized the hypertensive effect in POAG eyes was the D1 selective antagonist SCH23390, administered topically as a 1% solution. There was no change in mydriatic activity.

L-DOPA

The topical administration of *L*-DOPA, the precursor of dopamine, by means of an ocular bath of 0.25% concentration (the maximum obtainable in solution) induced no changes either in IOP or in pupillary diameter in both groups of eyes. Presumably the lack of activity was due to the low concentration used (1/8 that of dopamine) and to the poor transcorneal passage of this molecule.

Fenoldopam

Instillation of a 1% solution of fenoldopam (D1 selective dopaminergic agonist) induced no IOP changes in the 25 healthy eyes, whereas 45 min after administration there was a mean increase of 8.49 ± 1.46 (SD) mm Hg in the 20 POAG eyes. No modification of the pupillary diameter was noted. The drug was poorly tolerated because of conjunctival hyperemia, burning and ocular pain. Our data differ from those of other authors [39-43] who demonstrated a mean IOP increase of 3 mm Hg in healthy eyes following systemic administration of fenoldopam (5μg/kg/min as a slow intravenous infusion), leading to the conclusion that since D1 agonists cause vasodilatation, the IOP effect may have been the result of increased ocular blood volume.

3B90

Topical administration of 3B90 (D1 selective

dopaminergic agonist) induced no IOP changes in the 25 healthy eyes, whereas it caused a mean IOP increase of 10.2 ± 2.05 mm Hg in POAG eyes. Unlike ibopamine, this drug is similar to fenoldopam since it induces no pupillary diameter changes. The lack of mydriatic activity demontrates that these two drugs possess no α-agonistic effects.

Bromocryptine

This is a dopaminergic agonist with higher affinity for D2 receptors. Its ocular hypotensive effect has been observed both in animals [44] and in humans [45-47] after either topical or oral administration. We administered a 0.8% concentration by ocular bath and observed a mean IOP decrease of 2.9 ± 1.55 mm Hg in healthy eyes and 3.2 ± 1.26 mm Hg in POAG eyes.

Ibopamine

On the basis of the data already obtained, we plan to use ibopamine in the treatment of ocular post-surgical hypotony. Beacause of its lack of effect on IOP in healthy eyes [20, 21, 36], we attempted to induce an alteration of normal outflow pathways, by means of short-term corticosteroid administration, in 60 eyes of 30 patients suffering from mild inflammation of the ocular annexes.
Prior to entering the study the subjects were submitted to an ibopamine test [20]; thereafter 0.1% dexamethasone was administered topically four times daily for 10 days. Ibopamine treatment was repeated on the fourth, seventh and tenth day. In those eyes which showed a positive reaction to the test (IOP increase equal or greater than 3 mm Hg 45 min after instillation), the test was repeated 15 days after the interruption of the corticosteroid treatment.
As was expected, all the examinated subjects had a negative response to the ibopamine test before corticosteroid treatment started. At the end of the corticosteroid treatment ten patients (33%) became positive to the ibopamine test: these patients were considered as "responders". Such positivity did not occur 15 days after dexamethasone was discontinued (Fig. 6).
Considering IOP value prior to the instillation of ibopamine, we noticed a slight IOP increase, not statistically significant, during steroid treatment. A 2-ways ANOVA showed that there was a significant increase in IOP following ibopamine instillation.
The duration of dexamethasone treatment was a fundamental factor in the development of positivity to the ibopamine test. Actually, we found a significant trend in the increase of percent responders during treatment (Cochran Q = 9.93; $p = 0.0094$).

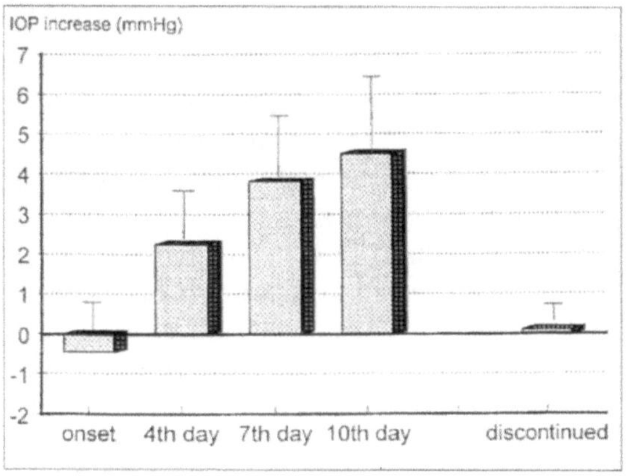

Fig. 6. Ibopamine (2%) is able to demonstrate the very early onset of hydrodynamic disorders induced by topical corticosteroids: throughout dexamethasone treatment (0.1%, 4 times daily), ibopamine induced a transitory increase of IOP in 33% of examined eyes before any changes in basal IOP were noticed. Such positivity did not occur 15 days after corticosteroids was discontinued

Treatment of Postsurgical Hypotony: A Pilot Study

A total of nine patients (seven males and two females; mean age: 40.78 years) suffering from ocular hypotony were selected.
The inclusion criteria were the following: (a) ocular hypotony following repeated surgical vitreoretinal procedures; (b) mean diurnal IOP not greater than 6 mm Hg; (c) diurnal IOP fluctuation not greater than 2 mm Hg; (d) stable IOP for at least 60 days; (e) topical corticosteroid treatment (β-methasone or dexamethasone) in progress; and (f) anatomic success of surgery.
Patients having a history of glaucoma or ocular hypertension, narrow irido-corneal angle, increase of IOP during corticosteroid treatment, phthysis or pre-phthysis of the eye and any other cause of ocular hypotony were excluded from the study.

As basal IOP, the mean value of three measurements (9 a.m., 2 p.m. and 7 p.m.) taken on the first day of the study was used.
A solution of 2% ibopamine (1 drop, 4 times daily) was added to the topical corticosteroid treatment (0.1%-0.2% dexamethasone or β-methasone 4 times daily).
Controls were performed every 15 days and IOP values were taken at the same time (9 a.m., 2 p.m. and 7 p.m.).
The ibopamine was administered for 30 days at least.
As final IOP, the mean value of three measurements (9 a.m., 2 p.m. and 7 p.m.) taken on the last day of ibopamine treatment was used.
Each IOP measurement was taken no earlier than 180 min after ibopamine instillation.
One month after ibopamine was discontinued, a measurement of IOP (average of three measurements (9 a.m., 2 p.m. and 7 p.m.) was performed again (Fig. 7).
The results of this study confirmed that, after treatment with 2% ibopamine (4 times daily, added to 0.1%-0.2% dexamethasone or β-methasone), a mean increase of IOP of 3.24 ± 3.333 mm Hg was obtained. The increase was statistically significant (paired $T = 2.5$; $p = 0.035$). One month after ibopamine was discontinued the mean IOP (4.34 ± 2.74) was similar to that of pre-treatment (4.08 ± 1.96; p = n.s.)
In four patients the IOP increase was greater than 3 mm Hg, in four patients the increase was between 1 and 3 mm Hg, and in one patient there was an IOP decrease of 2 mm Hg. No local or systemic adverse effects were ever observed in long-term ibopamine treated patients.

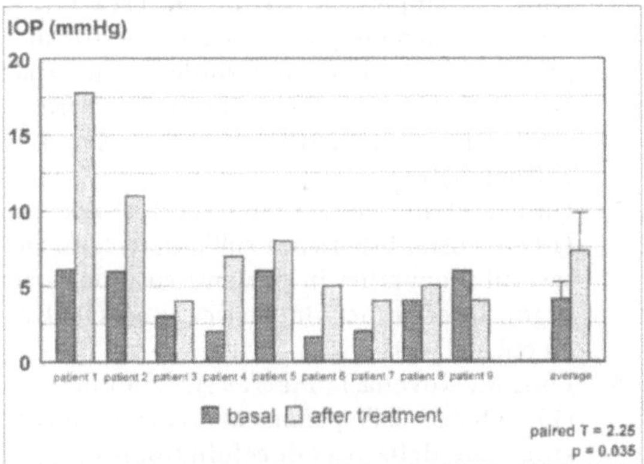

Fig. 7. Our preliminary results in treatment of ocular hypotony: we found a mean IOP increase of 3.24 mm Hg by means of 2% ibopamine added to topical corticosteroid (dexamethasone) administration. The IOP increase seems to be transitory and lasted 1 month after the ibopamine was discontinued. We suppose that treatment can be more effective, as there is less anatomic damage at the level of the ciliary body

Conclusion

The D1 dopaminergic agonists (dopamine, ibopamine, fenoldopam, 3B90), administered topically, were shown to induce an IOP increase only in eyes with intraocular hydrodynamic disorders. This hypertensive response does not change when pre-treatment, either by means of nonselective antagonists (haloperidol, sulpiride) or commonly used, topical, tension-lowering drugs (adrenergic, adrenolytic, cholinergic), is carried out. Complete inhibition of the hypertensive effect was obtained only by a pre-treatment with the D1 selective antagonist SCH23390: hence, the ocular hypertensive effect of the dopaminergic drugs is due to a stimulation of the D1 receptors.
As far as the mechanism of action is concerned, fluorophotometric studies showed that the stimulation of D1 receptors at the level of the ciliary body induces an increase in aqueous humor production both in healthy and glaucomatous eyes. In the eyes with altered outflow structures, the increased production of aqueous humor would involve a transient IOP increase.
Among the dopaminergic agonists considered, ibopamine seems to be the most interesting in terms of future clinical application, because of its good transcorneal permeability and lack of both systemic and topical side effects.
The ibopamine provocative test proved to be a valid pharmacological method to demonstrate an intraocular hydrodynamic disorder, even in a tonometric compensatory stage, and to reveal the very early onset of hydrodynamic disorders induced by topical corticosteroids. Furthermore, preliminary results obtained in the treatment of postsurgical ocular hypotony open a new field of application. Recent clinical studies [48] have also shown that ibopamine could be useful after trabeculectomy. Since the success of glaucoma surgery depends on rapid formation of the filtering bleb, ibopamine might aid such a process by stimulating D1 dopaminergic receptors and consequently increasing aqueous humor production.

References

1. Langer SZ (1973) The regulation of transmitter release elicited by nerve stimulation through a presynaptic feeed-back mechanism. In: Usdin E, Snyder SH (eds), Frontiers in catecholamines research. Pergamon, London, pp 543-549
2. Shannon RP, Mead A, Sears ML (1976) The effect of dopamine on the IOP and pupil of the rabbit eye. Inv Ophthal Vis Sci 15:371
3. Macri FJ, Cevario SJ (1978) The inhibitory action of dopamine, hydroxyamphetamine and phenilephrine on aqueous humor formation. Exp Eye Res 26:85-89
4. Mc Laughlin MA, Chiou GCY (1985) A synopsis of recent developments in antiglaucoma drugs. J Ocular Pharmacol 1:101-121
5 Cooper RL, Constable IJ, Davidson L (1984) Catecholamines in aqueous humor of glaucoma patients. Aust J Ophthalm 12:345-349
6. Chiou GCY, Chiou FY (1983) Dopaminergic involvement in intraocular pressure in the rabbit eye. Ophthalmic Res 15:131-135
7. Chiou GCY (1984) Treatment of ocular hypertension and glaucoma with dopamine antagonists. Ophthalmic Res 16:129-134
8. Chiou GCY (1984) Ocular hypotensive action of haloperidol, a dopaminergic antagonist. Arch Ophthalmol 102:143-145
9. Chiou GCY, Chiou FY (1989) Effects of dopaminergic antagonists injected through vortex veins on intraocular pressure. J Ocular Pharmacol 5:281
10. Leopold IH, Duzman E (1986) Observations on the pharmacology of Glaucoma. Ann Rev Pharmacol Toxicol 26:401-426
11. Hariton C (1991) Implication des recepteurs dopaminergiques dans la regulation de la pression intraoculaire. Clinique Ophtalm 1:97-102
12. Virno M, Taverniti L, Taloni M, Ioppolo A, Pellegrino N (1986) Studio sperimentale degli effetti locali e sistemici dell'ibopamina, farmaco dotato di attività adrenergica e dopaminergica. Boll Ocul 65:1169
13. Visioli O (1986) Ibopamine, a new drugs for heart failure. Arzneim-Forsch / Drug Res 36:285
14. Lodola E, Borgia M, Longo A, Pocchiari F, Pataccini R, Sher D (1986) Ibopamine kinetics after a single oral dose in healthy volunteers. Arzneim-Forsch / Drug Res 36:345
15. Pocchiari F, Pataccini R, Castelnovo P, Longo A, Casagrande C (1986) Ibopamine, an orally active dopamine-like drug: Metabolism and pharmacokinetics in rats. Arzneim-Forsch / Drug Res 36:334
16. Pocchiari F, Pataccini R, Castelnovo P, Longo A, Paro M, Casagrande C (1986) Ibopamine, an orally active dopamine-like drug: Metabolism and pharmacokinetics in dogs. Arzneim-Forsch / Drug Res 36:341
17. Virno M, Taverniti L, Motolese E, Taloni M, Bruni P, Pecori Giraldi J (1986) Ibopamina: nuovo midriatico non cicloplegico. Boll Ocul 65:1135
18. Soldati L, Gianesello W, Galbiati I, Gazzaniga A, Virno M (1993) Ocular pharmacokinetics and pharmacodynamics in rabbit of ibopamine, a new mydriatic agent. Exp Eye Res 56:247-254
19. Virno M, Pecori Giraldi J, Taverniti L, Taloni M, Bruni P (1987) Effetti ipertensivi oculari dell'ibopamina somministrata per via locale in soggetti con turbe idrodinamiche endoculari. Boll Ocul 66:833
20. Virno M, Pecori Giraldi J, Taverniti L, Taloni M, Pannarale L (1990) Intraocular hypertensive effects of topically administered ibopamine in eye with hydrodynamic disorders: a new provocative test for glaucoma. Glaucoma 12:88
21. Virno M, De Gregorio F, Grechi G, Da Dalt S (1991) Comportamento della pressione oculare e della motilità pupillare dopo somministrazione topica di ibopamina 2% in soggetti sani. Atti VI riunione AISG, 239
22. Rolle T, Brogliatti B, Valvo G, Boles Carenini B (1991) Uso dell'ibopamina collirio nell'iter diagnostico del glaucoma ad angolo aperto. Boll Ocul 70 (suppl 1):247
23. Boles Carenini B, Brogliatti B, Boles Carenini A, Valvo G, Sibour G (1994) The ibopamine test in diagnosis of POAG. 1st Joint Meeting of American Glaucoma Society and European Glaucoma Society, Reykjavik July 1993. New trends in ophthalmology IX: 2: 75-79
24. Nuti A, Ciappetta R, Diadori A, Frezzotti R (1992) Ibopamine provocative test in the diagnosis of hydrodynamic disorders. X international Congress of Eye Research, Stresa. September 20th-25th 1992. Exp Eye Res 55(suppl 1):185
25. Nuti A, Menicacci F, Ciappetta R, Diadori A (1993) Nostra esperienza sull'utilizzazione del test all'ibopamina in pazienti sottoposti ad argon laser trabeculoplastica. Boll Ocul 72 (suppl 2):92-102
26. Lodi M, Novella L, Marras A, Cambiaggi A (1992) Il test all'ibopamina in occhi portatori di sindrome della pseudoesfoliatio, Boll Ocul (suppl 2)50:111
27. Genitti G, Di Staso S, Blasi MA, Balestrazzi A (1995) The effect of N-methyl dopamine 3-4 butyryl ester on eyes with pseudoexfoliation syndrome. Inv Ophthalmol Vis Sci 36:3395
28. Virno M, Gazzaniga A, Taverniti L, Pecori Giraldi J, De Gregorio F (1992) Dopamine, dopaminergic drugs and ocular hypertension. Int Ophthalmol 16:349-353
29. Virno M, De Gregorio F, Taverniti L, Pannarale

L (1992) Azione sulla pressione oculare dei farmaci attivi sui recettori della dopamina, Acta III Congresso Nazionale di Farmacologia Oculare. Venice, pp 73-80
30. Virno M, Taverniti L, Matteocci G, De Gregorio F, Voccia L (1992) Dopaminergic drugs and intraocular pressure, 7th International Ophthalmological Symposium Genoa - Odessa, Genoa, May 1991. Boll Ocul 71 (suppl 6):185-189
31. Virno M, Pecori Giraldi J, Taverniti L, Taloni M, Gazzaniga A (1992) Ibopamine, dopamine and IOP. New Trends in Ophthalmol 7:275-280
32. Virno M, Taloni M, Taverniti L, Pannarale L, De Gregorio F (1994) Azione sulla IOP nell'occhio glaucomatoso del SCH23390, un antagonista selettivo dei recettori dopaminergici D1. Boll Ocul 73 (suppl 2):159-167
33. Virno M, De Gregorio F, Pannarale L, Taverniti L (1993) Ibopamine, a valuable pharmacological method for diagnosis of glaucoma. Oral presentation at 1st Joint Meeting of American Glaucoma Society and European Glaucoma Society, Reykjavik, Iceland
34. Pecori Giraldi J, Casali M, Cori MA, Maggi R, Scalvati M, De Gregorio F (1995) Analisi clinico -statistica del valore predittivo del test dell'ibopamina nel GAA: studio retrospettivo. Boll Ocul 74 (suppl 2):379
35. Pecori Giraldi J, De Gregorio F, Carbone F, Pica R, Scalfati M (1994) Curva tonometrica e positività al test dell'ibopamina nella prima diagnosi di glaucoma. Boll Ocul 73 (suppl 2):319
36. De Gregorio F, Pannarale L, De Stefano C, Virno M (1993) Azione di dosi ripetute di ibopamina (agonista dopaminergico) sulla IOP. Acta LXXIII Congress of Italian Society of Ophthalmology, Rome, Italy, pp 287-291
37. Virno M, De Gregorio F, Grechi G, Sedran L, Trimarchi M (1992) Azione dell'ibopamina sulla dinamica dell'umore acqueo: indagine fluorofotometrica. Boll Ocul 71 (Suppl 2):103
38. De Gregorio F (1993) Azione dell'ibopamina sulla produzione dell'umore acqueo. Personal communication presented at the National Meeting of Ocular Pharmacology, Rome, Italy
39. Virno M, Pannarale L, Arrico L, De Gregorio F (1994) Increase in aqueous humour production by topical administration of ibopamine, a dopaminergic agonist, in glaucomatous and healthy eyes. Inv Ophthal Vis Sci 35:2052
40. Karnezis TA, Murphy MB, Weber RR, Nelson KS, Tripathi BJ, Tripathi RC (1988) Effect of selective dopamine-1 receptor activation on IOP in man. Exp Eye Res 27:615
41. Karnezis TA, Tripathi BJ, Dawson G, Murphy MB, Tripathi RC (1989) Effects of dopamine receptors activation on the level of c-AMP in trabecular meshwork. Inv Ophth Vis Sci 30:1090
42. Karnezis TA, Murphy MB (1988) Dopamine receptors and intraocular pressure. Trends Pharmacol Sci 9:389-390
43. Piltz JR, Stone RA, Audet P, Boike S, Everitt D, Shusterman NH, Jordansky D (1992) Fenoldopam, a selective dopaminergic-1 receptors agonist, raises IOP in man. ARVO Abstract 33 (4):1121
44. Potter DE, Burke JA, Chang FW (1984) Ocular hypotensive action of ergoline derivatives in rabbits: effects of sympathectomy and domperidone pre-treatment. Curr Eye Res 3:307
45. Mekki QA, Hassan SM, Turner P (1983) Bromocriptine lowers intraocular pressure without affecting blood pressure. Lancet i:1250-1251
46. Costagliola C, Carella C, Amato G, Winkler NR, Scibelli G, Iaccarino G, Mastropasqua L (1995) Effect of oral bromocriptine administration on intraocular pressure in normotensive and glaucomatous human subjects. J Glaucoma 4:386
47. Costagliola C, Cotticelli L, Russo S, Iaccarino G, Acampora A, Rinaldi M (1992) Variazioni della pressione oculare dopo somministrazione orale di bromocriptina. Proceedings of LXXII National Congress of the Italian Society of Ophthalmology 1:997
48. Frezzotti R, Ciappetta R, Frezzotti P, Nuti A (1995) Use of ibopamine eye drops for the treatment of hypotony after trabeculectomy. International Symposium on Experimental and Clinical Ocular Pharmacology, Geneva, Switzerland, October 1995. Abstract, p 64

Concomitant Ocular Effects of Hypotensive Antiglaucomatous Drugs

B. Boles Carenini and A. Boles Carenini

Eye Clinic of the University of Turin, Via Juvarra 19, 10122 Turin, Italy

Introduction

The term "side effects" refers to the ensemble of mainly undesirable–though sometimes favourable–experiences which accompany the taking of drugs. Those experiences seem to be more accentuated the longer the therapy is continued. Regarding treatment of glaucoma, this aspect should not be ignored, since antiglaucomatous therapy, by its very nature, is long and drawn-out. The substances used to lower the intraocular pressure almost all produce as many systemic as local side effects, since almost all glaucoma medication acts on the autonomic nervous system.

Here we shall deal only with ocular local side effects, leaving aside the systemic effects. The principal groups of antiglaucomatous drugs and their side effects will be examined. We must, however, remember that topical side effects are always much less numerous and less important than systemic ones. Moreover, it is not always possible to distinguish true and proper drug-provoked side effects from those caused by preservatives and other added ingredients of the trade preparations [1].

Parasympathomimetics

The principal drug of this group is pilocarpine, the doyen of antiglaucomatous drugs. Others to be mentioned are aceclidine and carbachol. All these drug, beside their desired miotic and antihypertensive action, have, to a greater or lesser extent, ocular side effects which cannot be ignored (Table 1). These can be classified as:

Table 1. Parasympathomimetic and collateral ocular effects

Acetylcholine	No collateral effects
	Small loss of endothelial cells if injected into the anterior chamber
Pilocarpine	Cloudy vision
	For myosis
	For pseudomyopia
	Conjunctival toxicity
	Corneal toxicity
	Cytoplasmic vacuolization
	Decrease of endothelial regeneration
	Cataract
	Less frequent than anticholinesterases
	Retinal alterations
	For contraction of ciliary muscle and possible retinal traction (high myopia)
	Acute attack in closed angle glaucoma
Aceclidine	Like pilocarpine but fewer side effects
	Slight myopic effect
	Slight decrease in anterior chamber
	Less cataractogenic
	Conjunctival effects
	Hyperemia after first administration
Carbachol	Like pilocarpine but fewer side effects
	Corneal effects
	Possible formation of corneal opacity
	Cytotoxic
	Effects on accomodation
	Possible accomodative spasm
	Effects on the lens
	Less cataractogenic

Table 2. Aniticholinesterases (all have the same effects)

Reversible

- Neostigmine
- Demecarium
  - Effects on the lids: depigmentation of lid edge (in coloured people)
  - Effects on conjunctiva: allergic follicular conjunctivitis
  - Effects on the cornea: epithelial keratopathy, pseudotracomatous opacity
  - Effects on accomodation: spasm
  - Orbital myoclonus
- Carbachol

Irreversible

- DFP
- Mintacol (paraoxon)
- Phospholineiodide
  - Effects on conjunctiva: hyperemia; perikeratic injection
  - Effects on the cornea: superficial epithelial lesions with small endothelial depots
  - Effects on the anterior chamber: increased barrier permeability; increase in aqueous proteins; increase in IOP
  - Effects on the iris: hyperemia and vascular dilatation; anterior and posterior synechiae; edge cystis (children); fibrinous iritis; cataract and anterior undercapsular vacuoles
  - Effects on ciliary muscle: spasm; superorbital sense of weight; myopization; ciliary body congestion and possibility of acute glaucomatous attack (myotics paradoxical effect)
  - Effects on the retina: detachments from ciliary muscle contraction

Table 3. Epinephrine drugs

- Epinephrine
- Dipivefrin
  - Burning
  - Effects on conjunctiva: hyperemia; allergic reactions; adrenochrome pigmentation, also on lacrimal drainage system
  - Effects on the retina: cystoid macular edema

1. Concerning the conjunctiva and cornea, cell toxicity with corneal cell cytoplasmic vacuolation [2]; diminished epithelial regenerative capacity [3]; irreversible, conjunctival, cupola-shaped cell damage [4].
2. Concerning the ciliary muscles, contraction with possible pain.
3. Concerning the crystalline lens, opacity (cataract) only in response to strong miotics (anticholinesterases) [5-7], and ascribable to diminished lens respiration and diminished glucose-6-phosphate dehydrogenase activity [8].
4. Concerning the retina, in elevated myopia, reported cases of retinal detachment probably due to anomalous retinal tractions resulting from ciliary muscle contractions. Thus, careful examination of the retinal periphery before prescription of miotics to treat glaucoma in elevated myopia has been advised [9].

A "paradoxic effect of miotics" has also been reported in which there is an acute glaucoma attack in subjects with narrow-angle glaucoma [10, 11]. The subjective symptoms, caused by the miosis and pseudomyopia, due, in their turn, to the drugs also should not be disregarded [13].

Finally, a last side effect, albeit a useful one, is the choroidal blood flow improvement recorded after miotic therapy, especially with pilocarpine 4% [14].

α-Blockers and α-Agonist

These agents include thymoxamine, dapiprazole and clonidine. Thymoxamine has no local side-effect, except in high doses (5%), when it gives rise to a form of Horner's syndrome [15]. As regards dapiprazole, the more frequent side effects are conjunctival hyperemia and a temporary sensation of smarting and tearing, with no signs of any more serious side effects [16]. Clonidine has only transitory effects of conjunctival hyperemia from vasodilatation, followed, however, by clear and lasting vasoconstriction [17].

β-Blockers

This is the largest group and certainly the most complex. It includes various substances with different characteristics, such as, intrinsic sympathomimetic activity (ISA), which seems to influence in no small way the local and general effect of the drug and its selectivity or nonselectivity on β-receptors. All these agents have the great merit of not causing the characteristic undesirable reactions of the miotics (such as accommodation paralysis and "tight" miosis). Thus they are considered to be the better-tolerated drugs, with less compliance problems for the patient [18].

Among the undesirable side effects common to all β-blocking eye-drops but differing in extent depending upon the agent used, are erythema of the eyelid and conjunctival hyperemia, with allergic blepharoconjunctivitis, corneal edema with fogging of vision, sensation of foreign bodies, photophobia, tearing, conjunctival discharge and superficial punctate keratitis. These symptoms are often found together with corneal anesthesia, an effect confirmed by many authors [19] and linked with diminished lacrymal secretion due to the action of β-blockers on the tear gland [20]. This side effect is also to be found in subjects undergoing general β-blocking treatment [21]. While most of the studies refer to timolol, this is because it is the agent most often used in clinical practice; however, the same side effects are reported as possible for all the other β-blocking eye-drops.

Also to be included for the sake of completeness are the possibilities of reactive uveitis [22] during metipranolol treatment and the controversial observation of the appearance of macular edema in aphakic eyes treated with β-blockers.

Finally, of interest is the clearly demonstrated negative action on the choroidal circulation of β-blocking drugs, with the exception only of those possessing ISA (carteolol) or β-selectivity (betaxolol) [14].

Epinephrine Drugs

See Table (3) regarding the side effects of epinephrine and dipivefrin.

Prostaglandins

These drugs (latanoprost) have only recently been introduced into local use.

The only local side effects so far reported seem to be transitory conjunctival hyperemia, smarting, tearing and possible iatrogenic pigmentation of the iris (which can take on a brownish coloration).

Carbonic Anhydrase Inhibitors

One group of these substances, which includes acetazolamide, methazolamide, ethoxozolamide, dichlorphenamide and monochlorphenamide and which has long been used in general therapy, has recently been introduced in the form of eye drops (Dorzolamide - Trusopt). As far as local side effects are concerned, we can therefore distinguish between: (1) those connected with general usage, in which, despite the numerous and sometimes serious drawbacks, the local side effects are limited to an infrequent variation of refractive power of the lens, with consequent myopia (index variation) [23] and (2) side effects connected with local administration, such as itching and smarting, inflammation and irritation of the eyelids, conjunctivitis, tearing, a sensation of clouded vision, and headache. Rare cases of iridocyclitis have also been reported.

It should also be remembered that there is a positive, if transitory, effect on choroidal flow after oral administration of acetazolamide [14].

Osmotic Diuretics

These can be briefly differentiated into intravenous-administered diuretics, i.e., urea, mannitol, and ascorbate, and orally administered diuretics, i.e., glycerol, and isosorbide. These pharmacologically inert substances posses a weak tendency to pass through the semimpermeable membrans to reach specific regions. Therefore, their dehydrating effect in humans occurs above all in those anatomic areas where the hematic system is divided by semipermeable membranes [24], as in the cerebral and ocular regions. Fishman [25] has explained the mechanism of action of these drugs as lying in their inability to cross the hematoencephalic and hemato-ocular barriers. This leads to an osmotic imbalance with the formation of a concentration gradient between the blood (which becomes hypertonic) and the aqueous/vitreous (which become hypotonic), with subsequent active attraction of fluid to the point of isotonicity. Osmotic diuretic action on the vitreous is the result of a reduction in weight and volume together with a lowering of the viscosity [26-

29]. Consequently, there is an increase in depth of the anterior chamber because of the anterior hyaloid backing or, in aphakic eyes, the backing movement of the zonulo-lenticular diaphragm and the subsequent intraocular pressure drop [30-34]. Since osmotic diuretics are systemically administered drugs, the greatest number of side effects are systemic, while at the ocular level there have only been rare cases of hyphema [35] and of choroidal detachement due to the drastic tonometric drop. Following use of isosorbide only, there may be transitory myopia, due to accomodative spasm, and resolution can be brought about by instillation of a cycloplegic [36].

Conclusions

From this discussion of the possible side effects in use of antiglaucomatous hypotensive drugs, the following appears evident. First, topical side effects consist for the most part of symptoms which are significant only for the parasympathomimetics, while the effects of β-blockers and of other substances of more recent acquisition are limited to phenomena concerning eyelid and conjunctival reactions. Second, particular attention must nonetheless be given to the effect that each hypotensive drug can have on the ocular blood flow, considering the importance of that factor in the pathogenesis of the glaucomatous damage. Third, with respect to systemic side effects (which we have not dealt with here, but for which an imposing literature exists), the β-blockers are certainly the most dangerous of all the antiglaucomatous drugs. Finally, it would be in the better interest of the patient, if ophthalmologists, who prescribe a drug with greater enthusiasm the newer it is, and general practitioners, who often do not recognize the capacity of a local therapy to influence (even seriously) important systemic parameters, were aware of these issues.

References

1. Broadway D, Hitchings R, Grierson I (1995) Topical antiglaucomatous therapy: adverse effects on the conjunctiva and implications for filtration surgery. J Glauc 4:136-148
2. Coles WH (1975) Pilocarpine toxicity. Effects on the rabbit corneal endothelium. Arch Ophthalmol 93:36-40
3. Ziesmer W, Kaskel D (1975) Regenerative ability on the corneal epithelium under the action of various pressure reducing eyedrops. Ber Dtsch Ophth Ges 73:393-397
4. Naveh N, Wysenbeerk Y, Blumenthal M (1989) The morphological changes in the conjunctiva of the chick embryo caused by antiglaucoma drugs. Glaucoma meeting, Budapest
5. Axelsson U, Holmberg A (1966) The frequency of cataract after myopic therapy. Acta Ophthalmol 44:421-425
6. Axelsson U (1969) Glaucoma miotic therapy and cataract. Acta Ophth, (suppl) 102:1-10
7. Shaffer RN, Hetherington J Jr (1966) Anticholinesterase drugs and cataracts. Am J Ophthalmol 62:-613-620
8. Laties AM, (1969) Localization in cornea and lens of topically applied irreversible cholinesterase inihibitors. Am J Ophthalmol 68:848-850
9. Reibaldi A. Cantatore F, Asciano F (1980) Particolari orientamenti in tema di terapia medica di alcune forme di glaucoma. Atti 60° Congresso SOI, pp 437-440
10. Mapstone R (1970) Safe mydriasis. Br J Ophthalmol 54:690-695
11. Mapstone R (1981) Acute shallowing of the anterior chamber. Br J Ophthalmol 65:446-450
12. Hallden U (1973) Diffraction and visual resolution. The resolution of Landolt's ring. Acta Ophth 52:242-248
12. Poinoosawmy D, Nagasubramanian S, Brown NAP (1976) Effect of pilocarpine on visual acuity and on the dimension of the cornea and anterior chamber. Br J Neurol 105:583-585
13. Abramson DH, Coleman DJ, Forbes M, Franzen LA (1972) Pilocarpine. Effect on the anterior chamber and lens thickness. Arch Ophthalmol 87:615-620
14. Boles Carenini A (1995) Flusso ematico oculare: il Langham ocular blood flow system. Monografia S.O.I. I.N.C. Ed. Roma pp 31-52
15. Pau H (1955) Sympathikolise durch lokale konjunctivale pilonapplikation am auge. Kl Mbl Augen 126:171-180
16. Brogliatti B, Rolle T, Messelod M, Boles Carenini B (1985) A new alpha-blocking agent in the treatment of glaucoma: dapiprazole. Glaucoma 7:232-237
17. Heilmann K (1971) Untersuchungen uber die wirking von catpresan auf den intraokularen druck. 2. Klin Mbl Augen 158:493-499
18. Worthen DM (1979) Patient compliance and the "usefulness product" of timolol. Surv Ophth 23:403-407
19. Zimmermann TJ, Boger WP The beta adrenergic blocking agents and the treatment of glaucoma. Surv Ophth 23:347-350
20. Bonomi L., Zavarese C, Noya A, Michieletto S (1979) Effetti del trattamento locale con timo-

lolo sulla secrezione lacrimale. Boll Ocul 9:531-535
21. Almog Y, Monselise M, Almog C, Barishak YR (1982) The effect of oral treatment with beta blockers on the tear secretion. Metab Pediatric Syst Ophth 6:343-346
22. Kessler C, Crist T (1993) Incidence of uveitis in glaucoma patients using metipranolol. J Glaucoma 2:166-170
23. Back M (1956) Transient myopia after use of acetazolamide (diamox). Arch Ophthalmol 55: 546-550
24. Galin MA, Davidson R, Shachter N (1966) Ophthalmological use of osmotic therapy. Am J Ophthalmol 62:629-635
25. Fishman RA (1975) Brain edema. New Engl J Med Vol 293, pp 706-711
26. Bucci MG, Santillo C, Pecori-Giraldi J (1968) Determinazione quantitativa (microlitri/min) della partecipazione vitreale alla ipotonizzazione oculare da sostanze osmotiche. Boll Ocul 47:638-642
27. Kapetansky FM, Higbee JW (1969) Vitreous deturgescence. Eye Ear Nose Thr Monthly 48:313
28. Robbins R, Galin MA (1969) Effect of osmotic agent on the vitreous body. Arch Ophthalmol 82:694-700
29. Preste E, Traverso G (1966) Il meccanismo d'azione del mannitolo: ricerche viscosimetriche sul vitreo di coniglio. Ann Ottal: 92:827-832
30. Leone Jr CR, Callahan A (1967) Restoration of the anterior chamber with glycerol 50% and mydriasis. Am J Ophth 63:1686-1690
31. Takahashi T, Kawamura Y (1968) Use of 20% mannitol for absent anterior chamber following cataract surgery. Jap J Clin Ophthalmol 22: 1307-1317
32. Quon DK, Worthen DM (1981) Dose response of intravenous mannitol on the human eye. Ann Ophth 13:1392-1398
33. Grabrie MT, Gipstein MR, Adam DA (1981) Controindication for mannitol in aphakic glaucoma. Am J Ophthalmol 91:266-270
34. O'Keefe M, Nabil M (1983) The use of mannitol in intraocular surgery. Ophth Surg 14:55-60
35. Seeger FL, Meriwether PL (1964) Ophthalmological use of mannitol. Arch Ophthalmol 72:219-222
36. Dangel ME, Weber PA, Leier CB (1983) Transient myopia following isosorbide dinitrate. Ann Ophthalmol 15:1156-1159

Role of Carrier Substances in Hypotensive Drug Activity

A. Reibaldi, M.G. Uva, J.P. Ott, and A. Longo

Institute of Ophthalmology, Catania University, Via Bambino 32, 95124 Catania, Italy

Introduction

Ocular availability of topical drugs is strongly affected by several factors, i.e., tear fluid dynamics, corneal layers penetration, scleral and conjunctival absorption, blinking, binding with lacrimal proteins, and enzymatic disactivation [1].

Eye drops, traditionally the most widely used way to deliver ophthalmic drugs, are far from being optimal, with respect to bioavailability [2].

Some Authors [1, 3, 4] showed that only a minimal amount (<5%) of the active ingredient of topical eye drugs becomes available to ocular tissues. Normal tear turnover and drainage remove up to 90% of conventional eye drops, before the active drug can enter the eye. Excess drug can cause local side effects or may pass through the tear drainage ducts and cause adverse systemic reactions.

As for topical drugs, the "main entry way" into the eye is the cornea, a very selective barrier [5-9]. Thus, when aiming to increase the bioavailability of the drug, one of the most important parameters to be considered is the time the ophthalmic solution remains in contact with the surface of the eye. An increase in the corneal contact time will cause an increase in the ocular availability of the drug and a decrease in its systemic toxicity.

These concepts assume even greater importance in a chronic pathology such as glaucoma, in which the role played by carrier substances greatly conditions both the effectiveness of the hypotensive drug (from a pharmacokinetic and pharmacodynamic point of view) and patient compliance.

In aiming to improve topical hypotonizing therapy and to avoid compliance problems, some attempts have been made to improve the drug delivery systems.

Although drug delivery systems such as inserts, ointments, soft contact lenses, collagen shields, and suspensions have been investigated [10-14], it is a common experience that administration of a desired drug in the form of eye drops still remains preferable to assure the best patient compliance [15, 16].

The addition of soluble polymers (such as methylcellulose, polyvinylalcohol, hydroxypropylcellulose, polyvinyl-pyrrolidone) to eye drop solutions to increase the tear viscosity has showed minimal clinical effect [17, 18].

The Ocusert device, an ocular insert acting as a diffusion system for pilocarpine and made of unerosible hydrophobic polymer membranes (ethylene/vinyl acetate) was designed to release the drug at fixed rates of 10 μg/h or 40 μg/h for 1 week [10-19].

Notwithstanding the ingeniousness and elegance of such an idea (it is the only commercially available hypotonizing drug delivery system that works at a true constant, controlled rate), in time, it has fallen short of expectations owing to discomfort caused [16, 20-23].

Fewer problems plague the gel form of pilocarpine (Pilogel, Alcon, Forth Worth, TX), in which 4% pilocarpine is contained in an aqueous gel vehicle containing more than 90% water and employing Carbopol 940, a synthetic, high molecular weight, cross-linked polymer of acrylic acid, to impart high viscosity [16, 20-24].

Other long-acting drug delivery systems are still being investigated and involve nanocapsules [25, 26], cyclodextrins [27, 28], microemulsions [23, 29-31], and liposomes [32-34]. Here we update information on carriers either currently in use or in advanced experimentation. Our report is based on ophthalmic literature and on our own experience.

Gelrite

This novel ophthalmic drug delivery system (Kelco division of Merk and Co., USA) consists of a gellan gum, which is an anionic heteropolysaccharide produced by the microorganism *Pseudomonas elodea*. This material gels on contact with mono- and bivalent cations in the tear film. Several active drugs can be absorbed on the surface of the polymeric particles of this ion-activated, in situ, gelling vehicle. The resulting transition sol-gel is expected to prolong corneal residence time of the active drug (with other advantages, such as easier auto-application and less blurring of vision). Scintigraphic studies in volunteer subjects with technetium-99m-labelled Gelrite carried out by Greaves et al. [35], showed a significant increase in the clearance rates of Gelrite compared to hydroxyethylcellulose ($p < 0.006$) or saline ($p < 0.009$).

These data were confirmed by experimental and clinical studies performed with different drugs:

1. Timolol (0.25%-0.50%) carried with Gelrite (Timoptic-XE, MSD) once daily is equivalent to 0.25%-0.50% timolol (0.25%-0.50% Timoptic) twice daily [36-42] with a similar safety profile and a slightly higher incidence of transient blurred vision following instillation of Timoptic-XE. Similar results were reported in a multicentric study performed in Italy [43].
2. Two topical carbonic anhydrase inhibitors, sezolamide (MK-417) and dorzolamide (MK-507), formulated in Gelrite vehicle, were compared [22]. There was a slight increase in the duration of action of both compounds using this carrier as compared to conventional vehicle.
3. Chastaing et al. [44] reported an increased bioavailability of 1% pilocarpine in a Gelrite vehicle compared to a slightly viscous, commercially available solution of 1% pilocarpine (Chibro-Pilocarpine, MSD) containing 0.3% hydroxyethyl cellulose.

Amberlite

This drug delivery system (Alcon Lab., Fort Worth, TX) is an ion exchange polymeric resin developed to carry the vehicle 0.25% betaxolol (0.25% Betoptic S, Alcon). This ophthalmic suspension also contains Carbomer 934 P, an acrylic polymer that enhances the physical stability and viscosity of the suspension and increases the corneal residence time of the carried drug. Amberlite binds active drug molecules to resin particles and releases them once in the conjunctival cul-de-sac, by ion exchange with tear film. This delivery system optimizes the bioavailability of 0.25% betaxolol in 0.25% Betoptic S ophthalmic solution (equivalent to Betoptic 0.50% sterile ophthalmic solution at half the concentration of drug), with a comparable hypotonizing effect but a more uniform dosage, increased ocular comfort and less side effects, as shown by experimental studies and clinical trials [45-51].

Durasite

This is an eye drop based system (In Site Vision Alameda, CA) which delivers drugs in a cross-linked acrylic acid polymer formulation. Once in the conjunctival cul-de-sac, the polymer forms a soft molded insert with a mucoadhesive property. According to the manufacturer, unlike the material in conventional eye drops, the Durasite polymer swells in water rather than dissolving and, at physiologic pH and tonicity conditions, the particles expand and extend side chains. Inter-particle attraction creates an integrated insert, trapping the active drug by physical entrapment or reversible ionic interaction. Over time, the drug undergoes sustained release by diffusion and bioerosion from eyelid movements and tear flow. Together with the corneal residence time, the bioavailability of the drug is also increased, whereas the eroded polymer particles, which are insoluble, are eliminated through the nasolacrimal duct and leave the body via the GI tract without causing side effects. Harper et al., at ARVO '94 [52] showed the results of a study comparing 2% pilocarpine carried by Durasite b.i.d. (2% Pile Site), with 2% pilocarpine q.i.d. (2% Pilocar) in subjects with primary open-angle glaucoma (POAG) or ocular hypertension, demonstrating a similar efficacy and safety and a better acceptability of the b.i.d. vs the q.i.d. drug.

Hyaluronic Acid

Last but not least, this carrier substance is a polysaccharide repeating unit of glucoronic acid and *N*-acetylglucosamine with β-1-3 glycosidic bonds. Hyaluronic acid (HA) has mucoadhesive and pseudoplastic properties, which presents a well-known biocompatibility [53]. It also shows a bioavailability-enhancing activity for several active drugs [54-56].
It was speculated and experimentally demonstrated [56] that, owing to the mucoadhesive property of HA, there is a prolonged retention of active drug in the precorneal area, which is greater than what occurs by the sole effect of viscosity.
The ionically bound active drug is de-livered to the target tissue at a sustained rate, in analogy with the sustained release of drugs bound to ion-exchange resin [54].
Previously [57], we have evaluated the capabilities of this carrier to enhance both the bioavailability and the hypotonizing effect of 0.5% timolol and 2% pilocarpine, associated in a fixed combination in sodium hyaluronate vehicle.
We compared this new formulation (FI-SER C 301, Fidia-Oftal CT) with the commercially available product Timpilo 2 (MSD). The following parameters were evaluated:

1. Precorneal residence time (PRT) of timolol by spectroscopic UV reflectance method.
2. Bioavailability in the aqueous humor (AUC concentration/time of both drugs in the acqueous) in albino rabbits by HPLC.

Moreover, we evaluated the IOP lowering effect on POAG patients after single instillation. The PRTs of timolol were 450 ± 50 s for FISER C 301 and 120 ± 20s for Timpilo 2.
Bioavailability of timolol and pilocarpine in the aqueous after instillation of FISER C 301 increased, respectively, by 273% ($p < 0.05$) and 420% ($p < 0.05$) compared to Timpilo 2. Regarding IOP lowering effect in glaucomatous patients, both the peak effect and the duration of action of the active drugs, as determined by round-the-clock maintenance of IOP, were improved with the mucoadhesive association.

Discussion

As shown here for glaucoma (but actually regarding any disease), advances in medical therapy stem not only from the introduction of new drugs. An alternative way is to improve the drug therapeutic index (TI), i.e., the desired effect of the drug divided by its undesired (side) effect. Increasing attention has been devoted to improving the forms by which new and old drugs are administered. Important therapeutic advances have been realized through the control of drug delivery within the patient.
Poor drug delivery into the eye necessitates higher concentrations and/or more frequent applications in order to achieve adequate therapeutic responses. These higher concentrations and rates of application increase the risk of systemic side effects and systemic drug interactions with other medications [58, 59]. Conversely, optimized drug delivery will improve the TI of the active drug, requiring less frequent administration than conventional dosage forms, thus improving patient compliance and permitting utilization of drugs having very short biological half-lives [24].
If we consider the factors affecting the ocular availability of a topical applied drug, they coincide with protection mechanisms of the eye from exogenous chemical substances, i.e., drainage, lacrimation, induced blinking, conjunctival and scleral absorption, lacrimal protein binding, corneal penetration, and metabolism [1].
Moreover, if we consider the characteristics of an ideal-perfect carrier, i.e., acceptability (without interference with vision, irritation, aesthetic problems, painful sensations), patient self-medication feasibility, provision of sustained/controlled drug release, no interaction with the components, stability, possibility of industrialization of the finished products, we can stress the therapeutic advances obtained in this area of research.

References

1. Lee V, Robinson J (1979) Mechanistic and quantitative evaluation of precorneal pilocarpine disposition in albino rabbits. J Pharm Sci 68:673-683
2. Boles Carenini B, Brogliatti B, Gremmo E (1991) Le nuove modalità di somministrazione dei farmaci antiglaucomatosi. Boll Agg Farm Ocul

1,5:1-4
3. Benson H (1974) Permeability of the cornea to topically applied drugs. Arch Ophthalmol 91:313-319
4. Patton T (1980) Ocular drug disposition. In: Robinson (ed) Ophthalmic drug delivery systems. Am Pharm Assoc, Washington DC pp 28-42
5. Brewitt H, Honegger H (1982) Morphologische Befunde des Hornhautepithels bei Störung des präcornealen Films und nach Applikation von Augenmedikamenten. In: Marquard (ed) Chronische Conjunktivitis, Trockenes Auge. Springer, Wien, pp 641-647
6. Shell J (1982) Pharmacokinetics of topically applied ophthalmic drugs. Surv Ophthalmol 26:207-219
7. Maurice M, Mishima S (1984) Ocular pharmacokinetics. In: Sears M (ed) Pharmacology of the eye. Springer, Berlin Heidelberg, New York, pp 433-439
8. Maurice M (1987) Kinetics of topically applied ophthalmic drugs. In: Ophthalmic drug delivery, Liviana, Padova, pp 263-272
9. Benet L, Mitchell J, Sheiner L (1990) Pharmacokinetics: the dinamics of drug absorption, distribution and elimination. In: Gilman, Rall, Nies, Taylor (eds) The pharmacological basis of therapeutics. Pergamon, New York, pp 105-113
10. Montrone F, Balestrazzi E, Reibaldi A (1977) L'ocusert P40 nella terapia medica del glaucoma cronico semplice ad angolo aperto. Ann Ottal & Clin Ocul CIII 3:191-202
11. Uva MG, Scalia G, Gagliano C, Panta G (1988) Pilocarpina Gel e glaucoma. In: Drago F (ed) Farmacologia oculare - Attualità e prospettive, Cappelli Ed, Bologna, pp 17-27
12. Uva MG, Panta G, Biondi P, Randazzo D, Nicoletti G (1993) Sul ruolo di un nuovo veicolo nella terapia del glaucoma. Boll Ocul 73 (Suppl) 1:247-255
13. Reibaldi A, Avitabile T (1990) La Farmacologia del glaucoma. Medical Books, Palermo
14. Reibaldi A, Uva MG, Gagliano C, Panta G, Ott J (1993) Farmacologia antiglaucomatosa: up to date. In: Acts of the XXVII Congr SOM, Tipografica, Bari, pp 241-268
15. Lee V, Robinson J (1986) Review, topical ocular drug delivery: recent developments and future challenges. J Ocul Pharmacol 2:67-108
16. Hurvitz L, Kaufman P, Robin A, Weinreb R, Crawford K, Shaw B (1991) New developments in the drug treatment of glaucoma. Drugs 41:514-532
17. Adler C, Maurice D, Paterson M (1971) The effect of viscosity of the vehicle on the penetration of fluorescein into the human eye. Exp Eye Res 11:34-42
18. Chrai S, Patton T, Mehta A, Robinson J (1973) Lacrimal and instilled fluid dynamics in rabbit eyes. J Pharm Sci 1112-1121
19. Ros F, Greve E, Dake C, Miller W (1976) Experiences with Ocusert. Doc Ophthalmol 12:43-60
20. Goldberg I, Ashburn F, Kass M, Becker B (1979) Efficacy and patient acceptance of pilocarpine gel. Am J Ophthalmol 88:843-846
21. Johnson D, Epstein D, Allen R (1984) A one year multicenter clinical trial of pilocarpine gel. Am J Ophthalmol 98:723-729
22. Gunning F, Greve E, Bron A, Bosc J, Royer J, George J, Lesure P, Sirbat D (1993) Two topical carbonic anhydrase inhibitors sezolamide and dorzolamide in Gelrite vehicle: a multiple-dose efficacy study. Graefe's Arch Clin Exp Ophthalmol 231:384-388
23. Naveh N, Muchtar S, Benita S (1994) Pilocarpine incorporated into a submicron emulsion vehicle causes an unexpectedly prolonged ocular hypotensive effect in rabbits. J Ocul Pharmacol 10:-509-520
24. Shell J (1984) Ophthalmic drug delivery systems. Surv Ophthalmol 29:117-128
25. Sirbat D, Marchal-Heussler L, Maincent P (1992) Nanocapsules. The future drug administration system in ophthalmology? Their application in the treatment of experimental glaucoma. Ophthalmol 6:383-384
26. Umemoto M, Takahashi K, Higashi K (1993) Evaluation of ophthalmic suspension containing pilocarpine microcapsules: pharmacodynamic and pharmacokinetic studies. Inv Ophthalmol Vis Sci 34:1488
27. Freedman K, Klein J, Crosson C (1993) Betacyclodextrins enhance bioavailability of pilocarpine. Curr Eye Res 12:641-647
28. Jarho P, Urtti A, Järvinen T (1995) Hydroxypropyl-beta-cyclodextrin increases the aqueous solubility and stability of pilocarpine prodrugs. Pharmac Res 12:1371-1375
29. Boles Carenini B, Gremmo E, Brogliatti B, Gasco M (1989) Microemulsion and ion-pairs in topical administration of timolol. New Trends Ophthalmol 4:177-179
30. Gasco M, Gallarate M, Trotta M, Bauchiero L, Gremmo E, Chiappero O (1989) Microemulsions as topical delivery vehicles: ocular administration of timolol. J Pharm Biomed Analysis 7:433-439
31. Bar-Ilan A, Aviv H, Friedman D, Vered M, Belkin M, Amselem S, Baru H, Beilin M, Wellner E, Wolf Y, Shwarz J, Neumann R (1993) Improved performance of ocular drugs formulated in submicron emulsions. Inv Ophthalmol Vis Sci 34:1488
32. Stratford R, Yang D, Redell M, Lee V (1983) Effects of topically applied liposomes on disposition of epinephrine and insulin in the

albino rabbit eye. Int J Pharmaceutics 13:263-272
33. Fitzgerald P, Hadgraft J, Wilson C (1987) A gamma scintigraphic evaluation of the precorneal residence of liposomal formulations in the rabbit. J Pharm Pharmacol 39:487-490
34. Meisner D, Pringle J, Mezei M (1989) Liposomal ophthalmic drug delivery III. Pharmacodynamic and biodisposition studies of atropine. Int J Pharm 55:105-113
35. Greaves L, Wilson C, Rozier A, Grove J, Plazonnet B (1990) Scintigraphic assessment of an ophthalmic gelling vehicle in man and rabbit. Curr Eye Res 9:415-420
36. Levy N, Alsbury C (1993) Timolol-in-gelrite once daily in glaucoma. Inv Ophthalmol Vis Sci 34:927
37. Shedden A, Laibovitz A, Lepass R, Vogel R, Neafus R, Laurence J (1993) 24 hours diurnal variation of IOP following administration of Timoptic-Xetm(TXE)QD as compared to Timoptic (TS) bid. Inv Ophthalmol Vis Sci 34:927
38. Shedden A, Hommer A, Sharma D, Laurence J, Vogel R (1994) 3 month open label study of 0.25% timoptol-XE qd following 3 month double masked study of timoptol (TS) bid or timoptol-XE tm qd. Inv Ophthalmol Vis Sci 35:2176
39. Shedden A, Laurence J, Klotzbuecher C, Tipping R (1995) Multi-clinic studies of 0.25% timolol solution (Timoptol, TS) twice daily and 0.25% timolol gellan solution (Timoptol-XE,TXE) once daily. Abstr Int Symp on Exp & Clin Ocul Pharmacol & Pharmaceutics, Geneva 28/9-1/10, pp 56
40. Elena P, Polzer H, Khosravi E (1993) Bioequivalence between timolol maleate formulated in ophthalmic solution (Timoptol) and in a novel gel vehicle (T-gel). Inv Ophthalmol Vis Sci 34,4:1490
41. Laibovitz R (1995) Systemic pharmacokinetics of topical timolol maleate in a gellan gum formulation. Abstr Int Symp on Exp & Clin Ocul Pharmacol & Pharmaceutics, Geneva 28/9-1/10, pp 38
42. Rozier A, Chastaing G, Grove J, Plazonnet B (1995) Gelrite: a promising ophthalmic vehicle. Abstr Int Symp on Exp & Clin Ocul Pharmacol & Pharmaceutics, Geneva 28/9-1/10, pp 41
43. Studio Policentrico (Milano, Roma Cattolica, Roma Tor Vergata, Torino, Verona) (1995) Timololo in soluzione Gellan per la terapia dell'ipertono oculare. XI Riunione AISG, Rapallo 24/3-25/3
44. Chastaing G, Rozier A, Plazonnet B, Grove J (1995) Gelrite enhances the ocular penetration of pilocarpine in the pigment rabbit. Inv Ophthalmol Vis Sci 36:S159
45. Pfeiffer N (1992) New development in medicamentous treatment of glaucoma. Ophthal 89:W1-W13
46. Weinreb RN, Cadwell D, Goode S, Horwitz B, Laibovitz R, Shader C, Stewart R, Williams T (1990) A double-masked three-month comparison between 0.25% betaxolol suspension and 0.50% betaxolol ophthalmic solution. Am J Ophthalmol 110:189-193
47. Weinreb RN, Jani R (1992) A novel formulation of an ophthalmic beta-adrenoreceptor antagonist. J Parenter Sci Technol 46:51-53
48. Denis P, Demally P, Saraux IL (1993) Evaluation clinique du betaxolol en suspension ophtalmique avec ou sans conservateur chez des patients glaucomateux ou hypertones. J Fr Ophtalmol 16:297-303
49. Brogliatti B, Boles Carenini A, Protti R, Bolla N (1994) Confronto delle curve tensionali in pazienti affetti da POAG trattati con Betaxololo "S" vs. Betaxololo 0.5%. In: Drago F (ed) Farmacologia Oculare vol IV, Mediconsult, Catania, pp 385-391
50. Mastropasqua L, Ciancaglini M, Verdesca G, Carpineto P, Costagliola C, Gallenga P (1994) Betaxololo 0.25% sospensione vs betaxololo 0.50% soluzione: studio comparativo degli effetti sulla curva tonometrica giornaliera. In: Drago F (ed) Farmacologia Oculare vol IV, Mediconsult, Catania, pp 401-405
51. Jani R, Gan O, Ali Y, Rodstrom R, Hancock S (1994) Ion exchange resins for ophthalmic delivery. J Ocul Pharmacol 10:57-67
52. Harper D, Eto C, Lee P, PilaSite Study Group (1994) A 3-month study to compare the efficacy, safety, and acceptability of 2% Pilasite bid and 2% Pilocar qid. Inv Ophthalmol Vis Sci 35:2176
53. Camber O, Edmann P (1989) Sodium hyaluronate as an ophthalmic vehicle: some factors governing its effect on the ocular absorption of pilocarpine. 8:563-570
54. Saettone M, Monti D, Torracca M, Chetoni P, Giannaccini B (1989) Muco-adhesive liquid ophthalmic vehicles-evaluation of macromolecular ionic complexes of pilocarpine. Drug Dev & Indust Pharmacy 15:2475-2489
55. Ludwig A, Van Ooteghem M (1989) Evaluation of sodium hyaluronate of viscous vehicle for eye drops. J Pharm Belg 44:391-399
56. Mangiafico S, Spadaro A (1993) Ocular bioavailability of two new mucoadhesive topical drugs: pilocarpine hyaluronate, timolol hyaluronate. Inv Ophthalmol Vis Sci 34:1489
57. Uva MG, Panta G, Canino E, Cro M, Spadaro A, Reibaldi A (1995) A new mucoadhesive antiglaucoma association of timolol and pilocarpine, FISER C301. Abstr Int Symp on Exp & Clin Ocul Pharmacol & Pharmaceutics, Geneva 28/9-1/10, pp 31

58. Havener W (1978) Ocular Pharmacology. CV Mosby, St. Louis

59. Salminen L, Huupponen R (1989) Systemic effects of ocular drugs. Adv Drug React Acute Poisoning Rev 8:89-96

The Effect of Topical β-Blockers on Plasma Lipids and Lipoproteins

Y. Kitazawa[1], T. Yamamoto[1], A. Noma[2], T. Ido[3], and Y. Goto[4]

[1]Department of Ophthalmology, Gifu University School of Medicine, 40 Tsukasa-machi, Gifu-shi 500, Gifu, Japan
[2]Department of Laboratory Medicine, Gifu University School of Medicine, Gifu-shi 500, Gifu, Japan
[3]Department of Ophthalmology, Gifu Municipal Hospital, 7-1 Kashima-machi, Gifu-shi 500, Gifu, Japan
[4]Department of Ophthalmology, Gifu Prefectural Hospital, 4-6-1 Noisshiki, Gifu-shi 500, Gifu, Japan

Introduction

Topical adrenergic β–blockers are the drugs of choice for the treatment of glaucoma. However, they have systemic adverse effects, including increased airway resistance in the respiratory system, decreased pulse rate, and weakened myocardial contractility. In addition, oral β–blockers cause changes in plasma lipids and related compounds, including decreased high-density lipoprotein cholesterol (HDL-C), increased ratio of total cholesterol (TC) to HDL-C (TC/HDL-C), and increased triglyceride (TG). These changes in the plasma lipid profile are major risk factors for coronary heart disease and systemic atherosclerosis.

Several investigators have attempted to clarify the effects of topical β–blockers on the plasma lipid profile in normolipidemic normal volunteers, in subjects suspected of having glaucoma, and glaucoma patients. The results, however, have been conflicting: Coleman et al. and Freedman et al. reported that topical β–blockers unfavorably altered the lipid profile, but West and Longstaff found no significant changes [1-3].

In their studies Coleman and West and Longstaff used timolol and obtained conflicting results [1-3]. Freedman evaluated the effects of timolol and carteolol [2]. Although timolol and carteolol are nonselective β–blockers, carteolol possesses intrinsic sympathomimetic activity (ISA) and acts as a partial agonist; in contrast timolol does not possess ISA. There is some evidence that β–blockers with ISA affect the plasma lipid profile differently than those without ISA [4].

We conducted a prospective, randomized study to compare the effects of timolol and carteolol on plasma lipids and lipoproteins. The aim of the present report is to briefly summarize the results of the study and the practical implications of our results.

Materials and Methods

A prospective study involving three centers and patients with primary open angle glaucoma (POAG) or ocular hypertension (OHT) was carried out. Exclusion criteria included history of hyperlipidemia, use of drugs that could affect plasma lipid levels, history of β–blocker administration, abnormal plasma lipids level, and contraindications for β–blockers.

A total of 36 patients with either POAG or OHT were randomly allocated to bilateral therapy with 0.5% timolol, 1% carteolol, or 2% carteolol twice daily for 16 weeks.

The enrolled patients were treated and followed up prospectively at three medical centers. Twelve hour fasting venous blood samples were drawn at about 9:00 a.m. three times before β–blocker therapy was initiated and every 4 weeks during the 16 week treatment period. The blood samples were centrifuged for 15 min at 2500 rpm. Plasma lipids and lipoproteins–including TC, HDL-C, TG, lecithin-cholesterol acyl transferase (LCAT), and apoproteins A-I, A-II, B, C-II C-III, and E–were measured at the Department of Laboratory Medicine, Gifu University School of Medicine.

Intraocular pressure (IOP) was measured by a Goldmann applanation tonometer, and perimetry using the central 30-2 program of the Humphrey Field Analyzer was done prior to and following the 16 week administration.

Results

Of the 36 patients enrolled, one dropped out because of systemic discomfort of unknown origin, and two because they were unable to visit the clinic regularly. Thus, 33 (92%) of the patients originally enrolled in the study completed the entire treatment schedule.

Twelve were treated with 0.5% timolol, nine with 1% carteolol, and 12 with 2% carteolol. The pretreatment lipid levels and demographics of the three groups were basically the same.

The changes over time in plasma lipoproteins are summarized in Table 1.

Changes in HDL-C and the ratio of (TC-HDL-C) to HDL-C changes were significantly associated with use of 0.5% timolol ($p = 0.002$ and 0.022, respectively by repeated ANOVA: Fisher's protected least significant difference). The changes indicate an increased risk for coronary diseases.

The changes were not significantly associated with use of either 1% or 2% carteolol (repeated ANOVA), although the ratio of (TC-HDL-C) to HDL-C was significantly decreased at 8 weeks, as compared with the baseline value in the 1% carteolol group by the Wilcoxon signed-rank test. Changes in TG were not significantly associated with use of any β–blockers.

LCAT values did not change during the treatment period, with the exception of a significant decrease (although still within normal limits) following 16 weeks of treatment with 1% carteolol. However, the LCAT value for apoprotein A-I decreased in the 1% carteolol group at 4, 8, and 16 weeks after treatment ($p < 0.05$, Wilcoxon signed-rank test). Apoprotein C-II increased in the 0.5% timolol group after 16 weeks ($p < 0.05$, Wilcoxon signed-rank test). Apoproteins A-II, B, C-III, and E did not change during the study period.

Pulse rate significantly decreased in the 0.5% timolol treatment group, and systolic blood pressure significantly decreased in the 1% carteolol treatment group. IOP significantly decreased in the three treatment groups. There were no significant changes in visual acuity or visual field.

Discussion

The present study shows that topical β–blockers, particularly timolol, adversely affect the plasma lipid profile in normolipidemic Japanese glaucoma patients. HDL-C decreased and the ratio of (TC-HDL-C) to HDL-C increased following 16 weeks of topical β–blocker therapy. Plasma lipid profile changes reported previously and those found in the present study are summarized in Table 2.

Our results are consistent with those of Coleman and associates [1] and Freedman and associates [2], but not with those of West and Longstaff [3]. It is difficult to satisfactorily explain this discrepancy. However, considering our results together with previous ones, it seems likely that even short-term (i.e., 8/16 weeks) use of a topical β–blocker may alter the plasma lipid profile in Japanese glaucoma patients in the same way that it does in Western glaucoma patients. More importantly, the changes are ones that increase the risk of coronary heart disease, namely, a decrease of HDL-C and an increases of the ratio of (TC-HDL-C) to HDL-C.

It may be that the differential effect of these two nonselective β–blockers on HDL-C results

Table 1. Changes in lipids and lecithin-cholesterol acyltransferase

	0.5% Timolol		1.0% Carteolol		2.0% Carteolol´	
	Baseline mean	16 weeks	Baseline mean	16 weeks	Baseline mean	16 weeks
HDL-C	54.5±3.8	51.5±3.7	52.1±3.7	54.4±4.7	49.6±3.7	48.5±4.9
(TC-HDL-C)/HDL-C	3.0±0.2	3.3±0.4	3.2±0.3	2.9±0.4	3.2±0.4	3.4±0.4
TC	92.8±6.6	108.3±8.4	91.0±12.3	101.3±13.2	121.6±17.9	124.9±31.5
LCAT	719.8±73.4	646.2±84.5	754.4±32.9	542.9±66.2	654.8±42.2	565.8±69.9

HDL-C, high-density lipoprotein cholesterol; (TC-HDL-C)/HDL-C: ratio of total cholesterol minus high-density lipoprotein cholesterol to high-density lipoprotein cholesterol; TC, total cholesterol; LCAT, lecithin-cholesterol acyl transferase.

Values are mean ± standard error (nmole/ml/h for LCAT; mg/dl for others).

Table 2. Summary of plasma lipid changes caused by topical β-blockers

Authors Treatment duration	Coleman et al. 11 weeks (mean)	Freedman et al. 8 weeks		West and Longstaff 15 weeks	Present study 16 weeks		
Type of ß-blocker	0.5%T	0.5%T	1.0%C	0.5%T	0.5%T	1.0%C	2.0%C
Percent change in							
HDL-C	-9	-8.0	-3.3	-4.1	-4.8	4.3	-3.3
TC/HDL-C [a]	8	10.0	4.0	No data	13.8	-12.8	4.8
TG	12	7.1	6.0	7.3	19.2	14.3	6.5

HDL-C, high-density lipoprotein cholesterol; TC, total cholesterol; TG, triglyceride; T, timolol; C, carteolol.
[a] (TC - HDL-C)/HDL-C for the present study.

from the fact that carteolol possesses ISA and timolol does not. In fact, oral β–blockers with ISA affect plasma lipids unfavorably, but less than those without it [4].

One possible mechanism by which β–blockers decrease HDL-C is by decreasing LCAT activity, thereby decreasing the level of HDL-C However, in the present study, we were unable to demonstrate deceased LCAT activity, especially in the timolol-treated patients, in whom significant decreases in HDL-C were found. Thus, it seems unlikely that the differential effect of the two β–blockers is mediated by changes in LCAT activity.

Another possible mechanism is decreased activity of lipoprotein lipase (LPL) present in capillary endothelium caused by the constriction of peripheral vessels induced by β–blockers. Since LPL mediates hydrolysis of TG-rich lipoproteins and increases high-density lipoproteins, decreased activity of the enzyme may decrease the level of HDL-C. ISA may play a role in counteracting the vasoconstrictive effect of β–blockers, and therefore carteolol may have a lesser effect on HDL-C.

A third possible explanation is that, because HDL-C and cholesterol ester transfer protein are closely related, the changes in protein induced by β–blockers decrease HDL-C.

The degree of alteration in plasma lipids caused by β–blockers may not be large enough to warrant advising individual glaucoma patients to discontinue their use because of the increased risk of coronary heart diseases they may pose. However, since the prevalence of glaucoma or ocular hypertension is estimated to be 4.93% in Japan [5], changes in the lipid profile induced by topical β–blockers may have significant adverse effects on the population of Japanese glaucoma patients as a whole.

Timolol is metabolized by the hepatic cytochrome P-450 enzyme CYPD6, which is polymorphically distributed in the population. Interethnic differences in the distribution of CYPD6 results in less than 1% of Japanese and Chinese individuals being of the poor metabolizer phenotype [6]. In contrast, about 8% of the US white population lacks normally active CYP2D6 [5]. Hence, any systemic effect of timolol observed in the Japanese population must occur more often in the white population. However, CYPD6 plays a lesser role in metabolizing carteolol in the liver and about 70% of carteolol is excreted unchanged in the urine [6]; about 30% of carteolol is metabolized mainly in the liver [6]. Hence, the observed difference in the effect on lipid metabolism may be more distinct in the white population than in Japanese.

References

1. Coleman AL, Diehl DLC, Jampel HD et al. (1990) Topical timolol decreases plasma high-density lipoprotein cholesterol level. Arch Ophthalmol 108:1260-1263
2. Freedman SF, Freedman NJ, Shields MB et al. (1993) Effects of ocular carteolol and timolol on plasma high-density lipoprotein cholesterol level. Am J Ophthalmol 116:600-611
3. West J, Longstaff S (1990) Topical timolol and serum lipoproteins. Br J Ophthalmol 74:663-664
4. Van Brummelen P (1983) The relevance of intrinsic sympathomimetic activity for β-blocker-induced changes in plasma lipids. J Cardiovascular Pharmacol 5:s51-55
5. Shiose Y, Kitazawa Y, Tsukahara S et al. (1991) Epidemiology of glaucoma. A nationwide glaucoma survey. Jpn J Ophthalmol 35:133-155
6. Edeki T, He H, Wood JJ (1995) Pharmacological explanation for excessive, β-blockade following timolol eye drops. JAMA 27:1611-1618

The Effect of Anti-Glaucoma Medication on Ocular Blood Flow

C. Migdal

The Western Eye Hospital, Marylebone Road, London W1P 5LP, UK

Introduction

The pathogenesis of optic nerve damage in glaucoma is attributed to a combination of mechanical and vascular factors [1-3], with intraocular pressure (IOP) also playing a major role. The part played by each of these may vary according to the type of glaucoma (i.e., primary open-angle glaucoma or normal tension glaucoma). The efficacy of any anti-glaucoma medication will obviously be enhanced if it favourably influences the above, i.e., not only reducing IOP, but also improving perfusion of the optic nerve head.

The anatomy of the blood supply of the retrolaminar portion of the optic nerve head has been well described [4]. Measurement of blood flow in this region is, however, difficult due to poor visualisation of what are essentially very small vessels, which in addition have a fair amount of anatomical variability. There are limitations to the currently available techniques used to measure retrolaminar optic nerve head blood supply [5].

Patients with raised IOP due to primary open angle glaucoma have reduced ophthalmic artery blood flow velocity [6, 7] and reduced macular blood cell velocity proportional to disease severity [8]. Following surgical treatment of open angle glaucoma, central retinal artery and posterior ciliary artery flow velocities increase, probably related to the IOP lowering [9]. In normal tension glaucoma, patients have been shown to have an age-related increase in ophthalmic artery resistance [10]. Patients with glaucoma have also been found to have reduced blood flow velocity in the optic nerve head capillaries as measured by laser Doppler velocimetry, and increased erythrocyte aggregability [11].

Blood Flow Alterations with Therapy

Both α and β adrenergic receptors are present in the eye. This is of therapeutic use in glaucoma because of the effect of adrenergic stimulation or blockade in IOP. ß-Blockers and sympathomimetics may effect blood flow by producing an imbalance between the influence of the α and β receptors on the ocular vasculature. However, it is often difficult to determine whether these effects on measurements relevant to ocular blood flow are beneficial or harmful to the eye, the interpretation of results being confounded by effects of these agents on systemic blood pressure, IOP and the untreated fellow eye [5].

Vasoconstriction may be produced by both sympathomimetics and β-blockers, such as in the ciliary body following administration of topical phenylephrine, timolol and betaxolol in rabbit eyes [12]. In humans, vasoconstriction of the retinal arterioles was detected with timolol [13], which may be due to the compensatory autoregulatory effect resulting upon the increased perfusion pressure caused by the lowering of the IOP. Other β-blocker studies have detected no changes in blood flow, such as in the cross-over study comparing timolol, betaxolol and levobunolol [14], while timolol was found to have no effect on blood flow in rabbit eyes [15] or on pulsatile ocular blood flow [16, 17].

Studies using laser Doppler velocimetry have shown that carteolol (a β-blocker with intrinsic sympathomimetic activity) has no effect on retinal blood flow [18], although both timolol [19] and betaxolol [20] increase the retinal blood flow. However, with colour Doppler imaging, timolol had no effect on blood velocities in the ophthalmic or central retinal arteries, but did produce a reduction in the mean resistive indices [21].

Pilocarpine, with its parasympathomimetic action, has no direct effect on pulsatile ocular blood flow (POBF) [22]. Studies on the POBF following treatment with β-blockers vary. In one study, timolol did not alter POBF [17], while in another, levobunolol had a similar effect on both normal and glaucoma patients, decreasing IOP by about 30% and increasing POBF by about 12% [23]. In the same study, the pulse volume amplitude increased with levobunolol by 42% in normals, but was unchanged in glaucomatous eyes. POBF has been found to decrease in timolol-treated eyes over a 1 year period, but was stable in betaxolol-treated eyes [24].

When the IOP is lowered by topical hypotensive therapy, vasoconstriction may occur to compensate for the resultant increased perfusion pressure, thereby stabilising the blood flow. Changes in perfusion pressure may not always be detected [25]. No change in retinal or ciliary perfusion pressures were found with timolol, betaxolol, pilocarpine or acetazolamide [26]. Acetazolamide used systemically both reduces IOP and has been shown by laser Doppler velocimetry to cause vasodilatation and to increase retinal blood flow [27]. This effect may be mediated via local alterations of the partial pressure of carbonic dioxide. The effects on the ocular circulation of endothelin-1 and nitric oxide, which are derived from vascular endothelium and cause, respectively, vasoconstriction and vasodilatation, is an exciting area of research [28, 29]. The relationship of antiglaucoma drugs to these factors remains to be seen.

Systemic Factors

Nocturnal arterial hypotension may play a role in the pathogenesis of optic neuropathies (including glaucoma), by reducing optic nerve head blood supply below the critical level [30]. β-blockers used in systemic hypertension reduce IOP but may also exacerbate nocturnal hypotension, causing further damage to the optic nerve.

The systemic effects of topical therapy may be minimised by using a selective agent such as betaxolol that predominantly blocks β-1 receptors, sparing the β-2 receptors responsible for many side effects. On the downside, the reduction in IOP achieved with ß-1 selective β-blockers is not as great as that achieved with the nonselective β-blockers.

Further research will determine the effect on ocular blood flow of the newer ocular hypotensive agents, such as the prostaglandins (e.g., latanoprost), topical carbonic anhydrase inhibitors (e.g., dorzolamide), and the α agonists (e.g., brimonidine).

Conclusion

Many studies have investigated the effects of anti-glaucoma drugs on ocular blood flow. However, the clinical relevance of the findings is, as yet, unclear, especially as regard topical β-blockers. The methodology of each study must be carefully examined before the conclusions are accepted, or, indeed, a comparison made with other studies.

References

1. Quigley HA, Addicks EM (1981) Regional differences in the structure of the lamina cribrosa and their relationship to optic nerve damage. Arch Ophthalmol 99:137-143
2. Quigley HA, Addicks EM, Green WR, Maumenee AE (1981) Optic nerve damage in human glaucoma II. The site of injury and susceptibility to damage. Arch Ophthalmol 99:635-649
3. Quigley HA, Holman RM, Addicks EM (1984) Blood vessels of the glaucomatous optic disk in experimental primate and human eyes. Invest Ophthalmol Vis Sci 25:918-931
4. Hayreh SS (1989) Blood supply of the optic nerve head in health and disease. In: Lambrou GN, Greve EL (eds) Ocular blood flow in glaucoma. Kugler and Ghedini, Amsterdam, pp 3-48
5. Williamson TH, Harris A (1994) Ocular blood flow measurement. Br J Ophthalmol 78:939-945
6. Rojanapongpun P, Drance SM, Morrison BJ

(1993) Ophthalmic artery flow velocity in glaucomatous and normal subjects. Br J Ophthalmol 77:25-29
7. Michelson G, Groh MJ, Groh ME, Grundler A (1995) Advanced primary open angle glaucoma is associated with decreased ophthalmic artery blood flow velocity. German J Ophthalmol 4:21-24
8. Sponsel WE, De Paul KL, Kaufman PL (1990) Correlation of visual function and retinal leukocyte velocity in glaucoma. Am J Ophthalmol 109:49-54
9. Trible JR, Sergott RC, Spaeth GL, Wilson RP, Katz LJ, Moster MR, Schmidt CM (1994) Trabeculectomy is associated with retrobulbar hemodynamic changes. A color Doppler analysis. Ophthalmology 101:340-351
10. Butt Z, McKillop G, O'Brien C, Allan P, Aspinall P (1995) Measurement of ocular blood flow velocity using colour Doppler imaging in low tension glaucoma. Eye 9:29-33
11. Hamard P, Hamard H, Dufaux J, Quesnot S (1994) Optic nerve head blood flow using a laser Doppler velocimeter and haemorheology in primary open angle glaucoma and normal tension glaucoma. Br J Ophthalmol 78:449-453
12. Van Buskirk EM, Bacon DR, Fahrenbach WH (1990) Ciliary vasoconstriction after topical adrenergic drugs. Am J Ophthalmol 109:511-517
13. Martin XD, Rabineau PA (1989) Vasoconstrictive effect of topical timolol on human retinal arteries. Graefes Arch Clin Exp Ophthalmol 227:526-530
14. Harris A, Shoemaker JA, Burgoyne J, Weinland M, Cantor LB (1995) The acute effect of topical beta-adrenergic antagonist on normal perimacular haemodynamics. J Glaucoma 4:36-40
15. Green K, Hatchett TL (1987) Regional ocular blood flow after chronic topical glaucoma drug treatment. Acta Ophthalmol 65:503-506
16. Pillunat LE, Stodtmeister R, Wilmanns I, Metzner D (1986) Effect of timolol on optic nerve head autoregulation. Ophthalmologica 193:146-153
17. Trew DR, Smith SE (1991) Postural studies on pulsatile ocular blood flow: II Chronic open angle glaucoma. Br J Ophthalmol 75:71-75
18. Grunwald JE, Delahanty J (1992) Effect of topical carteolol on the normal human retinal circulation. Invest Ophthalmol Vis Sci 33:1853-1856
19. Grunwald JE (1990) Effect of timolol maleate on the retinal circulation of human eyes with ocular hypertension. Invest Ophthalmol Vis Sci 31:521-526
20. Gupta A, Chen HC, Rassam SM, Kohner EM (1994) Effect of betaxolol on the retinal circulation in eyes with ocular hypertension: a pilot study. Eye 8:668-71
21. Baxter GM, Williamson TH, Mc Killop G, Dutton GN (1992) Color Doppler ultrasound of orbital and optic nerve blood flow: effects of posture and timolol 0.5%. Invest Ophthalmol Vis Sci 33:604-10
22. Claridge KG (1993) The effect of topical pilocarpine on pulsatile ocular blood flow. Eye 7:507- 510
23. Bosem ME, Lusky M, Weinreb RN (1992) Short-term effects of levobunolol on ocular pulsatile flow. Am J Ophthalmol 114:280-286
24. Boles Carenini A, Sibour G, Boles Carenini B (1994) Differences in the long-term effect of timolol and betaxolol on the pulsatile ocular blood flow. Surv Ophthalmol 38:S118-124
25. Grunwald JE, Furubayashi C (1989) Effect of timolol maleate on the ophthalmic artery blood pressure. Invest Ophthalmol Vis Sci 30:1095-1100
26. Pillunat LE, Stodtmeister R (1988) Effect of different antiglaucomatous drugs on ocular perfusion pressures. J Ocular Pharmacol 4:231-242
27. Rassam SMB, Patel V, Kohner EM (1993) The effect of acetazolamide on the retinal circulation. Eye 7:697-702
28. Granstam E, Wang L, Bill A (1992) Ocular effects of endothelin-1 in the cat. Curr Eye Res 11:325-332
29. Granstam E, Wang L, Bill A (1993) Vascular effects of endothelin-1 in the cat; modification by indomethacin and L-NAME. Acta Physiol Scand 148:165-176
30. Hayreh SS, Zimmerman MB, Podhajsky P, Alward WL (1994) Nocturnal arterial hypotension and its role in optic nerve head and ocular ischemic disorders. Am J Ophthalmol 117:603-624

Ocular Vasospasm and Calcium Channel Blockers in Glaucoma

L. E. Pillunat[1], G. B. Kuba[2] and A. Harris[3]

[1]University Eye Hospital and Clinic Hamburg, Martinistrasse 22, 20246 Hamburg, Germany
[2]University Eye Hospital and Clinic Ulm, Prittwitzstrasse 43, 89075 Ulm, Germany
[3]Department of Ophthalmology, Indiana University, Indianapolis, IN, USA

Introduction

An increased intraocular pressure (IOP) has to be regarded as one of the most important risk factors in the pathogenesis of glaucomatous optic nerve damage; but beside an increased IOP other factors have to be involved. Already in 1862, von Graefe [28] observed a glaucomatous cupping of the optic nerve without any elevation in IOP, and Magitot (1908) put forward the theory that glaucomatous optic nerve damage has a vascular origin [37]. Since then it has become more and more obvious that vascular factors are of pathogenic importance, at least in some types of glaucoma, i. e., normal pressure glaucoma.

Vasospasm in Glaucoma

In 1985 Phelps and Corbett [45] observed an increased incidence of migraine and headaches in patients suffering from normal pressure glaucoma compared to age matched controls. They found that 47% of their normal pressure glaucoma patients suffered from migraine. Migraine, however, is often associated with other vasospastic diseases such as Prinzmetal angina and Raynaud's disease. Based on these findings it was obvious that a vasospastic disorder may be of pathogenic importance in some glaucoma patients and has to be regarded as one pathogenic vascular factor. Since Phelps' findings, many authors, using different methodes, have proved this theory. Flammer and coworkers were the first to investigate vasospastic disorders systematically and were able to correlate peripheral vasospasm to ocular findings in normal pressure glaucoma [13-22].

In 1986, Gasser described an ocular vasospastic syndrome in which patients with unexplained scotomas had abnormal capillaroscopic responses to cold in the nailfold of the finger. These findings in some of these patients resembled findings in patients suffering from normal pressure glaucoma. Many of these patients also had a history of cold hands and their visual field deteriorated by the immersion of one hand in cold water [15, 19]. In another study Guthauser, Flammer and Mahler found a statistically significant association between the capillaroscopic cold response and a history of cold hands and feet. The history of cold hands and feet was also related to the visual field change produced by the immersion of the hand in cold water. Additionally, the visual field deterioration was correlated with the abnormal digital response to cold in capillaroscopy [25].

In 1991 Gasser and Flammer showed that patients suffering from normal pressure glaucoma had a more pronounced and statistically significant decrease in the nailfold capillary blood cell velocity than found in high pressure glaucoma patients and controls. The most striking finding, however, was the difference in nailfold blood flow standstill after immersing one hand in cold water. In this respect, patients with high tension glaucoma and control subjects were essentially the same. The patients with normal pressure glaucoma, however, showed a clear and significantly higher occurrence of blood flow standstill [21].

Drance and coworkers [10] measured finger tip blood flow by laser-Doppler flowmetry in healthy volunteers, in subjects suffering from classical migraine headache, in normal pressure glaucoma patients and in normal pressure glaucoma patients additionally suffering from migraine. After immersion in warm water, control subjects with migraine showed a significantly greater flow than those without migraine. The mean baseline flow and the flow after cold exposure were found to be significantly lower in normal pressure glaucoma patients than in controls.

The results showed that 26% of healthy subjects without migraine showed a vasospastic response, and in subjects with migraine 64% reacted in this manner. In normal pressure glaucoma patients with and without classical migraine a vasospastic response was found in approximately 65%.

In a similar study, Usui and Iwata [62] measured finger blood flow by means of laser Doppler flowmetry in controls, normal pressure glaucoma and primary open angle glaucoma patients. In this study a vasospastic response to cold was found in 25% of patients suffering from normal pressure glaucoma, in 17% of the primary open-angle glaucoma patients and in 25% of the controls. There was no overall difference between the groups examined.

Pillunat and coworkers [47, 50, 51] showed a significant increase of ocular pulse amplitudes, after applying increasing carbon dioxide concentrations, in some normal pressure glaucoma patients compared to healthy controls. In these patients the visual field significantly improved during inspiration of increased carbon dioxide concentrations. An increased carbon dioxide reactivity in some normal pressure glaucoma patients, i.e., a significant increase of ocular pulse amplitude and a significant improvement of the central visual field during exposure to increased inspiratory carbon dioxide concentrations, may be due to an initial ocular vasospasm in these patients which can be released by induced vasodilation due to carbon dioxide exposure.

In a similarly designed study, Harris and coworkers [29] measured ocular and retrobulbar hemodynamics in normal pressure glaucoma patients by means of colour Doppler imaging. Compared with controls, normal pressure glaucoma patients had significantly lower end-diastolic velocities and higher resistance indices in the ophthalmic artery at baseline. Applying the very potent vasodilator carbon dioxide resulted in no change in controls, whereas it increased end-diastolic velocity in patients and abolished the difference in resistance index between the two groups.

Morphological evidence of ocular vasospasm was found by Rader and Anderson [55]. In a masked analysis of optic disc photographs they found a peripapillary vasoconstriction of retinal vessels in 48% of patients with severe normal pressure glaucoma, in 40% of patients with moderate normal pressure glaucoma, in approximately 40% of patients suffering from primary open-angle glaucoma, but only in 3% - 4% in controls and ocular hypertensives. These findings suggest that in about 40% - 50% of glaucoma patients there is some morphological evidence of ocular vasospasm and that no difference exists between primary open angle glaucoma and normal pressure glaucoma.

In 1992, Pillunat and coworkers [50] showed similar results. During exposure to the potent cerebral vasodilator carbon dioxide the central visual field improved in approximately 30% of patients suffering from normal pressure glaucoma but also in approximately 15% suffering from primary open angle glaucoma. These results suggest that a reversible ocular vasospasm might be also of pathogenic importance in some patients with primary open angle glaucoma with increased IOP and not only in normal pressure glaucoma patients.

Vasospastic Syndrome-Vasospasm

Functional vasospasm is defined as a reversible constriction of the vascular smooth muscle cells without any anatomical alterations. The cause of the vasospastic syndrome is not yet known but it might be the result of more than one mechanism. As already mentioned, it might be caused by exposure to cold, by emotions or by vasoconstrictive agents like caffeine or nicotine and can be released by vasodilators like carbon dioxide or heat. Women are more often affected than men and the patients tend to be younger than other glaucoma patients. Vasospasm can be local or more or less generalized. Such spasms can occur in individuals with arteriosclerotic vessels as well as in otherwise healthy subjects [11]. Anderson [2] describes a close link between the occurrence of an ocular vasospasm and a deficient autoregulation of optic nerve circulation. As shown in

different experimental studies [12, 46, 48, 56, 64, 65], there is some evidence that the vessels of the optic nerve head, as in some other tissues of the body, demonstrate autoregulation.
Vascular autoregulation is defined as the ability of a circulatory system to maintain local blood flow relatively constant in the face of a changing perfusion pressure [58]. A deficient autoregulation, however, might occur when some of the autoregulatory capacity has already been used up. Furthermore it might happen when the vessels are under the influence of a vasoconstricting agent or when there is a hyperconstrictive state such as occurs in vasospastic syndrome. The vessels are unable to dilate fully when the circulation is challenged. Such a challenge to the circulation is an elevation of IOP which reduces ocular perfusion pressures. In this case optic nerve vessels dilate to maintain local blood flow, but in patients suffering from ocular vasospasm these vessels are not able to dilate because they are under the influence of a vasoconstrictive factor. Therefore an elevation of IOP becomes harmful whereas it is not harmful in the absence of a vasoconstrictive influence.
From a mechanistic point of view, an increased blood pressure should protect the optic nerve from the influence of increased IOP. Anderson [59, 60] showed, however, that the optic nerve was much more sensitive to increased IOPs after elevation of arterial blood pressure induced by angiotensin. These results were explained by a diffusion of the vasoconstrictive agent angiotensin from the chorioid to the optic nerve. Anything that leakes out of the chorioid can leak into the disc but not into the retina and may cause a spasm of the vessels so that they cannot relax. This kind of spasm induced by a vasoconstrictive agent causes a lack of autoregulation and might be interpreted as some kind of local vasospasm.
Regarding the vascular concept of glaucomatous optic nerve damage and especially presumed ocular vasospasm or deficient autoregulation, factors derived from the vascular endothelium may be of pathogenic importance, either due to an excess of vasoconstrictive factors or a lack of vasodilators.
Endothelin, a peptide produced by the endothelial cells and a potent vasoconstrictor, was found to be elevated in vasospastic diseases and in some normal pressure glaucoma patients [33].
Nitric oxide, which was previously known as "endothelium derived relaxing factor", has recently been identified in the vascular endothelium where it promotes vasodilation [5, 7]. Glutamate causes calcium to enter the postsynaptic cell and nitric oxide to be synthesized there. Once inside the cell, calcium activates the enzyme nitric oxide synthase, which generates nitric oxide from *L*-arginine [36]. Therefore an excess of endothelin or a lack of nitric oxide may play a pathogenic role in ocular vasospam [61].

Calcium Channel Blockers

By acting on vascular smooth muscle cells, calcium channel blockers can lead to vasodilation or relief from vasospasm. Furthermore calcium channel blockers may also act, in part, by reducing intracellular calcium levels, by altering the metabolism of target nerve cells, or by acting on receptors. Elevation of intracellular calcium is likely to be neurotoxic for a number of reasons, including activation of catabolic enzymes, phospholipases, superoxide or other free radicals, protein kinases, and positive feedback stimulation of the release of additional glutamate (see nitric oxide).
There are two main types of calcium channels, i.e., voltage-operated channels, requiring membrane depolarization for functioning, and receptor operated channels, requiring a specific ligand, such as NMDA (*N*-methyl-*D*-aspartate), to bind a receptor molecule. Within the class of voltage operated channels, there are four main types of channels [3, 43, 9]: T-type, L-type, N-type and P-type. Only the L-channels, however, seem to be sensitive to organic calcium antagonists [38]. Each of these channel types can also function in at least three different modes. Mode 0 refers to the state in which the channel is unavailable for calcium flux. In mode 1 there is a flickering type of activity in which the channels seem open and shut rapidly. Mode 2 demonstrates a long period of opening [31].
There are four major groups of calcium channel blockers currently available [23]:

1. Dihydropyridines: nifedipine, nimodipine, nisoldipine and felodipine
2. Phenylalkylamines or papaverine derivates such as verapamil

3. Benzothiazepine derivatives such as diltiazem
4. Miscellaneous drugs: bepridil, piperazine derivates, chlorpromazine, phenytoin.

A special characteristic of calcium channel blockers is their tissue selectivity. The cardiovascular system in general is sensitive to these drugs but there exist different affinities. The dihydropyridines act preferentially on the vascular network causing vasodilation at doses which have no effect on heart rate or cardiac contractility. Within the vascular system itself some dihydropyridine based calcium channel blockers act preferentially on coronary vessels (nisoldipine) whereas nimodipine acts preferentially on cerebral vessels. The benzothiazepine diltiazem acts preferentially on the coronary vessels, and verapamil, a phenylalkylamine, is more selective for the Av node.

Calcium Channel Blockers in Glaucoma

Nimodipine

Nimodipine represents a centrally acting calcium channel blocker of the dihydropyridine group. It is mainly used in neurology and neurosurgery for the treatment of acute and chronic ischemic cerebrovascular damage. Nyborg [42] showed in animal experiments that nimodipine relaxes preconstricted bovine ciliary arteries significantly more than nifedipine and nimodipine crosses the blood-brain barrier much easier than nifedipine. In experimental studies the local cerebral blood flow, profoundly reduced after middle cerebral artery occlusion, was increased in animals treated with nimodipine [27]. Gelmers [26] and coworkers showed, in 1988, that nimodipine improves the functional recovery after ischemic stroke compared to placebo, and Bergener (1992) reported significant improvements after nimodipine treatment in senile dementia.

In 1990 Virno [63] and coworkers examined the influence of nimodipine on the visual field and retinal sensitivity in 18 patients suffering from primary open angle glaucoma. After a therapy with 60 mg nimodipine daily for 30 days, 45% of the eyes examined showed an improvement in visual function, 30% did not change and 24% of the eyes examined demonstrated a reduction of retinal sensitivity. The results suggest that in some patients suffering from primary open angle glaucoma, a therapy with calcium channel blockers might be beneficial.

Bose and coworkers [6] administered 60 mg nimodipine acutely, in a placebo controlled double-masked study, to healthy volunteers and to normal pressure glaucoma patients. Some 90 min after application of the drug spatial contrast sensitivity improved significantly in nimodipine treated subjects compared to the placebo group. The effect of nimodipine was observed in normal pressure glaucoma patients as well as in healthy volunteers, however, it was more pronounced in normal pressure glaucoma patients.

In another similarly designed study, Piltz and Bose [54] studied the effect of nimodipine on the central visual field, contrast sensitivity and on macular blood flow using the bluefield entoptic phenomenon. When corrected for performance, nimodipine improved overall visual function, while having little effect on localized scotomas and macular blood flow in normal pressure glaucoma patients and controls.

Pillunat [52] had shown that about 30% of normal pressure glaucoma patients had a significant increase of ocular pulse volumes and a significant improvement of their central visual field during breathing of increased carbon dioxide concentrations as a potent cerebral vasodilator. After 8 months of nimodipine therapy (60 mg daily) the visual field improved in those patients who also demonstrated a positive carbon dioxide reactivity. Those results suggest that an improvement in ocular pulse volumes and central visual field during carbon dioxide exposure can help identify those subjects in whom nimodipine therapy will improve visual function (Fig. 1A-C).

In a recent study 60 mg nimodipine was applied acutely to 16 healthy volunteers [53]. There was a significant improvement of contrast sensitivity but no change in capillary optic nerve head blood flow as measured by laser Doppler flowmetry according to Riva. These results suggest that an improvement in visual function after application of nimodipine at least in healthy volunteers, is not due to an improvement in optic nerve head blood flow and might be due to a change in retinal blood flow or a direct neuronal action (Fig. 2). These conclusions go along with the Doppler - sonographic findings of Michelson, who found an

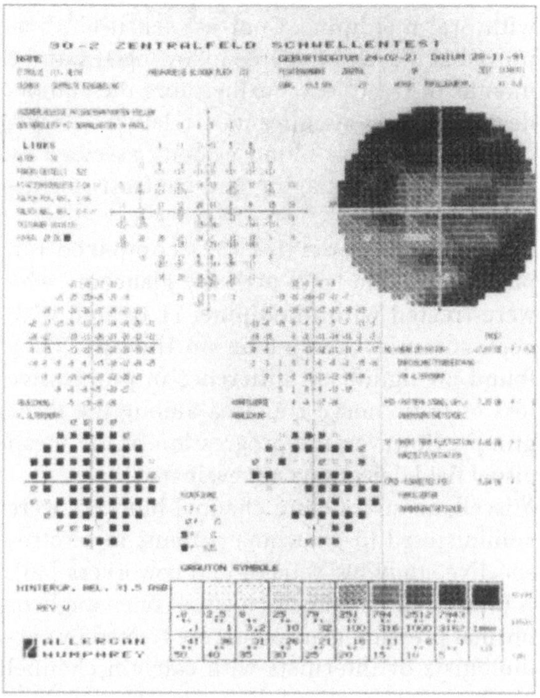

A

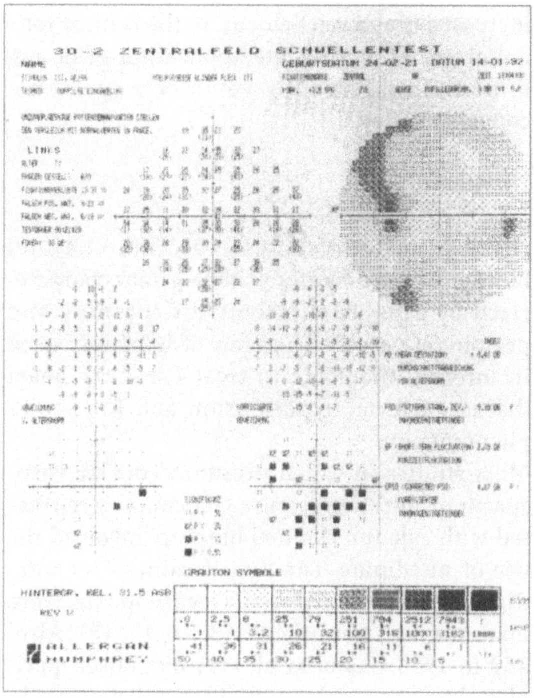

B

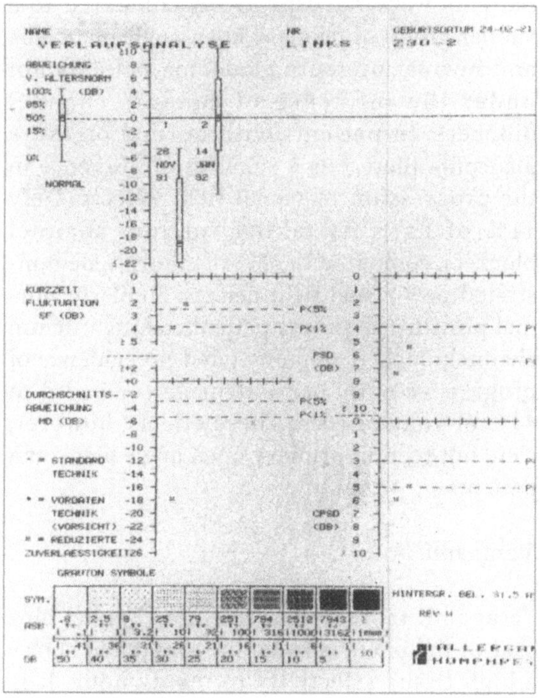

C

Fig. 1A-C. Central visual fields (Humphrey field analyzer, program 30-2) of a 70 year old woman suffering from normal pressure glaucoma and vasospastic symptoms. **A** Baseline central visual field. Mean deviation -17.9 dB; pattern standard deviation 7.3 dB, corrected pattern standard deviation 5.9 dB. **B** Central visual field after 3 month of nimodipine therapy with 3 x 30 mg/daily. Mean deviation -0.41 dB, pattern standard deviation 5.8 dB, corrected pattern standard deviation 4.87 dB. **C** Statistical comparison (Statpac program) of the baseline visual field and the visual field after nimodipine therapy

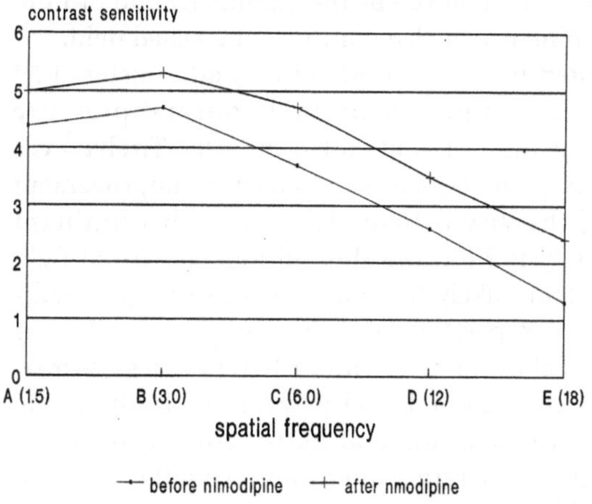

Fig. 2. Contrast sensitivity before and after an acute application of 60 mg nimodipine in 16 healthy volunteers

increased blood cell velocity in the central retinal artery after an acute application of 60 mg nimodipine in healthy volunteers (personal communication).

Nifedipine

Nifedipine represents a calcium channel blocker of the dihydropyridine group characterized by a tissue selectivity for coronary and peripheral vessels. Therefore it is mainly used in internal medicine to treat coronary heart disease, arterial hypertension and Raynaud's phenomenon.

Most studies in which presumed ocular vasospasm or normal pressure glaucoma were treated with calcium channel blockers involved the use of nifedipine. The first to administer nifedipine in presumed ocular vasospasm were Flammer and coworkers [13, 14, 17, 18]. Already in 1986 Gasser et al. [19] diagnosed peripheral vasospasm by nailfold capillaroscopy in patients with unexplained visual field loss, i.e., presumed ocular vasospasm. Patients who showed signs of peripheral vasospasm in nailfold capillaroscopy improved in visual function (Octopus visual field) after administration of nifedipine. These observations were confirmed in several studies [17, 18]. Furthermore Flammer and coworkers showed that some patients suffering from presumed vasospastic syndrome or normal pressure glaucoma demonstrated peripheral vasospasm and visual field loss after immersing the hands in cold water. This kind of provoked vasospasm could be relieved by the administration of nifedipine which also improved the visual field.

Kitazawa and coworkers [35] administered 30 mg nifedipine/daily in 25 normal pressure glaucoma patients for 6 months. Twelve eyes (six patients) showed a constant improvement of the visual field. By using a discriminant analysis Kitazawa showed that the visual field is more likely to improve with systemic nifedipine in patients who are young, have a higher initial mean defect, lower IOP, have less decrease in diastolic blood pressure with nifedipine administration, and better cold recovery of skin temperature after immersing the hands in cold water.

In a recent study, Harris [30] demonstrated an overall improvement in contrast sensitivity in normal pressure glaucoma patients treated with oral nifedipine. Contrast sensitivity improved at 6 cycles / degree following 1, 4 and 6 months of treatment. Furthermore the authors demonstrated a significant correlation between ophthalmic artery blood velocity assessed by colour Doppler imaging and contrast sensitivity.

Lumme and associates [32] compared ten patients with normal pressure glaucoma who were treated with nifedipine, 11 treated with acetazolamide and 11 on no therapy. They found no significant difference in progressive loss of optic nerve rim area among the three groups. However, the progression of the mean visual field defect was not evaluated.

Miscellaneous calcium channel blockers were administered to glaucoma patients in a retrospective study by Netland and coworkers [40]. A total of 56 patients with either open angle or normal pressure glaucoma were treated by cardiologists or internists with calcium channel blockers: 46% received diltiazem, 30% nifedipine and 24% were treated with verapamil. These patients were retrospectively compared to a similar group of primary open angle glaucoma and normal pressure glaucoma patients not under the influence of calcium channel blockers. In patients with normal pressure glaucoma there was a significant difference in the progression of visual field defects. Only 11% of patients taking calcium channel blockers, compared to 56% of controls, demonstrated new visual field defects. Similarly, normal pressure glaucoma patients taking calcium channel blockers demonstrated no evidence of progressive optic nerve damage compared to 44% of control eyes. These effects, however, were not seen in primary open angle glaucoma patients.

Verapamil

Verapamil represents a calcium channel blocker of the phenylalkylamine group and shows a high tissue selectivity to the Av node. It is therefore used mainly in cardiology to treat cardiac arrythmia. In a randomized, prospective double-masked study verapamil eye drops were administered once in healthy volunteers [41]. Retinal blood cell velocities were measured by colour Doppler imaging. The IOP dropped significantly compared to baseline and the mean systolic and diastolic blood cell velocities in the central retinal artery increased. Pourcelot's ratio, an index of vascular resistance, measured in the central retinal artery was significantly reduced after topical application of verapamil 0.0125%. These results suggest that topical verapamil-the only available topical calcium channel blocker-improves retinal blood flow, at least in healthy volunteers.

Calcium Channel Blockers and IOP

Calcium flux can have several effects on aqueous humor dynamics, including a hydrostatic component caused by an effect on arterial blood pressure and ciliary body perfusion, and an osmotic component caused by an effect on the active secretion of sodium and calcium [8]. Another possible effect is a modulation of aqueous outflow by decreasing episcleral venous pressure. Topical administration of calcium channel blockers in rabbits had either no effect or led to a mild increase in IOP [4, 44]. Schnell [57] reported that a single sublingual dose of nifedipine caused a sharp decrease in IOP in primary open angle glaucoma patients, whereas repeated doses had no effect.

Goyal [24] and Abelson [1] studied the effect of topical verapamil in patients with untreated ocular hypertension and found a marked decrease in IOP that persisted up to 2 weeks. Monica [39] similarly found a marked decrease in IOP after oral administration of nitrendipine in normotensive individuals. Kelly and Walley [34], however, found no effect of either oral or intravenous nifedipine on IOP in normal subjects.

References

1. Abelson MB, Gilbert CM, Smith LM (1988) Sustained reduction of intraocular pressure in humans with the calcium channel blocker verapamil. Am J Ophthalmol 105:155-161
2. Anderson DR (1992) Autoregulation in glaucoma. In: SM Drance (ed) Glaucoma, ocular blood flow and drug treatment. Williams and Wilkins, Baltimore, pp 82-89
3. Bean BP (1989) Classes of calcium channels in vertebrate cells. Ann Rev Physiol 51:367-384
4. Beatty JF, Krupin T, Nichols PF, Becker B (1984) Elevation of intraocular pressure by calcium channel blockers. Arch Ophthalmol 102:1072-1076
5. Beckman JS (1991) The double-edged role of nitric oxide in brain function and superoxide mediated injury. J Dev Physiol 15:53-59
6. Bose S, Piltz JR, Breton ME (1995) Nimodipine, a centrally active calcium channel blocker, exerts a benefical effect on contrast sensitivity in patients with normal tension glaucoma and in control subjects. Ophthalmology 102:1236-1241
7. Bredt DS, Snyder SH (1992) Nitric oxide: a novel neuronal messenger. Neuron 8:3-11
8. Brubaker RF (1984) The physiology of aqueous humor formation. In: Drance SM, Neufeld A (eds) Glaucoma: applied pharmacology in medical treatment. Grune and Stratton, Orlando, pp 35-70
9. Catterall WA, Striessnig J (1992) Receptor sites for calcium channel antagonists. Trends Pharmacol Sci 13:256-262
10. Drance SM, Douglas GR, Wijsman K, Schulzer M, Britton RJ (1988) Response of blood flow to warm and cold in normal and low-tension glaucoma patients. Am J Ophthalmol 105:35-39
11. Drance SM (1992) Possible implications of vasospasm as a risk factor in glaucomas. In: SM Drance (ed) Glaucoma, ocular blood flow and drug treatment. Williams and Wilkins, Baltimore, pp 78-81
12. Ernest JT (1975) Pathogenesis of glaucomatous optic nerve disease. Trans Am Ophthalmol Soc 73:366-372
13. Flammer J, Guthauser U, Mahler F (1987) Do ocular vasospasm help cause low tension glaucoma? Docum Ophthalmol Proc Ser 47:397-399
14. Flammer J, Guthauser U (1987) Behandlung chorioidaler Vasospasmen mit Kalziumantagonisten. Klin Mbl Augenheilk 190:299-300
15. Flammer J (1994) The vascular concept of glaucoma. Surv Ophthalmol 38:3-6
16. Gasser P (1989) Ocular vasospasm: a risk factor in the pathogenesis of low tension glaucoma. Int Ophthalmol 13:281-290
17. Gasser P, Flammer J (1989) Die dynamische-video-kapillarmikroskopische Beeinflußung akraler und okulärer Vasospasmen durch Kalzium und Serotoninantagonisten. Vasa 27:79-85
18. Gasser P, Flammer J (1990) Short and long-term effect of nifedipine on the visual field in patients with presumed vasospasm. J Int Med Res 18:334-338
19. Gasser P, Flammer J, Guthauser U, Niesel P, Mahler F, Linder HR (1986) Bedeutung des vasospastischen Syndroms in der Augenheilkunde. Klin Mbl Augenheilk 188:398-399
20. Gasser P, Flammer J (1987) Influence of vasospasm on visual function. Docum Ophthalmol 66:3-18.
21. Gasser P, Flammer J (1991) Blood-cell velocity

in the nailfold capillaries of patients with normal-tension and high-tension glaucoma. Am J Ophthalmol 111:585-588

22. Gasser P (1992) Nailfold capillary video microscopy for diagnosis of presumed ocular vasospasm. In: SM Drance (ed) Glaucoma, ocular blood flow and drug treatment. Williams and Wilkins, Baltimore, pp 70-77
23. Goldberg I (1992) Calcium channel blockers Are they an answer? In: SM Drance (ed) Glaucoma, ocular blood flow and drug treatment. Williams and Wilkins, Baltimore, pp 90-96
24. Goyer JK, Khilnani G, Sharma DP, Singh J (1989) The hypotensive effect of verapamil eye drops on ocular hypertension. Indian J. Ophthalmol 37:176-182
25. Guthauser U, Flammer J, Mahler F (1988) The relationship between digital and ocular vasospasm. Graefes Arch Clin Exp Ophthalmol 226:224-226
26. Gelmers HJ, Gorters K, de-Weerdt CJ, Wiezer HJA (1988) A controlled trial of nimodipine in acute ischemic stroke. New Engl J Med 318:203-207.
27. Gotoh O, Mohammed AA, McCulloch J, Graham DI, Harper AM (1986) Nimodipine and the hemodynamic and histopathological consequences of middle cerebral artery occlusion. J Cereb Blood Flow Metab 6:321-331
28. Graefe A, von (1862) Ueber die glaucomatoese Natur der Amaurose mit Sehnervenexkavation und ueber die Classifikation der Glaukome. Graefes Arch Clin Exp Ophthalmol, 8:271-297
29. Harris A, Sergott RC, Spaeth GL, Katz JL, Shoemaker JA, Martin BJ (1994) Color Doppler analysis of ocular vessel blood velocity in normal tension glaucoma. Am J Ophthalmol 118:642-649
30. Harris A, Cantor B, Edwards JD (1995) Long-term hemodynamical and visual function changes in normal tension glaucoma treated with oral nifedipine. Ophthalmology (Suppl) 102:90
31. Hess P, Lansman JB, Tsien RW (1984) Different modes of calcium channel gating behaviour by dihydropyridine calcium agonists and antagonists. Nature 311:538 547
32. Lumme P, Tuulonen A, Airaksinen PJ, Alanko HI (1991) Neuroretinal rim area in low tension glaucoma: Effect of nifedipine and acetazolamide compared to no treatment. Acta Opthalmol 69:293-298
33. Kaiser HJ, Flammer J, Wenk M, Luscher T (1995) Endothelin-1 plasma levels in normal tension glaucoma: abnormal response to postural changes. Graefes Arch Clin Exp Ophthalmol 233:484-488
34. Kelly SP, Walley TJ (1988) Effects of the calcium antagonist nifedipine on intraocular pressure in normal subjects. Br J Ophthalmol 72:216-221
35. Kitazawa Y, Shirai H, Go FJ (1989) The effecct of Ca-antagonists on the visual field in low tension glaucoma. Graefes Arch Clin Exp Ophthalmol 227:408 412.
36. Mayer B, Klatt P, Bohme E, Schmidt K (1992) Regulation of neuronal nitric oxide and cyclic GMP formation by calcium. J Neurochem 59:2024-2029
37. Magitot A (1908) Contribution à l'etude de la circulation artérielle et lymphatique du nerf optique et du chiasme. Thése, Paris
38. Miller RJ (1987) Multiple calcium channels and neuronal functions. Science 235:46-52
39. Monica ML, Hesse RJ, Messerli FH (1983) The effect of a calcium channel blocking agent on intraocular pressure. Am Ophthalmol 96:814-819
40. Netland PA, Chaturvedi N, Dreyer EB (1993) Calcium channel blockers in the management of low-tension and open-angle glaucoma. Am J Ophthalmol 115:608-613
41. Netland P, Grosskreutz C, Feke GT, Hart LJ (1995) Color Doppler ultrasound analysis of ocular circulation after topical calcium channel blocker. Am J Ophthalmol 119:694-700
42. Nyborg NCB, Nielsen PJ (1992) Comparison of the vasodilator effect of nifedipine and nimodipine in bovine isolated ocular arteries Abstracts of the European Glaucoma Society 1992:186
43. Pauwels PJ, Leysen JE, Janssen PAJ (1991) Calcium and natrium channels in neuronal cell death: protection by flunarizine. Life Sci 48:1881-1893
44. Payne FJ, Slagle TM, Cheeks LT, Green K (1990) Effects of calcium channel blockers on intraocular pressure. Ophthalmic Res 22:337-342
45. Phelps CD, Corbett JJ (1985) Migraine and low-tension glaucoma: A case control study. Invest Ophthalmol Vis Sci 26:1105-1108.
46. Pillunat LE, Stodtmeister R, Wilmanns I, Christ T (1985) Autoregulation of ocular blood flow during changes in intraocular pressure. Graefes Arch Clin Exp Ophthalmol 223:219-223
47. Pillunat LE, Lang GK (1992) Ocular carbon dioxide reactivity in normal pressure glaucoma. Invest Ophthalmol Vis Sci 33:1279
48. Pillunat LE, Stodtmeister R, Wilmanns I (1987) Pressure compliance of the optic nerve head in low tension glaucoma. Br J Ophthalmol 71:181-187
49. Pillunat LE, Lang GK (1993) Ocular carbon dioxide reactivity in healthy volunteers: Effect of age and CO_2 concentration applied. Germ J Ophthalmol 2:396
50. Pillunat LE, Lang G K (1993) Ocular carbon dioxide reactivity in normal pressure and high

pressure glaucoma. Germ J Ophthalmol 2:402
51. Pillunat LE, Lang GK, Harris A (1994) The visual response to increased ocular blood flow in normal pressure glaucoma Surv Ophthalmol 38:139-149
52. Pillunat LE, Lang GK, Harris A (1995) Ocular carbon dioxide reactivity and calcium channel blockers in normal pressure glaucoma. In: Drance SM (ed) Update to glaucoma, ocular blood flow and drug treatment. Kugler, Amsterdam, pp 67-71
53. Pillunat LE, Kuba GB, Baumert S (1996) Effect of nimodipine on contrast sensitivity and optic nerve head blood flow in healthy subjects. (submitted for publication)
54. Piltz J, Bose S, Grunwald JE, Petrig L, Riva CE (1993) Effect of nimodipine on automated threshold perimetry, spatial contrast sensitivity and macular blood flow in normal tension glaucoma and controls. Invest Ophthalmol Vis Sci 34:1287
55. Rader J, Feuer WJ, Anderson DR (1994) Peripapillary vasoconstriction in the glaucomas and anterior ischemic optic neuropathies. Am J Ophthalmol 117:72-80
56. Robert Y, Steiner D, Hendrickson P (1989) Papillary circulation dynamics in glaucoma. Graefes Arch Clin Exp Ophthalmol 227:436-439.
57. Schnell D (1975) Response of intraocular pressure in normal subjects and glaucoma patients to single and repeated doses of the coronary drug Adalat. In: Lochner W, Engel HJ, Lichtlen PR (eds). Second international Adalat symposium. Springer, Berlin Heidelberg New York, pp 290-302
58. Smith JJ, Kampine JP (1990) The peripheral circulation and its regulation. In: JP Kampine, JJ Smith, (eds) Circulatory physiology, Williams and Wilkins, Baltimore, pp 140-160
59. Sossi N, Anderson DR (1983) Blockage of axonal transport in optic nerve induced by elevation of intraocular pressure. Effect of arterial hypertension induced by angiotensin I. Arch Ophthalmol 101:94-97.
60. Sossi N, Anderson DR (1983) Effect of elevated intraocular pressure on blood flow. Occurence in cat optic nerve head studied with iodoantipyrine I 125. Arch Ophthalmol 101:98-101
61. Schumer RA, Podos SM (1994) The nerve of glaucoma! Arch Ophthalmol 112:37-44
62. Usui T, Iwata K (1992) Finger blood flow in patients with low tension glaucoma and primary open angle glaucoma. Br J Ophthalmol 76:2-4
63. Virno M, Pecori Giraldi J, Covelli GP, Grechi G, Appiotti A (1990) Effetti della nimodipina sulla sensibilità retinica nella neurotticopatia glaucomatosa. Boll Ocul 69:449-455
64. Weinstein JM, Duckrow B, Beard D, Brennan RW (1983) Optic nerve blood flow and its autoregulation. Invest Ophthalmol Vis Sci 24:1559-1565
65. Weinstein JM, Funsch D, Page RB, Brennan RW (1982) Optic nerve blood flow regulation. Invest Ophthalmol Vis Sci 23:640-647
66. White RP, Cunningham MP, Robertson JT (1982) Effect of the calcium antagonist nimodipine on contractile responses of isolated canine basilar arteries induced by serotonin, prostaglandin F2a,thrombin and whole blood. Neurosurgery 10:344-348

Discussion

Question:

A question for Dr. Virno. We have viewed systemic bromocriptine for glaucoma patients. It caused an enormous reduction in intraocular pressure but the main problem with this drug was tachiphilaxis. It worked in the first or second day, but the third time it didn't work anymore. What is your experience with the D1 antagonist, is it the same?

Answer: Virno

If I understood correctly, you treated a few patients with systemic bromocriptine. My question is: did you evaluated systemic blood pressure?

Question:

Yes, we measured systemic blood pressure and it was reduced.

Answer: Virno

Because when you are giving an hypotensive drug you may always have a reduction in the intraocular pressure. Concerning tacyphylaxis, I can't answer because I have no experience.

Question:

In studies in which we look at the effects of glaucoma, we most often try to see whether the disease progression has been altered. The data we presented today were whether the visual field improved or not. That was a rather interesting viewpoint, and of course it would be striking if glaucoma patients improved as much as the dramatic changes that we saw in the visual field. Those might simply be extreme examples and I would propose that we have much larger and long-term studies suggesting that beta-blockers should be used in glaucoma patients. This is particularly important because the American FDA have set controls on the use of nifedipine because it is leading to dramatic increases in heart disease in persons treated with this particular agent. So I think we must be very cautious in using these drugs.

Answer: Pillunat

I thank you very much for that comment and I agree on that, but first of all I think that what we showed before were some effects after nimodipine and not after nodipine. That's the first difference. The second one is that in the meantime we didn't have studies of about 18 months to 2 years where we could preserve the visual field like it was after the acute application of carbodioxide. You are absolutely right that all visual field improvements are not as striking as they were in the visual field I showed here. There was a 30% improvement in normal pressure glaucoma patients. All of the other 70% didn't change during the CO_2 provocation test, but they also didn't show any change during calcium channel blockers. I think somebody has to do something and at least we have good experience with nimodipine in those cases which show responsiveness to CO_2.

Question: Demailly

A question for Dr. Pillunat. I think that the effect of calcium channel blockers depends on the severity of glaucoma, the age of glaucoma and the type of calcium channel blockers. We experimented nimodipine with an antiaggregant in severe glaucoma patients and after 18 months we could improve the velocity and the resistance index in color imaging doppler, but we don't observe any significant difference between the control group and the group with glaucomatous patients.

Question: Hoste

Wouldn't it be more appropriate to apply a Ca^{2+} channel blocker topically instead of orally? When a Ca^{2+} channel blocker is administered orally, it will act on all arteries in the body. The subsequent general vasodilatation will induce a blood pressure fall. Blood pressure fall results in decreased ocular perfusion pressure and this will of course counteract or even exceed the local vasodilatatory effects of the Ca^{2+} channel blocker. Hence the outcome of such a treatment will be uncertain. But when we apply a Ca^{2+} channel blocker topically, we can achieve local vasodilatation without inducing systemic side-effects.
We have shown in the poster that we gave calcium channel blockers to patients with low tension glaucoma and we found a significant decrease in blood pressure. It is harmful because it reduces ocular perfusion.

Answer: Pillunat

I perfectly agree on that, therefore we didn't choose nifedipine since it is proved that it changes blood pressure; but we chose Nimodipine that is just a cerebral working calcium channel blocker. It has no peripheric side effects, so blood pressure is absolutely stable under that calcium channel blocker. I agree it would be better to have that one as a topical drug, but this is not available; at least we are sure we are not lowering blood pressure by this drug.

NORMAL TENSION GLAUCOMA

Pathogenetic Problems and Classification of Low Critical Tension Glaucoma

M. Miglior, P. Montanari, and P. Troiano

University of Milan, Ospedale Maggiore IRCCS, Via F. Sforza 35, 20122 Milan, Italy

Introduction

Glaucoma is a disease characterized by hydrodynamic disorders and by consequent critical intraocular pressure levels causing injury to the eye and including degeneration of the ganglion cell axons of the optic nerve head.

The occurence of a glaucoma-like disease not associated with significantly high IOP levels was first noted in 1857 by von Graefe [1]. Since then, this particular form of the disease has been the subject of numerous descriptions, interpretations and even conceptual reservations regarding its nosology.

General Aspects

Critical Ocular Pressure

Critical ocular pressure corresponds to the pressure level which, alone or together with other factors (risk factors), is apt to induce alterations of important morphological and sensorial parameters of the visual system [2].

The critical ocular pressure is strictly connected to the individual degree of vulnerability and may thus include pressure levels that are higher, equal to or lower than those considered statistically normal. Moreover, different pressure levels may be reached in particular circumstances; for example, they are low in high myopia, reaching 16 mm Hg in eyes with an axial length of 34 mm.

Four general classes of disease can be described based on pathologies due to pressure variations and different levels of critical pressure:

1. Diseases from IOPs higher than 30 mm Hg (very high critical pressure): acute angle-closure glaucoma, Posner-Schlossmann syndrome, in which the most typical alterations are corneal edema and anterior segment congestion
2. Diseases from IOP between 30 and 21 mm Hg (high critical pressure): primary open-angle glaucoma, in which the most typical damage is optical neuropathy
3. Diseases from IOP between 21 and 15 mm Hg (low critical pressure): low critical tension glaucoma
4. Diseases from IOP lower than 5 mm Hg (very low critical pressure): ocular hypotony.

Problems Regarding Nomenclature

The existing doubts about the characteristics of glaucoma not associated with ocular hypertension are responsible for the various names which have been applied in order to differentiate this form of glaucoma from the other forms. Von Graefe [1] named it simply "amaurose mit seh nerven excavation", avoiding any reference to the pressure level and any debate about a possible relation with glaucoma. De Wecker [3] used the term "pseudo-glaucoma" underlining therefore apparent analogies with glaucomatous disease. Duke Elder and Jay [4] called it "low tension glaucoma", thus confirming the glaucomatous nature of this disease and underlining the particular pressure level. Quaranta and Boles [5] named it "glaucoma sine ipertensione", a term which, although negative, stresses exactly that which is lacking. Other definitions have [6, 7] included mention of the progressive visual field loss or progressive optic nerve cupping. Drance [8] described it more precisely as "normal pressure glaucoma". We prefer the name "low-critical-tension glaucoma" (LCTG) [9] for two reasons: firstly, to emphasize the importance of the term "critical IOP" in classifying the glaucomas; secondly, to underline that in this form of glaucoma the pressure is able to induce damage even though it remains within the normal range.

Clinical Picture

Low-critical-tension glaucoma is a disease that begins deceitfully, has a cronic course and is generally diagnosed in an advanced stage. Its clinical picture is somehow similar to that of primary open-angle glaucoma. Nevertheless there are many characteristics that, while not specific, are more frequently associated with LCTG. These include:

1. Optic disc: marked pallor, excavation with sloping edges, marked thinning of the lamina cribrosa in the infero-temporal area, localized erosions of the neural rim with small and transient superficial hemorrhages
2. Peripapillary choroid: marked atrophy with characteristic hyperfluorescence
3. Trabecular meshwork: accumulation of extracellular material, particularly in the cribriform layer [10]
4. Visual field: deep defects, more frequent in the superior part, close to the fixation point
5. Bioelectric potentials: marked alterations both of the retinal potentials and the evoked visual potentials
6. IOP: constantly lower than 22 mm Hg
7. Outflow facility: often reduced
8. Provocative tests: often positive.

According to these data, LCTG can be defined, from a clinical point of view, as a disease characterized mainly by damage of the optic nerve head and visual field defects of evident glaucomatous nature. These defects develop in a normal pressure context (in spite of possible alterations of the aqueous humor circulation) and have nevertheless a pathologic potential due to the concomitant presence of risk factors.

Phatologic Associations (Risk Factors)

Many studies on LCTG have been devoted to finding pathologic associations, with the goal of identifying possible factors as well. The most significant data appear to be the following: (a) acute hemodynamic crisis in 40%-93% of the patients; (b) systemic hypotension in 31%-59% of the patients; and (c) systemic vascular diseases in 33%-80% of the patients.

Therapeutic Problems

The treatment of LCTG is problematic for many reasons:

1. The difficulty in determining the effective therapeutic benefits considering that the natural progression of the disease is very slow
2. The possibility that specific hypotensive drugs can compromise the blood supply of the optic nerve head which is already damaged by the disease
3. The effective risk that surgical treatments are complicated by a sudden worsening of visual field defects.

Glaucomatous Identity

Low critical tension glaucoma has to be considered as an autonomous clinical entity, whose glaucomatous specificity is nonetheless undoubtable. This is due to the presence of the following elements: hydrodynamic disorders; the critical character of the IOP (even normal) concomitant with the precarious condition of the ganglion fibers deficit of the blood supply, constitutional weakness of the lamina cribrosa); typical optic neuropathy; specific visual field defects; unanimous agreement on the therapeutical approach, which also corresponds to treatment of the glaucomas.

Epidemiological Aspects

Data on the frequency of LCTG have been reported in the literature.

The prevalence among the general population is 0.32% (0.05 0.52%) while the prevalence among primary open-angle glaucoma is 39.9% (6.3% 68.3%).

The disease is more frequent among patients 64-67 years old and more frequent among women. Regarding ocular laterality, bilaterality is more frequent, and regarding refractive defects, myopia is more frequent.

Etiopathogenetic Hypotheses

The etiopathogenetic analysis of LCTG should proceed in two separate directions: etiopathogenesis of the hydrodynamic disorders; etiopathogenesis of the subsequent damage.

Origin of the Hydrodynamic Disorders

Hydrodynamic disorders in LCTG seem to be represented by obstruction of the trabecular meshwork, as seen in the histological studies of Rohen and Lütjen-Drecoll [10]. The etiology of these alterations could be the same as those hypothesized for primary open-angle glaucoma (genetics, aging, etc.).

Given the presence of trabecular obstruction in LCTG, we should explain the reason for the absence of ocular hypertension. The various hypotheses include the constitutional presence of pressure values (10-12 mm Hg) at the lowest grade of the normal distribution of the IOP.

Thus, an IOP increase of 8-10 mm Hg could be detrimental for the optic nerve head, even if the resulting IOP is still in the normal range.

Origin of the Optic Neuropathy

In LCTG the most important damage is to the optic nerve head, choroid, and retina, causing visual field defects and visual acuity reduction.

Therefore it is evident that the marked presence of such damage is disproportional to the modest (at least apparently) presence of hydrodynamic disorders. Possible explanations for this discrepancy may be:

1. A concomitant interposition of important risk factors, such as systemic vascular diseases, that can affect the optic nerve head blood supply
2. A genetic predisposition
3. A loss of connective tissue of the lamina cribrosa
4. IOP levels in LCTG patients which are at the lower end of the normal distribution of IOP in the general population (11-12 mm Hg) and therefore possibility of optic nerve head damage when the IOP reaches 18-20 mm Hg
5. The possibility of recurrent pressure peaks over 20-21 mm Hg occurring at times IOP is not being measured.

Classification

Identification of Clinical Forms

Recent studies have increased our clinical knowledge concerning LCTG, particularly the circumstances of its appearance and the different forms it can assume. Geijssen [11], also on the basis of previous studies [12-14], has come to the conclusion that LCTG can be subdivided into the following forms: (1) focal ischemic normal pressure glaucoma, characterized by focal defects of the rim disc, more often at the inferior pole; (2) senile sclerotic normal pressure glaucoma, characterized by the pale, sloping cup of the disc, which has a "moth-eaten" appearance, and by the extensive peripapillary atrophy and choroidal sclerosis; (3) myopic normal pressure glaucoma, characterized by an obliquely implanted, shallow myopic disc with a myopic crescent and myopic choroid; (4) mixed normal pressure glaucoma, without any pathognomonic features.

Miglior and coworkers [2, 15, 16] claim that in LCTG two subgroups are distinguishable: (1) primary (idiopathic) LCTG, equivalent to the more common forms in wich the IOP level (not higher than 21 mm Hg) remains a constant characteristic following the first observation; (2) secondary (subsequent) LCTG, which takes place in the setting of a glaucoma with high critical pressure in which, in spite of the consolidated IOP normalization in response to treatment, further damage of the optic nerve head occurs.

Quaranta [17], on the basis of studies of the vascular ocular system, proposed the following subdivision: (a) normal pressure glaucoma with reduced ocular blood flow (of functional, anatomical, mixed origin); (b) normal pressure glaucoma with apparently normal ocular blood flow.

Table 1. Classification of low critical tension glaucoma

Level I	Level II	Level III	Level IV
General etiology	Type of hydrodynamic disorder	Etiology of the hydrodynamic disorder	Clinical aspects
Primary glaucomas	Trabecular meshwork obstruction	Degenerative origin	Focal ischemic Senile sclerotic Myopic Mixed With reduced ocular blood flow With normal ocular blood flow
Secondary glaucomas	Trabecular meshwork obstruction	Degenerative origin	Subsequent to primary open-angle glaucoma

Collocation in the General Classification of the Glaucomas

We have previously proposed a general classification of the glaucomas: (1) independence or not of the glaucoma from other diseases; (2) type of hydrodynamic disorder; (3) etiology of the hydrodynamic disorder; (4) clinical aspect [18]. In such a scheme, LCTG was placed among primary glaucomas, in the subgroup of the glaucomas due to trabecular meshwork obstruction of degenerative origin. Considering the most recent clinical findings mentioned above, the classification of LCTG should perhaps be amended (Table 1).
LCTG should thus be placed in the column of primary glaucomas and, separately, in that of secondary glaucomas. At level II, both the primary and secondary forms have to be placed among the types due to trabecular meshwork obstruction. At level III (etiology of the hydrodynamic disorder), the two forms of LCTG should be placed in the column of the primary glaucomas due to trabecular meshwork obstruction of degenerative origin. At level IV (clinical aspects), the primary form is subdivided into six subgroups: focal ischemic, senile sclerotic, myopic, mixed, with reduced ocular blood flow, with normal ocular blood flow.

Comments

Low critical tension glaucoma is actually a well-delimited disease, as regards many of its clinical aspects, and the glaucomatous identity of this disease has been proved. However, the real frequency of this disease has yet to be statistically determined and the relationship between hydrodynamic disorders and the optic nerve head damage are not yet clear enough.

References

1. Von Graefe A (1857) Amaurose mit Sehnervenexcavation. Archiv of Ophtalmol 3:484
2. Miglior M, Montanari P, Prandoni S (1991) Il glaucoma a pressione critica bassa: concetti di evoluzione. Atti della Società Oftalmologica Meridionale. Editrice Tipografica, Bari, pp 11-32
3. De Wecker L (1969) Glaucoma and hypotony. In: Duke-Elder S (ed) System of ophthalmology, vol 11. Henry Kimpton, London, p 379
4. Duke-Elder S, Jay B (1969) Glaucoma and hypotony. In: Duke Elder S (ed) System of ophthalmology, vol. 11. Henry Kimpton, London, p 484
5. Quaranta CA, Boles Carenini B (1977) La tonografia nel glaucoma cronico semplice. In: L'attendibilità dei mezzi semeiologici nella diagnosi del glaucoma cronico semplice. Relaz. al 58° Congr. della Soc. Oftalm. Italiana. La Stampa Editore, Genova, p 158
6. Chandler PA, Grant WM (1979) Glaucoma (2nd ed). Lea and Febiger, Philadelphia
7. Hoskins HD (1981 Definition, classification, and management of the glaucoma suspect. In: Transactions of the New Orleans Academy of Ophthalmology: symposium on glaucoma, Mosby, St Louis, pp 228-231

8. Drance SM (1985) Low-tension glaucoma, enigma and opportunity. Arch Ophthalmol 103:1131
9. Miglior M (1987) Low-critical tension glaucoma. Present problems. Glaucoma 9:77
10. Rohen JW, Lütjen-Drecoll E (1996) Morphology of aqueous outflow pathways in normal and glaucoma eyes. In: Ritch R, Shields M B, Krupin T (eds) The glaucomas, 2nd ed. Mosby, St. Louis, p 111
11. Geijssen HC (1991) Material, methods, definitions. In: Studies on normal pressure glaucoma, Kugler Publications, New York, p 36
12. Spaeth GL (1980) Low-tension glaucoma: its diagnosis and management. Glaucoma Symposium Amsterdam. Doc Ophthalmol Proc Ser 22:263
13. Greve EL, Furono F (1980) Myopia and glaucoma. Graefes Arch Clin Exp Ophthalmol 213:33
14. Geijssen HC, Greve EL (1987) The spectrum of primary open-angle glaucoma I: senile sclerotic glaucoma versus high tension glaucoma. Ophthalmic Surg 18:207
15. Miglior M, Bozzini S, Montanari P, et al. (1990) Formes particulières de glaucome à pression critique basse. In: Bechetoille (ed) Glaucomes à pression normale. Japperenard, Angers, pp 242-243
16. Miglior M, Montanari P, Troiano P (1995) Low critical tension glaucoma: clinical forms and epidemiological aspects. Greek Glaucoma Society Symposium, Athens (in press)
17. Quaranta L (1994) I pattern vascolari nel glaucoma a pressione normale. Atti del LXXIV Congresso SOI. Casa Editrice Mattioli, Fidenza, pp 217-224
18. Miglior M (1987) Classificazione dei glaucomi. Minerva Oftalmologica 29:37-50

Aspects of Normal Pressure Glaucoma

E.L. Greve, H.G.C. Geijssen, and H.F.A. Duijm

Academic Medical Center of the University of Amsterdam, Glaucoma Center, Meibergdreef 9, 1105 AZ Amsterdam, The Netherlands

I intend to discuss two aspects of normal pressure glaucoma (NPG). This condition is usually defined as a glaucomatous optic neuropathy, primary glaucoma, with typical glaucomatous cupping and accompanying glaucomatous visual field defects, an open chamber angle and intraocular pressures (IOPs) within the statistically normal limits. We will find that there is quite some variation in the combination of glaucomatous cupping and glaucomatous visual field defects, and that an IOP within the normal range by no means indicates that it is not a pathogenetic factor. A statistically normal IOP does not rule out a raised IOP within the normal range. For instance, about 12% of the population has an IOP of 12 mm Hg. A rise in pressure from 12 mm Hg to 20 mm Hg, which is quite substantial, would still not lead to an IOP that exceeds the limit of the mean plus one standard deviation in the normal population. We should not forget that a sizeable part of the so-called NPGs are nothing else but primary open-angle glaucomas (POAGs) with a raised IOP within the normal range. As we will indicate later, it may very well be that in this group of raised pressure NPGs the optic disc has an appearance that is indistinguishable from that of the other "pressure" POAGs. Apart from this group of POAGs with a statistically normal IOP, we have described three other types of NPG: myopic NPG, senile sclerotic NPG and focal ischemic NPG [1]. The latter type has been described earlier by Spaeth. Now, why bring up these types of NPGs again? It can not be overemphasized that there is no such thing as the NPG patient; rather, there are several types of NPG patients whose diseases presumably vary in their pathogenesis.

The existence of three subtypes of NPGs has been confirmed by the research groups of Drance and Jonas. We have described the typical optic disc appearance of these subgroups [1]. The focal ischemic type has a focal notch with an accompanying visual field defect which is often close to the center. The myopic type has a myopic disc with shallow excavation, nasal subtraction and myopic peripapillary atrophy. The senile sclerotic type has a pale, moth-eaten, sloping excavation with extensive peripapillary atrophy and choroidal sclerosis. Apart from these three types of discs, one finds the well known type with a concentric general enlargement. As we mentioned earlier, it is probable that this type of general enlargement is most comparable to the type of disc in POAG. Nicolela and Drance have demonstrated that, when patients are selected based purely on the appearance of the disc, patients with a general enlargement of the disc have higher pressures than those with focal, myopic, and senile sclerotic NPG [2]. The same group has also shown that localized visual field defects occur more frequently in focal ischemic and myopic glaucoma. The existence of senile sclerotic glaucoma was also confirmed and described by the group of Jonas.

The concept of different types of NPG is not only important for understanding the pathogenesis but also the progression and, possibly, the treatment of the disease. The risk factors for progression, amongst others are: myopia, disc hemorrhages, peripapillary atrophy and choroidal sclerosis, and slow venous and choroidal filling times as demonstrated in the extensive work of Geijssen [1], whose studies in the late 1980s used classical fluorescein angiography to measure venous and choroidal filling times. In the above mentioned list of risk factors for progression most of the factors are vascular. Geijssen demonstrated that progressive myopic and focal ischemic NPGs have long choroidal filling times. It should be noted that the calculated progression for different types of NPG may be quite different. Geijssen found a 35% progression for the senile sclerotic and miscellaneous types of NPG and 80% progression for the myopic NPGs.

From these data we may conclude that not only do the different types of NPG have different rates of progression, but also that this progression is often accompanied by vascular risk factors. In the late 1980s accurate quantifying methods for measurement of blood flow were hardly available. Nowadays we have a number of methods that claim to measure blood flow in a quantified way. As it seems that vascular risk factors are truly important for the pathogenesis and progression of glaucomatous disease, it is of great importance that we do indeed have accurate quantitative bloodflow measurements. The available methods include pulsatile ocular blood flow, scanning laser angiography of the peripapillary choroid and retinal circulation (arterio-venous passage time), scanning laser angiography using indocyanine green, (scanning) laser Doppler flowmetry, and colour Doppler imaging.

As we have spent many years developing software for the measurement of choroidal blood flow with the help of scanning laser angiography, we will limit the majority of our discussion to the results obtained with this technique. The scanning laser can be used for the simultaneous measurement of the retinal circulation and the choroidal circulation. This is one of the great attractions of this method. Furthermore, fluorescein angiography is a well known clinical method for assessing vascular problems. Scanning laser angiography has a high temporal resolution and the results can easily be further analysed using image processing techniques, enabling parametrization of, e.g., choroidal hemodynamics. A further advantage, besides the simultaneous measurement of retinal and choroidal circulation, is the large area of choroid and retina that can be investigated. The disadvantage of the method is that fluorescein has to be injected and that not all patients are suitable for this type of angiography. The arteriovenous passage time has been used as the subject of other studies [3, 4] (Fig. 1a). Based on a model we have described the mean choroidal blood refreshment time of the peripapillary choroid, also expressed as τ (Fig. 1b). Briefly, the intensity of dye in each pixel is measured over time resulting in an exponential curve. The steepness of this curve indicates the speed of passage of blood through the choroid. We have shown that this method for the measurement of choroidal refreshment time is well correlated, in the rabbit, with the microsphere method for measuring blood flow [5]. We have measured

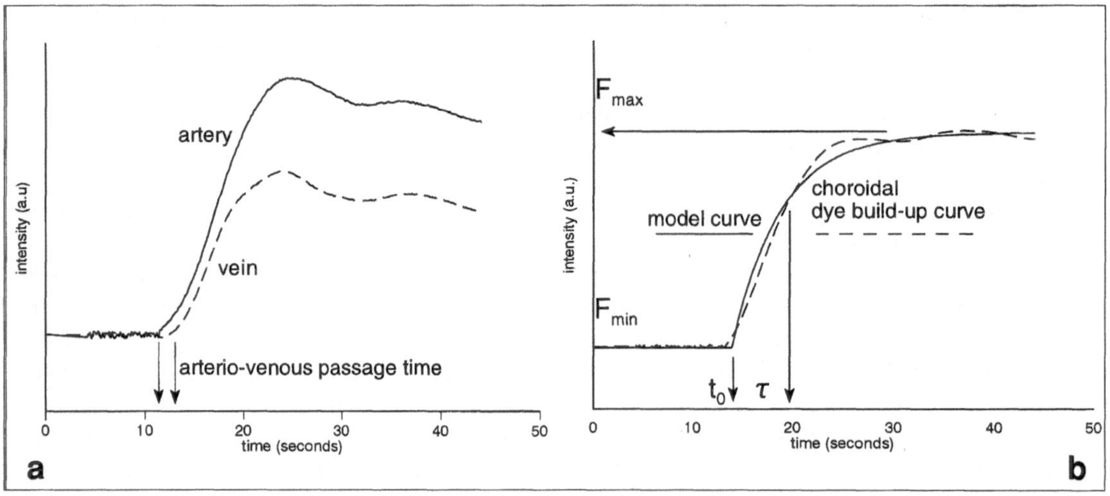

Fig. 1a, b. The retinal arteriovenous passage time is calculated from the difference between an arterial and venous dye build-up curve (**a**). The choroidal blood refreshment time, τ, is derived from the analysis of choroidal dye build-up curves using an exponential or a compartmental model (**b**)

the choroidal refreshment time and retinal arteriovenous passage time, both in seconds, in normals, in patients with ocular hypertension, with POAG and with NPG [6]. Before we discuss these results I would like to mention some selected findings by other authors. The group of Drance, using colour Doppler imaging, showed that the blood flow in senile sclerotic glaucoma is slower than in the other subgroups of NPG [7].

Using colour Doppler imaging, Galassi and colleagues showed that there is a reduction of systolic velocity in myopic glaucoma as compared to nonmyopic glaucoma [8]. Blood flow in glaucomatous patients can be improved; for example, Harris has shown improvements in NPG after carbon dioxide inhalation [9]. We have shown that after pressure reduction by trabeculectomy the slow choroidal blood refreshment time can become normal [10]. These findings indicate that blood flow disturbances are not irreversible and this gives us hope that they may be influenced by some form of treatment. The results of Harris show that reversible vasospasm is involved in at least some cases of NPGs.

Let me now get back to the results on choroidal refreshment time and arteriovenous passage time. Interestingly, the results of the measurements in POAG patients and in NPG patients are somewhat different. Whereas it is the retinal circulation that suffers most in POAG, it is the choroidal circulation that suffers most in NPG [6]. We propose that the raised IOP in POAG is accompanied by a defect in autoregulation, causing reduced perfusion pressure, particularly in cases of POAG with higher pressure. This, however, does not explain the reduced choroidal blood flow. It is known that the choroid has very limited autoregulation; however, if autoregulation is the explanation, one would expect the same phenomenon as observed for retinal arteriovenous passage time. In the case of the choroid, it is the NPG group of patients that suffers most. This means that in the group with the lower pressures and the supposedly better perfusion pressure the choroidal times are the longest. This indicates to us that there must be primary vascular choroidal or prechoroidal disease in the NPGs. Thus the explanations for the retinal findings and the choroidal findings may be different. We can add to this that we found no correlation between the retinal results and the choroidal results. It would be of interest to correlate these intriguing results with the findings of colour Doppler imaging.

We conclude that there is evidence for a vascular pathogenesis in at least some of the cases of NPG. This can now also be shown by quantitative methods for the measurement of blood flow. We also conclude that participation of the two ocular vascular systems that supply the eye with blood is different in POAG and NPG. It may very well be that it is also different in the different types of NPG. It is important to optimize our methodology for blood flow measurement, to have a long term follow-up of these measurements and to correlate the different type of measurements with each other. It is through these approaches that we will get a better insight into the vascular pathogenesis of glaucoma. Last, but not least, we may be able to find appropriate treatment for the vascular component of glaucomatous damage.

References

1. Geijssen HC (1991) Studies on normal pressure Glaucoma, Kugler, Amsterdam
2. Nicolela M, Drance SM. (1995) Vascular parameters in various glaucomatous disc appearances. Third European Professors Workshop on the Quantification of Ocular Blood Flow in Glaucoma, October 7, 1995, Edinburgh
3. Wolf S, Arend O, Sponsel WE, Schulte K, Cantor LB, Reim M (1993) Retinal hemodynamics using scanning laser ophthalmoscopy and hemorheology in chronic open angle glaucoma. Ophthalmol 100:1561-6
4. Riva CE, Feke GT, Ben-Sira I(1978) Fluorescein dye-dilution technique and retinal circulation. Am J Physiol 234:h315-22
5. Duijm HFA, Rulo AHF, Astin M, Mäepea O, Berg TJTPvd, Greve EL (1996) Study of choroidal blood flow by comparison of SLO fluorescein angiography and microspheres (submitted)
6. Geijssen HC, Duijm HFA, Berg TJTPvd, Greve EL(1996) Choroidal and retinal hemodynamics are different in POAG and NPG (ARVO)
7. Rankin SJA, Drance SM, Buckley AR, Walman BE (1995) Colour Doppler imaging and visual field correlations of the optic nerve head in glaucoma. Third European Professors Workshop on the Quantification of Ocular Blood Flow in Glaucoma, October 7, 1995, Edinburgh
8. Galassi F, Sodi A, Vielmo A, Saint Pierre F, Rossi MG, Ciardullo P (1995) Glaucoma and myopia. A study by means of color Doppler imaging.

Third European Professors Workshop on the Quantification of Ocular Blood Flow in Glaucoma, October 7, 1995, Edinburgh
9. Harris A, Sergott RC, Spaeth GL, Katz JL, Shoemaker JA, Martin BJ(1994) Color Doppler analysis of ocular vessel blood velocity in normal-tension glaucoma. Am J Ophthalmol 118:-642-9
10. Greve EL, Buimer R, Duijm HFA, Geijssen HC (1995) SLO Fluorescein angiography of the peripapillary choroid before and after trabeculectomy. Invest Ophthalmol Vis Sci 36:S436 (abstract)

Therapeutic Problems of Normal Tension Glaucoma

Y. Kitazawa and T. Yamamoto

Department of Ophthalmology, Gifu University School of Medicine, 40 Tsukasa-machi, Gifu-shi 500, Gifu, Japan

Introduction

The pathogenetic mechanism(s) of optic nerve damage of normal tension glaucoma (NTG) still remain to be clarified. However, it is unanimously accepted that the disease is most likely multifactorial and, therefore, a variety of treatment modalities should be considered in treating each individual patient.

The aim of this report is to briefly review the results of our two different, therapeutic attempts. The results of our clinical studies and their practical implications will be discussed.

Materials and Results

Ocular Hypotensive Therapy

In an attempt to determine the therapeutic value of surgery in NTG, we initiated a prospective study about 4 years ago in which we operated upon only one eye of NTG patients, leaving the contralateral fellow eye untreated. All patients had visual fields with either threat of fixation or progressive deterioration while followed up without medication. To be eligible for study enrollment, IOP and visual field changes had to be symmetrical: the mean diurnal IOP difference was less than 2 mm Hg and the difference in mean deviation (MD) was less than 10 dB in each individual. As a method of surgery, we chose trabeculectomy (TLE) with adjunctive intraoperative mitomycin C (MMC) administration, since, as we already noted, a large majority of high pressure glaucoma patients achieved IOPs ranging 5-12 mm Hg after MMC TLE [1].

Sixteen NTG patients were successfully followed up for at least 2 years and their clinical data were analyzed. Five were males and 11 were females; the mean age was 57.8 years. IOP and the mean deviation of Humphrey central 30-2 field were very similar between pairs of eyes (Table 1).

Table 1. Pretreatment IOP and mean deviation.

	Operated eyes	Unoperated eyes
IOP (mm Hg)	14.5 ± 1.8	14.8 ± 2.2
Mean deviation (dB)	-11.9 ± 5.8	-9.7 ± 6.9

Mean ± standard deviation.

The eye with the more severely affected visual field was operated upon.

The IOP was reduced by 4.8 mm Hg on average on the operated side at the last visit, while it remained identical on the unoperated side. The mean deviation of the visual field was not significantly changed regardless of surgery; the MD appeared to be at least stable in 15 operated eyes and in 13 unoperated eyes.

However, point by point comparison using Statpac II was more enlightening. Glaucoma change probability analysis determines the statistical significance of change of differential light sensitivity at each point. We subtracted the number of significantly worsened points from the number of significantly improved points in the latest field as compared with the field at the time of surgery.

On the average 3.5 points improved in the operated eye, while 1.8 points worsened in the unoperated eye.

The difference was statistically significant by

Wilcoxon signed-rank test ($P = 0.03$), indicating that when compared point by point the visual fields of the operated eyes did better than those of the unoperated, contralateral eyes.

Operative complications included shallow anterior chamber, bleb leakage and cataract progression. Lasting hypotonous maculopathy was noted in one eye. None of the complications required surgery. Visual acuity deteriorated by 2 lines or more in four of the operated eyes and in five of the unoperated eyes.

Systemic Administration of Ca^{2+} Blockers

A vascular, or rather microcirculatory, insufficiency independent of IOP level has been implicated in the development of optic nerve damage in glaucoma. The association of vasospastic syndromes with NTG is well known. Collagen diseases involving vessels are reportedly more prevalent [2] and disc hemorrhages are more frequently seen in NTG [3]. Disc hemorrhages are not only highly prevalent in NTG patients, but their location is closely correlated to that of retinal nerve fiber layer defect (NFLD) in NTG. The cause of disc hemorrhage remains to be clarified; however, undoubtedly, the loss of integrity of small vessels and NFLD go hand in hand.

The etiology of circulatory disturbances is likely to be divergent. The only reportedly promising therapeutic approach directed at the improvement of blood supply is systemic Ca^{2+} blockers. We reported beneficial effects of oral nifedipine in a subset of NTG patients in 1989 [4]. Patients who responded favorably to nifedipine were characterized by improvement of peripheral vasospastic response to cold exposure, by younger age and by lower visual field corrected pattern standard deviation (CPSD).

Recently we tested the therapeutic effect of brovincamine, a vincamine alkaloid, which dilates intracranial vessels as a Ca^{2+} blocker [5]. This was a prospective, randomized study in 28 eyes of 28 NTG patients matched for age, visual field, and past history of disc hemorrhages. Each patient was randomly allocated to either brovincamine fumarate 20 mg tid or placebo tid. In addition to routine eye examinations, perimetry was performed with a Humphrey Field Analyzer using the program central 30-2 at least every 6 months. The minimum follow-up was 30 months.

The significance of visual field changes was judged based on the Statpac II linear regression analysis. Also, when reproducible loss of threshold of 10 dB or greater was demonstrated for at least one point, the field was judged to have worsened regardless of MD slope. We found that in the brovincamine-treated group six eyes improved and eight were unchanged. In contrast, in the placebo-treated group two eyes worsened and 12 were unchanged (Table 2).

Table 2. Visual field outcome (number of cases)

Treatment group	Improved	Unchanged	Aggravated	Total
Brovincamine	6	8	0	14
Control	0	12	2	14
Total	6	20	2	28

The difference was statistically significant ($P = 0.012$, Fisher direct probability test).

Stepwise discriminant analysis was carried out by using 12 clinical factors. Significant contributing factors for favorable outcome were the use of brovincamine, better cold recovery rate, and higher systolic systemic blood pressure. Here again, reactivity of blood vessels was identified as a prognostic factor.

Comments

The two independent studies conducted in our department indicated that both surgical reduction of IOP and oral administration of Ca^{2+} blocker can be beneficial in preventing the progression of optic nerve damage in a substantial number of NTG patients. The beneficial effect of surgical reduction was recently reported by Hitchings et al. In their study, as in ours, only one eye was operated upon in 18 patients with NTG. Their results demonstrated less deterioration of visual field in the operated eyes than in the unoperated contralateral fellow eyes [6]. Using color Doppler imaging technique, a recent report indicated that topical verapamil, a Ca^{2+} blocker, reduced vascular resistance of the central retinal artery in normal subjects [7]. Thus, the beneficial effect of Ca^{2+} blockers seems to be due to the improvement of optic nerve blood flow. However, it remains to be elucidated how to determine the responsiveness of each individual NTG patient to a specific therapy. There is evidence that NTG can be classified into more than two subsets, based not only on the appearance of the disc but also on the vasospastic response of the peripheral vessels, immunological features, and ocular and systemic factors. Hence, further efforts must be made to clarify the pathogenetic mechanisms of optic nerve damage in NTG. Better understanding of the pathogenesis of the ailment will help us develop novel and effective therapeutic modalities.

References

1. Kitazawa Y, Kawase K, Matsushita H, et al. (1991) Trabeculectomy with mitomycin: a comparative study with fluorouracil. Arch Ophthalmol 109:1693-1698
2. Cartwright MJ, Grajewski AL, Friedberg ML, et al. (1992) Immune related disease and normal-tension glaucoma. A case-control study. Arch Ophthalmol 110:500-502
3. Kitazawa Y, Shirato S, Yamamoto T (1986) Optic disc hemorrhage in low-tension glaucoma. Ophthalmology 93:853-857.
4. Kitazawa Y, Shirai H, Go FJ (1989) The effect of Ca^{2+} antagonist on visual field in low-tension glaucoma. Graefes Arch Clin Exp Ophthalmol 227:408-412
5. Sawada A, Kitazawa Y, Yamamoto T, et al (1996) Brovincamine prevents progression of visual field defects in normal-tension glaucoma. Ophthalmology 103:283-288
6. Hitchings RA, Wu J, Poinoosawmy D, McNaught A (1995) Surgery for normal tension glaucoma. Br J Ophthalmol 79:402-406
7. Netland PA, Grosskreutz CL, Feke GT, et al. (1995) Color Doppler ultrasound analysis of ocular circulation after topical calcium channel blocker. Am J Ophthalmol 119:694-700

Discussion

Question: Di Tizio

My question is for Prof. Kitazawa. You said that following surgery, intraocular pressure should be around 12 mmHg to avoid damages to the optic nerve. My assumption then is that all patients shoud be operated, since with medical theraphy is not possible to reach 12 mmHg. I personally prefer the use of Mitomycin or 5-Fluorouracil. Can you make a comment on this?

Answer: Kitazawa

Yes, whenever I feel that ocular hypotensive therapy helps and that the visual field is very bad and is definitively progressing I certainly count on trabeculotomy.

Question:

To Prof. Kitazawa. I was very interested in your presentation of an apparent improvement in patients with normal pressure glaucoma. In the first study you showed that there weren't any differences in the main deviation between treated and untreated groups and finally after you did operations you found there wasn't any difference in the mean deviation. I think it's very important in this case that you show us those points that improved and those points that got worse. In fact, the amount of deviation those points had was the same. A likely scenario is that if you have a point that's more damaged, it will vary so much that you will not be able to show change. Yet a point which is relatively mildly damaged will more readily show the change.

Answer: Kitazawa

How to determine a progression or a stability of the visual field is a very difficult task at least for us, and what you have just pointed out could be that the cases in our study don't have a very solid evidence against or for what you have just commented on.

Question:

To Dr. Greve. You have got a very large collection of low tension glaucoma data. You think that disease in one eye is more frequent than in the other eye? I have a question to Dr. Kitazawa: Were actually these patients progressing before surgery? The other question is: The starting mean ocular pressure was 14 mmHg, which is rather low. I think it's probably because this is a characteristic of the

Japanese population and you actually lowered pressure down to 12 mmHg, which is only a 2 mm mercury drop. I think that it is quite difficult to say that 12 could be a sensible target pressure. Probably we should try quantifying in percentages, saying well in the normal tension glaucoma group a 30% IOP drop. I am sure that the Caucasian population would probably show a higher pressure than 14 mm of mercury; if we should say 30% that may be enough or may not be enough.

Answer: Greve

Your question was whether there was a general difference in our normal pressure glaucoma population. No simple answer.

Answer: Kitazawa

Most of them were definitively progressing in the sense that the point nearest to the center has been loosing its sensitivity; it is why we decided to operate or at least to do something.

Question:

And do you think 12 mmHg is actually a target IOP?

Answer: Kitazawa

Not in these cases, I said 12 mm mercury based on the data of our literature. I personally feel that in the group of patients we operated 12 mmHg is not a very good target pressure.

Question: Quigley

Perhaps the audience is not all familiar with the differences in the normal distribution of aplanation intraocular pressure in Japan compared to Europe. What definition did you use? Did you use a pressure criterion to define normal pressure glaucoma and if so, what did you use and why did you say that relative to Japanese versus European numbers?

Answer: Kitazawa

Let me answer your second question. A cut of pressure was 20 mmHg just as you do in the US. That cut of pressure reduced to 13, just to make our study compatible with yours. The papers from our Institutions would never be accepted by American journals, I mean, not American journals in general, I am saying American ophtalmological journals.

Question: Quigley

This is a very interesting point though, because if we say that normal glaucoma patients means that a person has glaucoma in a normal range of pressure, then the normal range of pressure for a Japanese person seems to be 18 instead of 20 and I think that, as you and another have reported, there seems to be a difference in the rate or proportion of normal pressure glaucoma patients when one does that.

Answer: Kitazawa

I will certainly convey those general comments to my collegues in Japan.

Answer: Quigley

I guarantee that one journal will do that if you send them the paper.

Answer: Kitazawa

In every western testbook, mean IOP is around 15 or 15.5 with a standard deviation of 2.5. A nationwide population survey in Japan showed it was not necessarily applicable to the Japanese. What we found was a mean IOP somewhere around 13.5 mm mercury and even lower. So if we take two standard deviations, the upper limit of normal IOP in the Japanese must be around 18 mm mercury. That's the result of the study.

Question: Virno

My question is to Dr. Kitazawa. Did you evaluate the hypotensive effect during treatment with nifedipine?

Answer: Kitazawa

We made that study more than 8 years ago, and at that time we knew much less and we paid much less attention to the systemic effects of nifedipine and certainly not to IOP; also nifedipine brings about many more systemic side effects including standing hypotension and facial flushing. After we recognized the side effects, while that particular study was in progress we stopped using nifedipine. So obviously a decrease in systemic blood pressure caused by nifedipine should not do any good at least theoretically, and at the moment I don't like to advocate the use of nifedipine as a therapeutic means to treat normal pressure glaucoma. I hope I have answered your question.

SURGICAL TREATMENT

Contact Transscleral Cyclophotocoagulation in the Treatment of Refractory Glaucoma

R. Brancato and R. Carassa

Department of Ophthalmology and Visual Sciences, University of Milan, S. Raffaele Hospital, Via Olgettina 60, 20132 Milano, Italy

Introduction

Contact transscleral cyclophotocoagulation (CTCP) with the Nd:YAG laser is an effective procedure in lowering intraocular pressure (IOP) in refractory glaucomatous eyes [1, 2]. In previous studies we demonstrated the possibility of producing thermal damage in the ciliary body using a semiconductor diode laser and we determined the best laser settings [3,4]. The aim of the present study was to assess the long-term clinical effectiveness of CTCP with a diode laser in eyes suffering from refractory glaucoma.

Materials and Methods

Eyes affected by glaucoma refractory to conventional medical, laser and surgical therapy were selected. All eyes had an uncontrolled IOP despite maximum tolerated medical therapy; laser trabeculoplasty had been performed when applicable and all eyes in which surgery was advisable had already undergone one or more filtering procedures.

Both seeing eyes, in which IOP reduction was indicated to preserve visual acuity, and blind (defined as no light perception) eyes, with IOP-related pain and in which IOP reduction was advisable to relieve pain, were included.

The eyes underwent CTCP using either an EOS-3000 (Optikon, Italy) or a VISULAS II (Zeiss, Germany) continuous-wave diode laser emitting 810 nm light. The lasers were coupled with a quartz optic fiber ending in a 3 mm focusing tip. At the end of the follow-up time, ultrasound biomicroscopic examination (UBM, Humphrey - Zeiss, San Leandro, CA) with a 50 MHz transducer was performed, according to previous studies [5], to evaluate the presence of alterations of the sclera and conjunctiva. Patients treated in the last 2 years of the study were examined before treatment to verify that the ciliary body position was consistent with the probe position chosen for CTCP.

Before treatment the patient was given retrobulbar anesthesia using 3 ml of 2% lidocaine and was placed in a supine position. Treatment was carried out by applying 16-20 laser spots over 360° (4-5 per quadrant). Spot energy was 4J using the EOS2000 or 2J using the VISULAS II diode laser due to geometric differences in the optic fiber and tip. The procedure was carried out by positioning the tip of the fiber 1.5 mm posterior to the CLJ (tip rim tangent to the CLJ) or at the distance measured by UBM.

Complete ocular examination was performed 1 h, 1 week and 1 month after the treatment and subsequent visits were scheduled depending on the conditions of the eye.

If the IOP reduction was not satisfactory at 1 month, the treatment was repeated using the same parameters until the cumulative number of spots delivered reached 80 (four treatments). Eyes in which IOP control was not achieved after four treatments were considered refractory to CTCP.

Glaucoma medications were tapered after IOP reduction following treatment.

Only patients with at least 6 months of follow-up were included in the study.

Success was defined as the achievement of an IOP > 2 and ≤ 21 mm Hg in seeing eyes and as the resolution of pain in blind eyes.

Table 1. Preoperative diagnosis

Diagnosis	Seeing eyes	Blind eyes
Neovascular glaucoma	10	16
Congenital glaucoma	11	1
Glaucoma secondary to retinal detachment surgery	9	4
Aphakic glaucoma	10	0
Primary glaucoma	18	3
Glaucoma secondary to uveitis	6	3
Traumatic glaucoma	6	2
Total	70	29

In order to compare pre- and postoperative ocular hypotensive therapies, a glaucoma medication score was defined. Topical drugs were assigned the following scores: dipivefrin = 1; ß-blocker, pilocarpine 2% and clonidine = 2; pilocarpine 3% = 2.5; pilocarpine 4% = 3. Oral carbonic anhydrase inhibitors were assigned 2 points per tablet/day.

The differences between initial and final IOPs and visual acuity were analyzed using Student's *t* test for paired samples, while differences between initial and final medication scores were evaluated using the Wilcoxon signed rank test.

Results

Seventy seeing eyes of 67 patients (41 males and 29 females) and 29 blind and painful eyes of 29 patients (13 males and 16 females) were treated. The mean age was 53.91 ± 20.1 years in seeing eyes and 57.1 ± 20.7 years in blind eyes. The follow-up time was 23.4 ± 12.7 months (range 6-50) in seeing eyes and 20.5 ± 10.9 months (range 6-39) in blind eyes.

In the seeing eye group, pre- and post treatment IOP values were 35.9 ± 10.7 and 18.47 ± 7.4 mm Hg respectively. The difference was statistically significant ($t = 11.16$; $p = 0.0000$). In the blind eye group, pre- and post-CTCP IOP values were 49.21 ± 12.7 and 23.62 ± 14.2 mm Hg, respectively, with a statistically significant difference ($t = 7.21$; p = 0.0000) (Table 2).

Table 3 reports the number of treatments carried out in both groups. The mean ± SD number of treatments was 2.25 ± 1.4 in the seeing eye group and 2.03 ± 1.3 in the blind eye group.

Success was achieved in 55 of the 70 seeing eyes (78.6%) and in 28 of the 29 blind eyes (97%). In the seeing eye group, success was achieved in six of the 11 congenital glaucomas, in four of the six glaucomas secondary to uveitis, in seven of the nine glaucomas secondary to retinal detachment surgery, in two of the six post-traumatic glaucomas, in nine of the ten neovascular glaucomas, in 17 of the 18 primary glaucomas and in all the aphakic glaucomas. In the blind eye group the only unsuccessful eye was a neovascular glaucoma. Statistical analysis of the differences among success rates in the various disease groups was not applicable due to the small sample size.

At the end of the follow-up, visual acuity (VA) was increased in two cases (2.8%), stable in 53 (75.8%), and reduced in 15 (21.4%), i.e., by two or more lines in ten eyes, from 2.5/10 to Count Finger (CF) in one eye, from CF to No Light Perception (NLP) in one eye, and from Light Perception (LP) to NLP in three eyes. Mean ± SD pre- and post-treatment VAs were 0.16 ± 0.22 and 0.13 ± 0.21, respectively.

The difference in VA before and after treat-

Table 2. Data related IOP (mm Hg)

	Patients (n)	Pre-treatment IOP (mm Hg)[a]	Post-treatment IOP (mm Hg)[a]	Percent decrease[a]	*t*	*p*
Seeing eyes	70	35.93 (10.7)	18.47 (7.4)	44.31 (24.6)	−11.16	0.0000
Blind eyes	29	49.2 (12.7)	23.62 (14.2)	49.55 (32.2)	−7.21	0.0000

[a] Mean (SD)

Table 3. Number of treatments

Number of treatments	Seeing eyes	Blind eyes
1	28	15
2	19	6
3	7	2
4	16	6

ment was not statistically significant ($t = 1.79$, $p = 0.08$).

At the end of the follow-up in the seeing eye group, the medication score was increased in 15 eyes (21.4%), unchanged in 26 eyes (37.2%) and reduced in 29 eyes (41.4%).

Median (25th, 75th percentile) pre- and post-treatment medication scores were 6 (4, 7) and 5 (3.75, 6), respectively, and the difference was significant ($U = 322$, $p = 0.04$). In the blind eye group, the medication score was increased in two eyes (6.9%), stable in 14 eyes (48.3%) and reduced in 13 eyes (44.8%). Median (25th, 75th percentile) pre- and posttreatment medication scores were 4 (2.5, 6) and 2 (2, 4), respectively, and the reduction was significant ($U = 3.63$, $p = 0.001$).

As for complications no conjunctival injuries were detected and no IOP spikes exceeding 8 mm Hg were measured within 2 h after laser treatment. Mild to moderate reactive iridocyclitis (1+ - 2+ Tyndall, flare and/or cells), was present in 32 (45.7%) seeing eyes and in 18 (62%) blind eyes; one seeing eye (1.4%), which had been characterized by the occurrence of several audible pops during the energy delivery, developed a vitreous hemorrhage and another seeing eye (1.4%), along with a blind eye (3.4%), developed a phthisis.

No scleral alteration and, in particular, no focal thinning were detected in the treated area neither on biomicroscopic nor on ultrasound biomicroscopic examination. All fellow eyes were carefully monitored and no sign of sympathetic ophthalmia was detected.

Discussion

CTCP has been proved to reduce IOP in refractory glaucomatous eyes[1, 2]. The Nd:YAG laser was employed for treatment because the 1064 nm wavelength is highly transmitted through the human sclera (75%), but poorly absorbed by melanin. The introduction of the 810 nm diode laser has raised interest in transscleral photocoagulation due to its higher absorption by melanin (twice that of 1064 nm Nd:YAG radiation). However, the lower scleral transmission of the 810 nm wavelength (35%) is largely overcome by using contact techniques which allow scleral indentation, as shown by Vogel et al. [6]. Based on these considerations, histologic studies were performed on rabbit [1], on cadaver [7] and on living human [2] eyes demonstrating ciliary body photocoagulation with the use of diode laser and allowing determination of the best laser settings.

On the basis of these experiences, an ongoing clinical study was started [8-11].

In the only other study of diode CTCP [12] 30 eyes affected by refractory glaucoma were treated using 16/18 contact applications evenly spaced over 270° and centered 1.2 mm posterior to the surgical limbus. Power was set at 1.5, 1.75 or 2 W and a duration of 2 s was used. All patients had a 6 week follow-up, while 22 had a 3 month follow-up. Mean IOP decreased from an initial value of 37 mm Hg to 21 mm Hg at 6 weeks and 23 mm Hg at 3 months. Out of 22 eyes, 17 had an IOP below or equal to 23 mm Hg. No major complication and, in particular, no hypotony were reported and VA changes were minimal (only one eye with neovascular glaucoma went from Hand Motion (HM) to NLP. In 21 eyes, one or more "pops" could be heard during the application. Mild superficial burns were reported in 12 eyes.

Hawkins and Stewart [13] presented a study of the noncontact technique. A total of 30 refractory glaucomatous eyes were treated with 40/45 100 μm spots over 360°, 1 mm from the limbus, defocused 1 mm posteriorly, using a 990 ms pulse duration and a 1200 mW power output. In the 19 successful patients, 12 months after surgery, IOP dropped from a preoperative value of 32.5 mm Hg to 20.8 mm Hg. As for complications, two eyes developed complete visual loss despite an effective IOP drop. Mild conjunctival hyperemia and uveitis were also reported in all cases.

In the present study, 70 seeing eyes were treated to reduce IOP to or below 21 mm Hg; success was achieved in 55 of them (78.6%).

In 29 blind and painful eyes treated to relieve

pain, success was achieved in 28 (97%). Mean percent IOP reduction, at the end of the follow-up period, was 44.3% in the seeing eye group and 49.5% in the blind eye group.

Due to the small sample size, statistical analysis could not be performed among the subgroups. Nevertheless glaucomas secondary to uveitis and to retinal detachment surgery, along with congenital and traumatic glaucomas, seemed less responsive to CTCP than the other glaucomas studied.

In order to minimize the risk of major complications reported using high total energy [5], we decided to use low total energies, with the possibility to repeat the treatment. This led to a relative high retreatment rate. By study design, the treatment was complete after four laser sessions, and therefore all unsuccessful cases underwent four treatments before failure could be affirmed.

VA did not show a significant difference before CTCP and at the end of the follow up. Three eyes affected by neovascular glaucoma secondary to advanced diabetic retinopathy went from LP to NLP despite controlled IOP (15 and 6 mm Hg). This late VA reduction was likely related to the worsening of an already severe retinal damage, though this statement cannot be confirmed due to the absence of a control group. One eye affected by glaucoma secondary to retinal detachment surgery went from CF to NLP after developing hypotony and phthisis. One eye went from 2.5/10 to CF despite controlled IOP (20 mm Hg) due to a late worsening of a preexisting bullous keratopathy. Ten eyes had a progressive VA reduction of two or more lines: among these, four were failures and six showed progression of a preexisting cataract.

The treatment allowed significant reduction of the medical therapy. As for complications, one of the major concerns with CTCP is the risk of sympathetic ophthalmia, since seven cases are reported in the literature, all following Nd:YAG treatment [14-19].

In this study, all fellow eyes were carefully monitored during the follow-up and no sign of such a complication was detected.

As concerns the onset of deep hypotony, which used to be a major risk with cyclocryotherapy, one blind eye suffering from glaucoma secondary to retinal detachment and one seeing eye affected by neovascular glaucoma became hypotonic and developed a phthisis.

No damage to conjunctiva, sclera or lens was detected. In particular no scleral thinning was revealed by ultrasound biomicroscopy. The absence of superficial burns, which were reported in one study [12], is probably related to the focalizing tip of the probe used in the present investigation.

Conclusions

According to this study diode laser CTCP is an effective procedure in lowering IOP in most refractory glaucomatous eyes and in relieving IOP-related pain in blind eyes, with minor side effects and minimal discomfort. The high success rate, with minor or no influence on VA, allows us to recommend CTCP as an effective procedure in eyes with glaucoma refractory to conventional therapies.

References

1. Brancato R, Leoni G, Trabucchi G, Pietroni C (1989) Contact transscleral cyclophotocoagulation with Nd:YAG laser in uncontrolled glaucoma. Ophthalmic Surg 20:547-551
2. Schuman JS, Puliafito CA, Allingham RR, et al. (1990) Contact transscleral continuous-wave Nd:YAG laser cyclophotocoagulation. Ophthalmology 97:571-580
3. Brancato R, Leoni G, Trabucchi G, Cappellini A (1991) Histopathology of continuous wave Nd:YAG and diode laser contact transscleral lesion in rabbit ciliary body. Invest Ophthalmol Vis Sci (Suppl) 32:1586
4. Verdi M, Brancato R, Trabucchi G, Carassa R, Gobbi P (1993) A comparative histopathologic study of contact transscleral cyclophotocoagulation performed on the human eye with Nd:YAG and diode lasers. Invest Ophthalmol Vis Sci (Suppl) 34:737
5. Pavlin CJ, Sherar MD, Harasiewicz K, Foster FS (1991) Clinical use of ultrasound biomicroscopy. Ophthalmology 98:287-295
6. Vogel A, Dlugos C, Nuffer R, Birngruber R (1991) Optical properties of human sclera and their consequences for transscleral laser applications. Laser Surg Med 11:331-340
7. Hennis HL, Assia E, Stewart WC, Legler UFC, Apple DJ (1991) Transscleral cyclophotocoagulation using semiconductor diode laser in cadaver eyes. Ophthalmic Surg 22:274-278

8. Carassa RG, Trabucchi G, Bettin P, Fiori M, Brancato R (1992) Contact transscleral cyclophotocoagulation (CTCP) with diode laser: a pilot clinical study. Invest Ophthalmol Vis Sci (Suppl) 33:1019
9. Carassa RG, Brancato R, Trabucchi G, Bettin P, Fiori M (1993) A 1-year follow-up study of contact transscleral cyclophotocoagulation with diode laser. Invest Ophthalmol Vis Sci (Suppl) 34:737
10. Brancato R, Carassa RG, Trabucchi G (1993) Contact transscleral cyclophotocoagulation with the diode laser. Ophthalmology 100:110
11. Brancato R, Carassa RG, Bettin P, Fiori M, Trabucchi G (1995) Contact transscleral cyclophotocoagulation with the diode laser in refractory glaucoma. Eur J Ophthalmol 5:32-39
12. Gaasterland DE, Abrams DA, Belcher CD, et al. (1992) A multicenter study of contact diode laser transscleral cyclophotocoagulation in glaucoma patients. Invest Ophthalmol Vis Sci (Suppl) 33:1019
13. Hawkins TA, Stewart WC (1993) One-year result of semiconductor transscleral cyclophotocoagulation in patients with glaucoma. Arch Ophthalmol 111:488-491
14. Edward DP, Brown SVL, Higginbotham E, Jennings T, Tessler HH, Tso MOM (1989) Sympathetic ophthalmia following Nd:YAG cyclotherapy. Ophthalmic Surg 20:544-546
15. Brown SVL, Higginbotham E, Tessler H (1990) Sympathetic ophthalmia following Nd:YAG cyclotherapy. Ophthalmic Surg 21:736-737
16. Tessler HH, Lam S, Wilensky J, Higginbotham E, Brown S (1992) Sympathetic ophthalmia after noncontact neodymium: YAG cyclotherapy. Presented at the Third International Symposium on Uveitis; May 27, 1992, Brussels, Belgium
17. Lam S, Tessler HH, Lam BL, Wilensky JT (1992) High incidence of sympathetic ophthalmia after contact and noncontact neodymium: YAG cyclotherapy. Ophthalmology 99:1818-1822
18. Pastor SA, Iwach A, Nozik RA, Hetherington J, Fellman R (1993) Presumed sympathetic ophthalmia following Nd:YAG transscleral cyclophotocoagulation. J Glaucoma 2:30-31
19. Bechrakis NE, Mueller-Stolzenburg MW, Helbig H, Foerster MH (1994) Sympathetic ophthalmia following laser cyclocoagulation. Arch Ophthalmol 112:80-84

A Controversial Decision: When to Operate on Chronic Glaucoma

F. Ponte

University Eye Clinic, Via Liborio Giuffrè 13, 90127 Palermo, Italy

The decision to perform surgery for chronic glaucoma depends on whether surgery has to be done early or is required only after medical treatment failure. Furtermore, consideration must be given not only to the patient's needs and the ophthalmologist's skill, but also to the answers to some more general questions:

1. What is the aim of the therapy?
2. How can that goal be achieved?
3. What are the therapy risks and benefits compared with the natural history of the disease? And, in the case of more than one therapy, which has the best risk/benefit relationship?

As far as the first question, the aim is to stabilize the clinical picture by blocking the disease or slowing its worsening as much as possible. This can be done only if we have enough sensible and specific clinical tools to detect early clinical signs of damage or disease worsening.

Today, computerized perimetry is the most reliable technique (and the most popular), even though media opacities, such as cataract, sometimes make identification of glaucomatous damage difficult. Other, more sophisticated, methods, such as study of the ganglion retinal fibers, the morphometric study of the optic nerve head, or the electrophysiological methods are not yet suitable at the routine clinical level.

As far the therapeutical outcome, the ideal treatment should reduce the ocular pressure under critical values for the extent of 24 hours. However, the current pharmacology of chronic glaucoma acts on only one risk factor of the disease: the ocular hypertension. Thus, it is not always followed by the arrest of the disease.

The answer to the third question arise from the knowledge of the disease natural history and from refined drugs available whose side effects and eventual complications have to be carefully evaluted. Moreover, the personal professional experience cannot be understated.

In the past, the standard in case of first therapy of open angle glaucoma was the medical treatment. In the last twenty years, such rule has been fighted.

In the early '80, the trabeculectomy get a so valid surgical option that the early surgery [1], or after a short minor medical treatment (ß-blockers, f.i.) [7], has been considered the best method to reduce the ocular pressure and arrest the visual field damage evolution. The following rationales are proposed in favour of such therapeutical direction:

1. If the drug daily administration has been twice a day, we obtain the control of the optic nerve and the visual field damage only in 1/3 of the cases [7]. If the frequency of administration is higher and we use miotics, the patients's compliance gets lower and the drugs can be irregularly utilised or definitely ceased.
2. The earlier the surgery is performed, the less serious the post-op complications [1], in particular, cataract and post-operative synechias. Prolonged medical treatment does not improve the post-trabeculectomy outcome. By contrast, short medical treatment prevents disease evolution and surgery can yield the best results.
3. The histologic studies of Grierson et al. [3] on the trabeculum in two groups of patients, one operated on early and the other after years of medical therapy, show a significantly higher loss of trabecular cells in the second group. However, many other studies disagree with these results. Indeed, from the point od view of tonometry, the success of filtering surgery in

glaucoma cannot be questioned (normalized ocular pressure in 75%-85% of cases) and the mean tonometric values are lower than those obtained with medical therapy. Nevertheless, the true problem is that glaucoma therapy has to be evaluated not only in terms of ocular pressure but also on the basis of optic disc cupping, visual field, and visual acuity, as well as job, compliance and life style of each patient.
Smith [6] reported a 18 year follow-up study of a group of chronic glaucoma patients. Randomly, 50% of patients underwent surgery and 50% were treated with medical therapy. The study showed no correlation between visual field and the ocular pressure. Moreover, surgery seems to have preserved the visual field, and medical therapy maintained the visual acuity.
Demailly's clinical review [2] of long-term functional prognosis agrees with Smith's point of view. Visual field deterioration is significantly delayed after an adequate trabeculectomy. However, visual acuity damage is already present 1 year after surgery, generally, due to cataract, ranging about 0.3-0.5.
Quigley [5] showed that post-surgical nicthemeral pressure control may be insufficient, even in the presence of a good filtering bleb. To some extent, this accounts for the 15% of operated eyes showing progression of visual field damage [4], and further evidence is given by the percentage of eyes needing medical treatment after surgery. The percentage increases with time after surgery, involving about one third of cases 2 years after surgery. In Demailly's opinion, 50% of eyes need additional medical theraphy 5 years after surgery.
In Watson's report [7] on the trabeculum, there was no evidence found of any lesion related to long-term medical therapy; other authors [2] demonstrated ultrastructural trabecular lesions in primate eyes after experimental trabeculectomy.
Moreover, even when performed early, trabeculectomy has a number of complication that are potentially dangerous for visual function. Atalamia (a shallow anterior chamber) and a cataract are the most frequent, with a mean incidence of 5% [5]; endophthalmitis is less frequent (0.5%-1%) [6, 8]. As mentioned above, cataract, due to hypotony and hypotalamia, (a shallow anterior chamber) is the main cause of visual acuity loss after trabeculectomy. A review [2] confirms the higher cataract risk of surgery compared with medical treatment.
For a glaucomatous patient without or with ± lens opacities at the beginning of the disease, the cataract risk (lens opacity: ++ or +++) is 46% 5 years after trabeculectomy vs 12.5% for a patient with medical therapy only ($P < 0.001$) [4]. However, there is no doubt that the cataract incidence is related to the age of the patient, with positive correlation after 55 years of age ($P < 0.001$).
In conclusion, early surgery as the best choice for treating glaucoma has still to be demonstrated. Today, it seems most rational to start treatment of a glaucoma patient with medical therapy because of at least two reasons: (1) we do not know the whole mechanism of the disease at the level of the trabeculum and optic nerve head; (2) no strong relationship exists between ocular pressure and visual field damage. However, progression damage, as shown by computerized perimetry, the need for maximal medical therapy with relatively poor compliance, the patient's life expectancy, and the eventual lens opacities support (alone or associated) a surgical resolution, which should be "cum grano salis", neither early nor too late and hence not useful.
Therefore, the ophthalmologist must decide when to operate on a patient by patient basis, relying not only on basic knowledge of the disease but also on own medical and surgical experience.

References

1. Cairns JE (1981) Indication for surgery in glaucoma. Glaucoma 3: 307-310
2. Demailly Ph (1989) Traitment actuel du glaucome primitif à angle ouvert. Masson, Paris
3. Grierson I, Lee WR, Abraham S (1978) The effects of pilocarpine on the morphology of the human outflow apparatus. Br J Ophthalmol 62: 302-313
4. Kidd MN, O'Conner M (1985) Progression of field loss after trabeculectomy: a five year follow-up. Brit J Ophthalmol 69: 827-831
5. Quigley HA (1984) A revaluation of glaucoma management. In: Zimmerman TL, Monica ML (eds) Controversies in glaucoma. Little Brown, Boston
6. Smith RJH (1986) The Lang lecture 1986. The enigma of primary open angle glaucoma. Trans Ophthalmol Soc UK 105: 618-633
7. Watson PG (1987) When to operate to open-angle glaucoma? Eye I: 51-54

8. Wilson R, Hertzmark E, Walker A, Childshaw K, Epstein DL (1987) A case-control study of risk factors in open-angle glaucoma. Arch Ophthalmol 105: 1066-1071

Antifibrosis Drugs in Filtration Surgery

H. D. Jampel

Department of Ophthalmology, Johns Hopkins University School of Medicine, Baltimore, MD 21287-9205, USA

Introduction

The two most important advances over the past 10 years in glaucoma filtration surgery are the introduction of antifibrosis drugs to improve the success rate and the development of flap suturing techniques to reduce the risk of hypotony and flat anterior chamber. The story of the development of antifibrosis drugs in trabeculectomy is one of both the logical application of scientific principles and good fortune. As with any new therapy, practitioners have been confronted with the complications of the use of these agents.

History

Researchers at the Bascom Palmer Eye Institute in the early 1980s borrowed from the experience of their colleagues who were using 5-fluorouracil to treat experimental proliferative vitreoretinopathy. They demonstrated, first in monkeys [1] and then in high risk glaucoma patients [2], that postoperative subconjunctival injections of 5-fluorouracil increased the success rate of filtration surgery. This led to the initiation of the multicenter, National Eye Institute funded Flourouracil Filtering Surgery Study (FFSS) [3]. The protocol of the study, limited to eyes that had undergone previous glaucoma or cataract surgery, required an intensive regimen of up to 21 injections of 5-fluorouracil over a 14 day period [3]. Smaller studies undertaken while the FFSS was in progress showed good results with many fewer injections [4, 5]. During this time the main drawbacks encountered were corneal epithelial defects from the inhibition of corneal epithelial migration and division, and the inconvenience of multiple injections.

Although Chen had published several years earlier [6] that mitomycin C given topically at the time of trabeculectomy had a beneficial effect upon the outcome of surgery, it was not until 1991, when Palmer published his paper [7], that the use of mitomycin C began in the United States. Theoretically it seemed unlikely that a single application of any agent would inhibit the wound healing response to a sufficient extent to result in lower intraocular pressure. Clinical results, however, proved theory wrong. Quickly there were two randomized trials demonstrating that a single intraoperative application of mitomycin C was as effective as multiple subconjunctival injections of 5-fluorouracil [8, 9]. The beneficial effects of mitomycin C [10] as well as 5-fluorouracil [11] have now been shown to last for at least 3 years.

It was not long, however, before enthusiasm for the use of mitomycin C became tempered by multiple reports of hypotony and hypotony maculopathy [12-14]. A literature grew up around how to avoid and reverse this sight threatening complication [15-17].

Knowing that an intraoperative application of mitomycin C was effective, investigators wondered if intraoperative 5-fluorouracil might be effective as well.

Although preliminary reports of intraoperative 5-fluorouracil have been encouraging [18, 19], its utility remains to be definitely demonstrated.

The Use of Antifibrosis Agents in Trabeculectomy Today

Why Use an Antifibrosis Agent?

Antifibrosis agents should be used in selected trabeculectomy surgery because they have been shown to increase the success rate. This is true for eyes that have undergone previous cataract or glaucoma surgery [8, 9, 11]. There is strong evidence from multiple case series that the use of these agents increases the success rate of trabeculectomy surgery in uveitic [20, 21] and neovascular glaucoma, and in eyes of young patients as well.

When to Use an Antifibrosis Agent?

Antifibrosis agents should be used when an eye is at high risk of having unsuccessful surgery. All eyes that have undergone previous incisional glaucoma surgery or cataract surgery, as well as eyes with inflammation or neovascularization, fall into the high risk category. Other types of eyes that may be at high risk for surgical failure include eyes of young patients [22], eyes of patients of African descent, eyes with a history of conjunctival scarring, and eyes with anterior segment abnormalities, such as the iridocorneal endothelial syndrome [23]. Fellow eyes of eyes that have had unsuccessful surgery may be at high risk for trabeculectomy failure.

Whether an antifibrosis agent should be used in eyes not considered at high risk for surgical failure is an open question. Even the best prognosis cases probably have no better than an 80%-90% chance of success, so it is possible that the use of antifibrosis agents could further increase the success rate. The use of an antifibrosis agent can result in a lower intraocular pressure than would otherwise be obtained from a trabeculectomy without an antifibrosis agent [24], and lower intraocular pressure, even within the normal range, may be more effective in preserving vision [25]. On the other hand, subjecting eyes likely to have a favorable surgical outcome to the additional risk of antifibrosis therapy may not have a favorable risk/benefit ratio.

Which Antifibrosis Agent Should be Used?

5-fluorouracil and mitomycin C are the only two agents in common clinical use. Mitomycin C is more potent [10]. The principal advantages of mitomycin C are its potency, ease of administration, and lack of corneal epithelial toxicity. Its effectiveness stems from its ability to inhibit cell proliferation, its activity against cells that are not actively proliferating, and its possible action against vascular endothelial cells as well as fibroblasts [26]. Its ease of administration derives from the observation that a single intraoperative application is effective. Because it is given subconjunctivally by sponge, the corneal epithelium is not directly contacted by the drug and no toxicity is seen. Mitomycin C has the disadvantage of resulting in hypotony in predisposed eyes. It is expensive.

The chief advantage of 5-fluorouracil is that it can be titrated. It can be administered intraoperatively, and then supplemented by postoperative injections. If the eye appears to be doing well, 5-fluorouracil can be witheld. If early toxicity is noted, the 5-fluorouracil can be discontinued. In contrast, with mitomycin C the dose can not be adjusted based on the clinical course of the eye. 5-fluorouracil is much cheaper than mitomycin C. The disadvantages of 5-fluorouracil include the need for postoperative injections and the substantial risk of corneal epithelial defects.

I use mitomycin C in all eyes that I consider at high risk for surgical failure. I reserve 5-fluorouracil for those eyes in which I think that the risk of hypotony from mitomycin C exceeds the benefits in terms of patient comfort and convenience. Currently I am using the algorithm in Fig. 1 for antifibrosis use.

How Should Antifibrosis Agents Be Administered?

5-fluorouracil was initially administered as a postoperative subconjunctival injection. In the Fluorouracil Filtering Surgery Study [3] it was given as 0.5 ml of a 10 mg/ml solution subconjunctivally with a 30 gauge needle 180° from the site of the trabeculectomy. It can also be given as 0.1 ml of a 50 mg/ml solution. The conjunctiva should be anesthetized with pro-

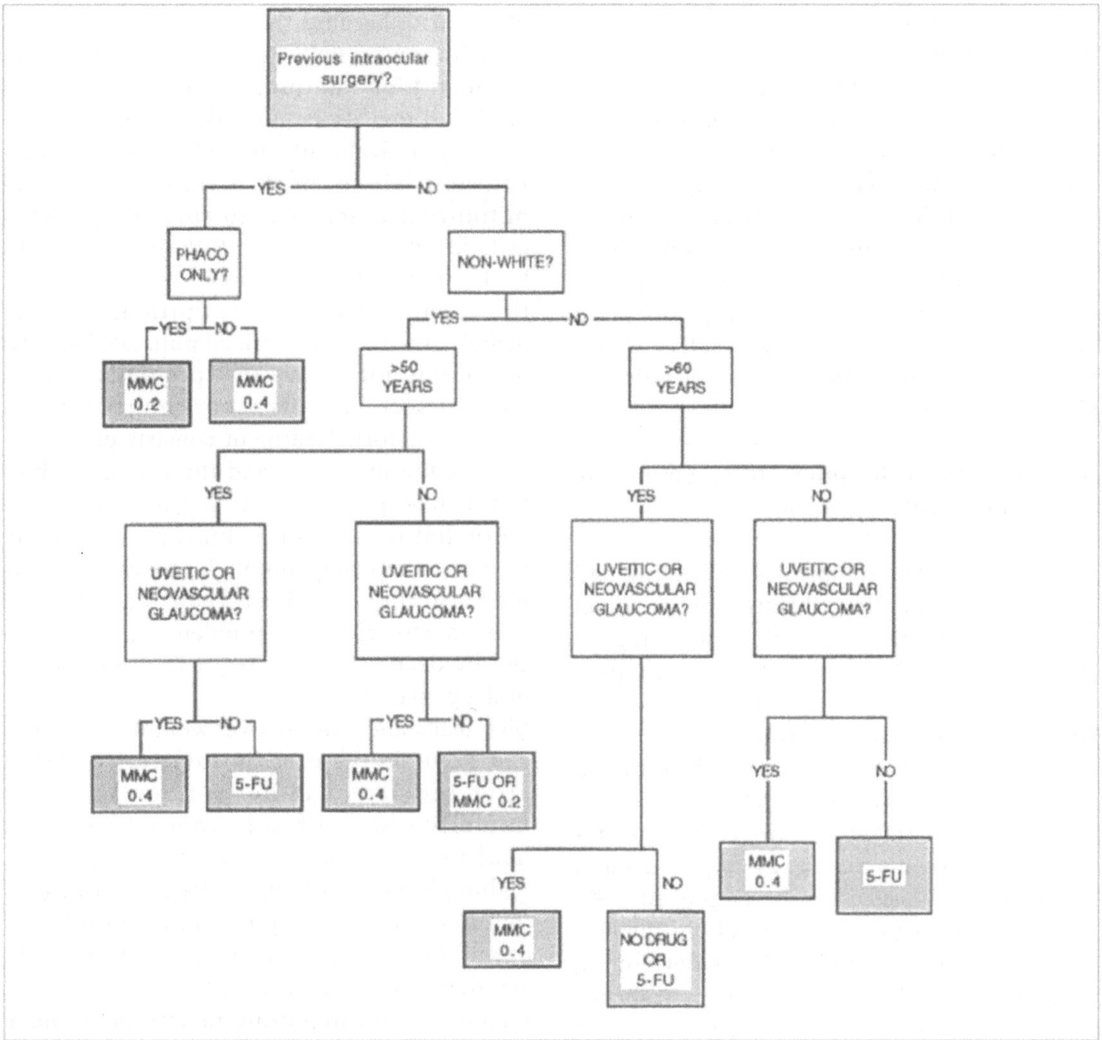

Fig. 1. Algorithm for the use of antifibrosis drugs. Concentrations of mitomycin C are in mg/ml. Duration of application may vary from 2 to 5 min. *MMC* mitomycin C; *5-FU* 5-fluorouracil, either intraoperative, postoperative, or both

paracaine or a similar topical anesthetic.
5-fluorouracil can also be administered intraoperatively in a manner similar to mitomycin C (see below). For intraoperative application the concentration is 50 mg/ml. I leave the 5-fluorouracil in place for 5 min. The intraoperative administration can be supplemented by postoperative subconjunctival injection.
The use of mitomycin C is restricted to intraoperative application. This is because of data suggesting significant toxicity to the corneal endothelium, iris, and ciliary processes [27]. After trabeculectomy, when a direct passageway exists from the subconjunctival space to the anterior chamber, mitomycin injected subconjunctivally might have ready access to the anterior chamber. For the same reason, mitomycin C is applied before the creation of the surgical fistula.
There are multiple variables to be considered when applying mitomycin C. Concentrations of mitomycin C commonly employed vary from 0.2 to 0.5 mg/ml. The length of application has been varied from 15 s to 5 min. The location of the application of the drug can be in the subconjunctival space or beneath the trabeculectomy flap as well. Mitomycin C is generally applied on a sponge, and the amount of drug delivered is influenced by the size and composition of the sponge. I currently use a round shield, designed for placement on the cornea to prevent retinal light toxicity, as my

delivery system. Other parameters to be considered in the use of mitomycin C include which tissues to expose to the drug, and how much irrigation is necessary after removal of the sponge. Some surgeons like to avoid exposing the conjunctival incision to the drug for fear of decreasing desirable healing of the conjunctival incision. Others like to treat the conjunctiva and avoid exposure of the sclera to the drug, out of concern for scleral penetration and intraocular toxicity. A protective shield has been devised for the purpose of reducing scleral exposure [28].

Altering Surgical Technique to Accommodate the Use of Antifibrosis Agents

Antifibrosis agents inhibit wound healing and increase aqueous flow through the surgical site. Therefore, the trabeculectomy surgical technique should be adjusted to anticipate complications that can arise from the inhibition of wound healing. Strong consideration should be given to using a limbus-based conjunctival flap, because most surgeons consider it to be a tighter closure than a fornix-based flap. If a fornix-based flap is used, a "water-tight" closure can be employed [29]. The use of a microvascular needle in the closure can reduce the risk of holes developing around the needle tracks. Tying the trabeculectomy flap down tightly with sutures that can be released manually or cut with a laser allows the surgeon some control postoperatively over the rate that aqueous humor leaves the eye.

Complications of Antifibrosis Drugs Used in Trabeculectomy

Although 5-fluorouracil and mitomycin C are highly toxic agents when used systemically for cancer chemotherapy, their ocular use has not been associated with systemic side effects. The complications from these agents appear to be solely ocular.

Corneal epithelial defects are the most common complication of subconjunctival 5-fluorouracil injections, but do not occur with intraoperative administration of either 5-fluorouracil or mitomycin C. Corneal surface problems arise because the 5-fluorouracil interferes with the normal process of corneal epithelial migration and proliferation. The corneal epithelial toxicity is most likely a result of the subconjunctival route of application of 5-fluorouracil, since both 5-fluorouracil and mitomycin C are toxic to corneal epithelial cells in vitro [30]. Excess 5-fluorouracil leaks back through the needle track and washes over the corneal surface. The epithelial defect usually starts as a superficial punctate keratitis in the inferior cornea that progresses into a frank defect. Patients report blurred vision and discomfort. Treatment consists of discontinuing the injections and the use of antibiotics. Patching is generally not necessary. The epithelial toxicity of 5-fluorouracil usually resolves completely, although rare cases of corneal scarring have been reported [31]. The incidence of epithelial problems can be reduced by decreasing the frequency and amount of drug given [4].

Bleb leaks and conjunctival wound dehiscence can occur in the early postoperative period after the use of either 5-fluorouracil or mitomycin C and result from inhibition of healing near the conjunctival incision. Although more difficult to treat than in eyes that have not been exposed to an antifibrosis agent, these complications usually respond to standard conservative therapy.

Hypotony and hypotony maculopathy have become a major consideration in the use of antifibrosis agents. Gass termed the phrase "hypotony maculopathy" to describe an infolding of the retina and choroid in the posterior pole that he observed in a series of patients with wound leaks after cataract surgery and full thickness filtration surgery [32] . Although hypotony maculopathy must have been occurring infrequently with trabeculectomy surgery with 5-fluorouracil, it was not until mitomycin C began to be used frequently that this complication was commonly recognized [13, 33]. Although initially attributed to overfiltration secondary to potent inhibition of wound healing in the subconjunctival space, there is a growing body of evidence that it may be related to toxicity of mitomycin C to the ciliary processes [34, 35]. Hypotony maculopathy is usually evident in the early postoperative period and rarely reverses spontaneously. Strategies to prevent its development, such as tying the trabeculectomy flap tightly, may reduce but will not eliminate this complication. There are numerous ways to elevate the intraocular pressure to reverse the hypotony, such as injection of autologous blood [36], resuturing of the scleral flap, and cryotherapy to the bleb. Although these techniques often will restore the intraocular pressure to a physiological range, in some eyes the anatomic changes can not be totally reversed and visual function can not be restored to the preoperative level. Hypotony maculopathy appears to be more common in myopic eyes of young patients, and antifibrosis agents must be used with extreme caution in such circumstances.

As we enter the next century, late onset endophthalmitis may become the most serious complication of our use of antifibrosis agents today. Although not proven, there is a strong clinical impression that the use of antifibrosis agents results in the production of thinner and more avascular blebs, more prone to leaks, than when trabeculectomy is performed without 5-fluorouracil or mitomycin C. This type of bleb appears to be more prone to bleb leaks and endophthalmitis [37]. Since endophthalmitis is often visually catastrophic, a significant increase in the incidence of endophthalmitis due to antifibrosis agents could radically alter the risk/benefit ratio for their use.

Role of Antifibrosis Agents in Combined Surgery

Logic would dictate that performing cataract surgery at the same time as trabeculectomy would be a risk factor for failure of the trabeculectomy. Most surgeons would agree that the success of combined procedures is lower than for a trabeculectomy alone. For this reason, antifibrosis agents have been tried in conjunction with combined cataract and glaucoma surgery to improve the success of the trabeculectomy. The results to date are mixed.

5-fluorouracil injections do not appear to dramatically improve the success rate of extracapsular cataract extraction, either with nuclear expression [38, 39] or phacoemulsification [40], when combined with trabeculectomy. Although clinical observation and uncontrolled series suggest that mitomycin C improves the success rate of combined surgery using either nuclear expression [41] or phacoemulsification [42], one randomized, controlled study showed no effect [43]. We need additional studies to clarify the role of mitomycin C in combined surgery.

The Future of Antifibrosis Agents in Filtration Surgery

The drawbacks of the antifibrosis agents in current use, are that trabeculectomies continue to fail despite their use and that they can cause or contribute to sight threatening complications. A more complete understanding of the mechanism of action of mitomycin C and of the pharmacokinetics of its administration might increase its effectiveness and decrease its complications. Alternatively, the development of new agents, along with novel drug carrier systems, may improve the therapeutic index of these agents.

The paradigm of an ordered sequence of glaucoma therapy starting with medicine may change over the next several years as the results of ongoing clinical trials become available. The establishment of a role for early surgery in the treatment of glaucoma, combined with the realization that surgery may be the only realistic alternative for treating glaucoma in the developing world, will make improving the success rate of filtration surgery in all patients more important. Antifibrosis agents will almost certainly have a prominent role to play in making filtration surgery as effective as possible.

References

1. Gressel MG, Parrish R Folberg R (1984) 5-fluorouracil and glaucoma filtering surgery: I. An animal model. Ophthalmol 91:378-383
2. Heuer DK, Parrish R, Gressel MG, Hodapp E, Palmberg PF, Anderson DR (1984) 5-fluorouracil and glaucoma filtering surgery. II. A pilot study. Ophthalmol 91:384-394
3. The Fluorouracil Filtering Surgery Study Group (1989) Fluorouracil Filtering Surgery Study one-year follow-up. Am J Ophthalmol 108:625-635

4. Weinreb RN (1987) Adjusting the dose of 5-fluorouracil after filtration surgery to minimize side effects. Ophthalmol 94:564-570
5. Rabowsky JH, Ruderman JM (1989) Low-dose 5-fluorouracil and glaucoma filtration surgery. Ophthalmic Surg 20:347-349
6. Chen C-W (1983) Enhanced intraocular pressure controlling effectiveness of trabeculectomy by local application of mitomycin-C. Trans Asia-Pacific Acad Ophthalmol 9:172-177
7. Palmer SS (1991) Mitomycin as adjunct chemotherapy with trabeculectomy. Ophthalmol 98:317-321
8. Skuta GL, Beeson CC, Higginbotham EJ, Lichter PR, Musch DC, Bergstrom TJ, Klein TB, Falck FJ (1992) Intraoperative mitomycin versus postoperative 5-fluorouracil in high-risk glaucoma filtering surgery. Ophthalmol 99:438-444
9. Kitazawa Y, Kawase K, Matsushita H, Minobe M (1991) Trabeculectomy with mitomycin. A comparative study with fluorouracil. Arch Ophthalmol 109:1693-1698
10. Katz G, Higginbotham E, Lichter P, Skuta G, Musch D, Bergstrom T, Johnson A (1995) Mitomycin C versus 5-fluorouracil in high-risk glaucoma filtering surgery: extended follow-up. Ophthalmol 102:1263-1269
11. The Fluorouracil Filtering Surgery Study Group (1993) Three-year follow-up of the Fluorouracil Filtering Surgery Study. Am J Ophthalmol 115:82-92
12. Costa VP, Wilson RP, Moster MR, Schmidt CM, Gandham S (1993) Hypotony maculopathy following the use of topical mitomycin C in glaucoma filtration surgery. Ophthalmic Surg 24:389-394
13. Jampel HD, Pasquale LR, Dibernardo C (1992) Hypotony maculopathy following trabeculectomy with mitomycin c. Arch Ophthalmol 110:1049-1050
14. Zacharia P, Depperman S, Schuman J (1993) Ocular hypotony after trabeculectomy with mitomycin C. Am J Ophthalmol 116:314-326
15. Geijssen HC, Greve EL (1993) Prevention of hypotony after trabeculectomies with mitomycin. Doc Ophthalmol 85:45-49
16. Wise JB (1993) Treatment of chronic postfiltration hypotony by intrableb injection of autologous blood. Arch Ophthalmol 111:827-830
17. Duker JS, Schuman JS (1994) Successful surgical treatment of hypotony maculopathy following trabeculectomy with topical mitomycin C. Ophthalmic Surg 25:463-465
18. Egbert PR, Williams AS, Singh K, Dadzie P, Egbert TB (1993) A prospective trial of intraoperative fluorouracil during trabeculectomy in a black population. Am J Ophthalmol 116:612-614
19. Dietze PJ, Feldman RM, Gross RL (1992) Intraoperative application of 5-fluorouracil during trabeculectomy. Ophthalmic Surg 23:662-665
20. Jampel HD, Jabs DA, Quigley HA (1990) Trabeculectomy with 5-fluorouracil for adult inflammatory glaucoma. Am J Ophthalmol 109:168-173
21. Patitsas CJ, Rockwood EJ, Meisler DM, Lowder CY (1992) Glaucoma filtering surgery with postoperative 5-fluorouracil in patients with intraocular inflammatory disease. Ophthalmol 99:594-599
22. Gressel MG, Heuer DK, Parrish R (1984) Trabeculectomy in young patients. Ophthalmol 91:1242-1246
23. Kidd M, Hetherington J, Magee S (1988) Surgical results in iridocorneal endothelial syndrome. Arch Ophthalmol 106:199-201
24. Wilson RP, Steinmann WC (1991) Use of trabeculectomy with postoperative 5-fluorouracil in patients requiring extremely low intraocular pressure levels to limit further glaucoma progression. Ophthalmol 98:1047-1052
25. Roth SM, Spaeth GL, Starita RJ, Birbillis EM, Steinmann WC (1991) The effects of postoperative corticosteroids on trabeculectomy and the clinical course of glaucoma: five-year follow-up study. Ophthalmic Surg 22:724-729
26. Smith S, D'Amore PA, Dreyer EB (1994) Comparative toxicity of mitomycin C and 5-fluorouracil in vitro. Am J Ophthalmol 118:332-337
27. Derick RJ, Pasquale L, Quigley HA, Jampel H (1991) Potential toxicity of mitomycin C. Arch Ophthalmol 109:1635
28. Mietz H, Addicks K, Krieglstein GK (1994) A scleral shield for the application of mitomycin C during trabeculectomy: a rabbit model. Ophthalmic Surg 25:466-470
29. Wise JB (1993) Mitomycin-compatible suture technique for fornix-based conjunctival flaps in glaucoma filtration surgery. Arch Ophthalmol 111:992-997
30. Ando H, Ido T, Kawai Y, Yamamoto T, Kitazawa Y (1992) Inhibition of corneal epithelial wound healing. A comparative study of mitomycin C and 5-fluorouracil. Ophthalmol 99:1809-1814
31. Knapp A, Heuer DK, Stern GA, Driebe WJ (1987) Serious corneal complications of glaucoma filtering surgery with postoperative 5-fluorouracil. Am J Ophthalmol 103:183-187
32. Gass J (1972) Hypotony maculopathy. In: Bellows J (ed) Contemporary ophthalmology: honoring Sir Stewart Duke-Elder. Williams & Wilkins, Baltimore, pp 343-366
33. Shields MB, Scroggs MW, Sloop CM, Simmons RB (1993) Clinical and histopathologic observations concerning hypotony after trabeculec-

tomy with adjunctive mitomycin C. Am J Ophthalmol 116:673-683

34. Kee C, Pelzek CD, Kaufman PL (1995) Mitomycin C suppresses aqueous humor flow in cynomolgus monkeys. Arch Ophthalmol 113:239-242
35. Mietz H, Addicks K, Diestelhorst M, Krieglstein GK (1994) Extraocular application of mitomycin C in a rabbit model: cytotoxic effects on the ciliary body and epithelium. Ophthalmic Surg 25:240-244
36. Nuyts RM, Greve EL, Geijssen HC, Langerhorst CT (1994) Treatment of hypotonous maculopathy after trabeculectomy with mitomycin C. Am J Ophthalmol 118:322-331
37. Wolner B, Liebmann JM, Sassani JW, Ritch R, Speaker M, Marmor M (1991) Late bleb-related endophthalmitis after trabeculectomy with adjunctive 5-fluorouracil. Ophthalmol 98:1053-1060
38. Wong PC, Ruderman JM, Krupin T, Goldenfeld M, Rosenberg LF, Shields MB, Ritch R, Liebmann JM, Gieser DK (1994) 5-fluorouracil after primary combined filtration surgery. Am J Ophthalmol 117:149-154
39. Hennis HL, Stewart WC (1991) The use of 5-fluorouracil in patients following combined trabeculectomy and cataract extraction. Ophthalmic Surg 22:451-454
40. O'Grady JM, Juzych MS, Shin DH, Lemon LC, Swendris RP (1993) Trabeculectomy, phacoemulsification, and posterior chamber lens implantation with and without 5-fluorouracil. Am J Ophthalmol 116:594-599
41. Joos K, Bueche M, Palmberg P, Feuer W, Grajewski A (1995) One-year follow-up results of combined mitomycin C trabeculectomy and extracapsular cataract extraction. Ophthalmol 102:76-83
42. Munden PM, Alward WL (1995) Combined phacoemulsification, posterior chamber intraocular lens implantation, and trabeculectomy with mitomycin C. Am J Ophthalmol 119:20-29
43. Shin D, Simone P, Song M, Reed S, Juzych M, Kim C, Hughes B (1995) Adjunctive subconjunctival mitomycin C in Glaucoma Triple Procedure. Ophthalmol 112:1550-1558

Trabeculectomy Utilizing Releasable Sutures, Combined with Phacoemulsification and Intraocular Lens Implantation: Efficacy and Safety*

T. Y. Chou, W. J. Stark, and K. W. Choy

Department of Ophthalmology, The Wilmer Ophthalmological Institute, The Johns Hopkins University, Baltimore, MD 21287-9238, USA

Introduction

Trabeculectomy in combination with cataract extraction and intraocular lens (IOL) implantation has been demonstrated to be effective with regard to both visual acuity and control of post-operative intraocular pressure (IOP) [1-4]. Advantages of combining surgery include avoiding a second operation, control of post-operative pressure elevation, and, potentially, long-term control of glaucoma with less dependency on chronic medical or laser therapy [5].
There remains controversy, however, concerning the best approach to maximize effectiveness and minimize risk. The development of laser to cut tight trabeculectomy flap sutures has facilitated the treatment of elevated pressures in the early postoperative period. Surgeons can fashion tighter flaps, thereby lessening postoperative hypotony complications [6].
Laser suture lysis has disadvantages as well. The suture must be seen in order to be lysed. Blood, chemosis, or thickening of Tenon's capsule may prevent visualization of the suture. The procedure itself may be both expensive and uncomfortable for a patient who has just undergone recent eye surgery. Bleb leaks and subconjunctival hemorrhage may be induced during the procedure. Time requirements and laser access may be additional hindrances.
As an alternative, this institution, in the past 2 years, has been performing combined phacoemulsification, IOL implantation, and trabeculectomy utilizing releasable scleral flap sutures. We have found releasable sutures in the setting of combined surgery to be relatively easy to place and exceptionally easy to remove safely. The technique of releasable sutures has been described for trabeculectomy [7-10], and its advantages would seem to hold as well for the combined procedure. In this retrospective review, we present our experience thus far with releasable sutures as applied to the combined phacoemulsification, IOL implantation, and trabeculectomy procedure, including data on its efficacy and safety.

Patients and Methods

Between January 5, 1994 and November 8, 1995, 69 patients underwent combined phacoemulsification, IOL implantation, and trabeculectomy with releasable scleral flap sutures. Eleven patients underwent bilateral surgery in that time period, resulting in data for 80 eyes in this study. All surgery was performed by one of the authors (WJS).
Patients selected for surgery all demonstrated visually significant cataracts interfering with activities of daily living. In addition, all had glaucoma, based on IOP elevation, increased cupping of the optic nerve, and/or glaucomatous visual field defects on automated perimetry. Many patients were on multiple glaucoma medications, including oral carbonic anhydrase inhibitors, and several had previous glaucoma-related laser procedures. Patients with mild glaucoma were often designated for "small" trabeculectomies. There were nine patients who preoperatively were not taking glaucoma medications. Seven of these were newly dia-

* Supported by research grants from Mr. and Mrs. Albert Brocolli and Mr. Ray Stark

gnosed with glaucoma preoperatively and underwent combined surgery at the recommendation of our glaucoma consultants. One patient was intolerant of multiple glaucoma medications. One uveitis patient was a strong steroid responder with elevated preoperative pressures.

Patients were counselled on the risks, benefits, and alternatives of surgery, and informed consent was obtained preoperatively. Surgery was performed under local anesthesia with monitored sedation. Patients were prepped and drapped in a sterile fashion.

A fornix-based conjunctival flap was created at the 11 o'clock position. A triangular, partial thickness scleral flap was grooved and then shelved forward onto clear cornea. Small trabeculectomies had smaller inner sclerectomies. The anterior chamber was entered from under the scleral flap, and standard phacoemulsification with IOL implantation was performed. A sector iridectomy was often cut in small pupil cases to facilitate cataract removal. A variety of lenses were utililized including polymethyl methacrylate (PMMA), silicone, and acrylic. Following IOL insertion, a posterior lip sclerectomy was accomplished, followed by peripheral iridectomy.

The trabeculectomy flap was closed next with interrupted 10-0 nylon sutures as follows: the apex of the triangular scleral flap was secured with a permanently tied 10-0 nylon suture (Fig. 1). The lateral sides of the triangle were reapproximated with an initial pass from outside to inside the triangle, bisecting the lateral side (Fig. 2). The needle was then passed from the base of the triangle into the anterior chamber, going full-thickness through the limbal tissue and exiting in clear cornea 1-2 mm anterior to the limbus (Fig. 3). The suture was then embedded within the corneal stroma perpendicular to the previous pass (Fig. 4). The proximal suture was then secured with a triple throw slip-knot (Fig. 5) and the distal ends cut flush against the cornea (Fig. 6). Usually, two of these sutures were tied as releasable slip knots. Occasionally, only one releasable suture was utilized, but in one case, three were placed. Finally, the conjunctival flap was pulled back over the scleral flap and secured with interrupted 10-0 vicryl suture.

Postoperatively, many patients were examined for IOP in the evening of the day of surgery. All were examined on the day following the day of surgery. The usual follow up schedule involved additional clinic visits at 5-7 days, 2 weeks, 3-4 weeks, 6-8 weeks, 3 months, 6 months, and 1 year postoperatively.

Excessively low IOPs were commonly treated with an injection of Healon through the surgi-

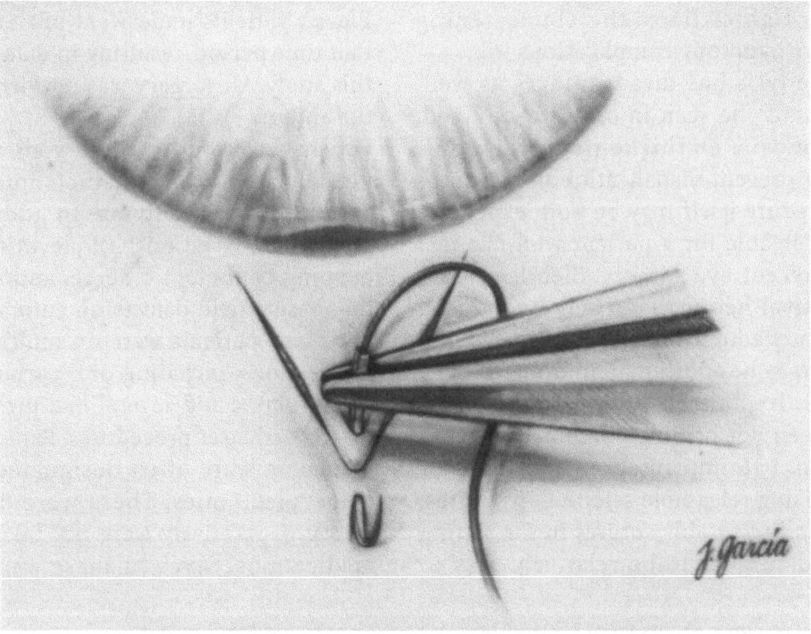

Fig. 1. Securing the apex of the scleral flap with a 10-0 nylon suture

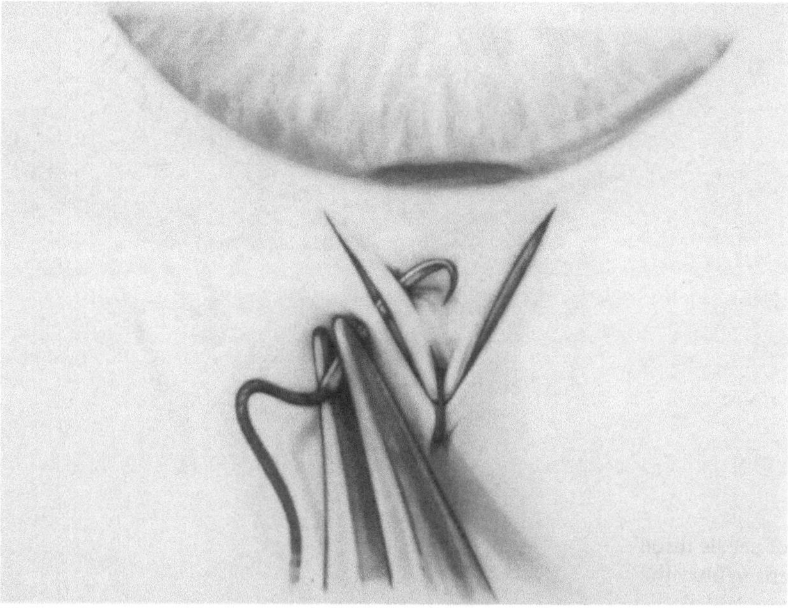

Fig. 2. Initial pass of needle to reapproximate lateral sides of triangular scleral flap

cal paracentesis site. Elevated IOPs were treated with gentle massage, pressure adjacent to the scleral flap, and/or by removal of one or more of the releasable sutures. Additional sutures were cut, if necessary, using argon laser.

All data were gleaned from careful chart review. Follow-up reports from other offices and clinics were incorporated when possible. Multiple eye pressure readings within a similar time period were averaged. If more than one method of tonometry was used on the same clinic visit (i.e., applanation tonometry, pneumotonometry, and Tonopen) then the applanation reading was the one used for data analysis. A clinically significant immediate postoperative IOP elevation was defined as an IOP of 8

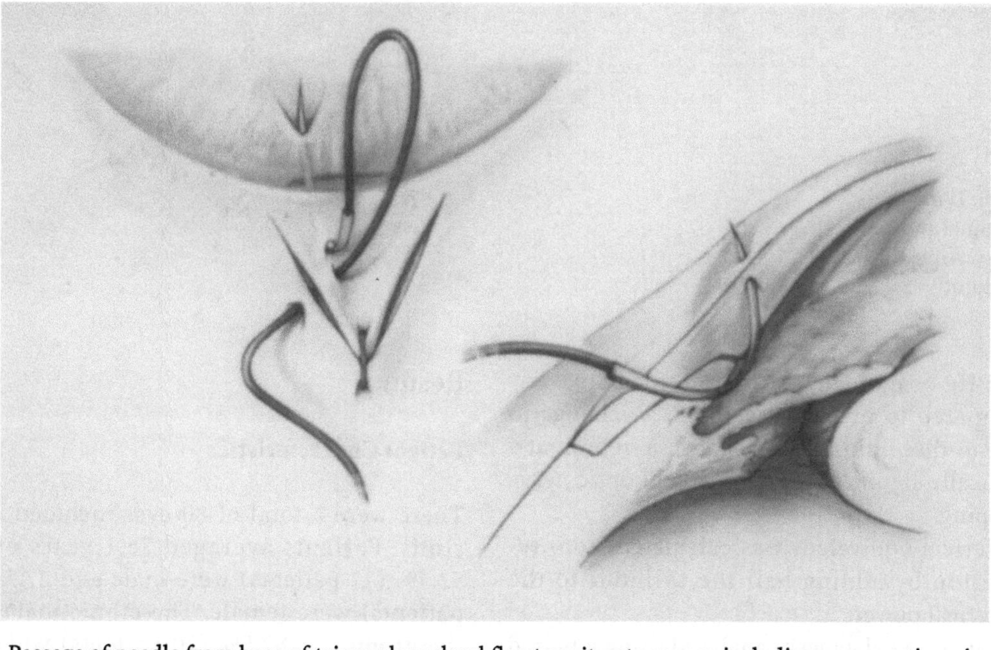

Fig. 3. Passage of needle from base of triangular scleral flap to exit onto cornea including cross section view demonstrating full thickness path through limbal tissue

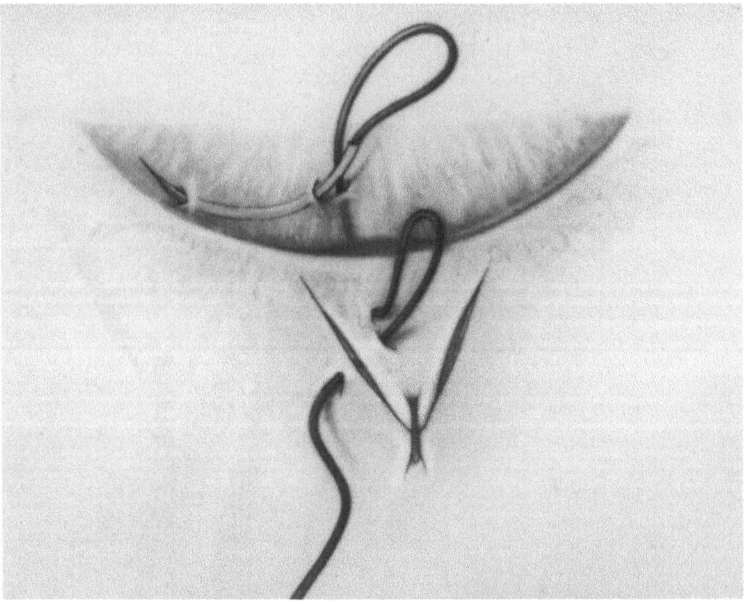

Fig. 4. Passage of needle through corneal stroma to bury the suture

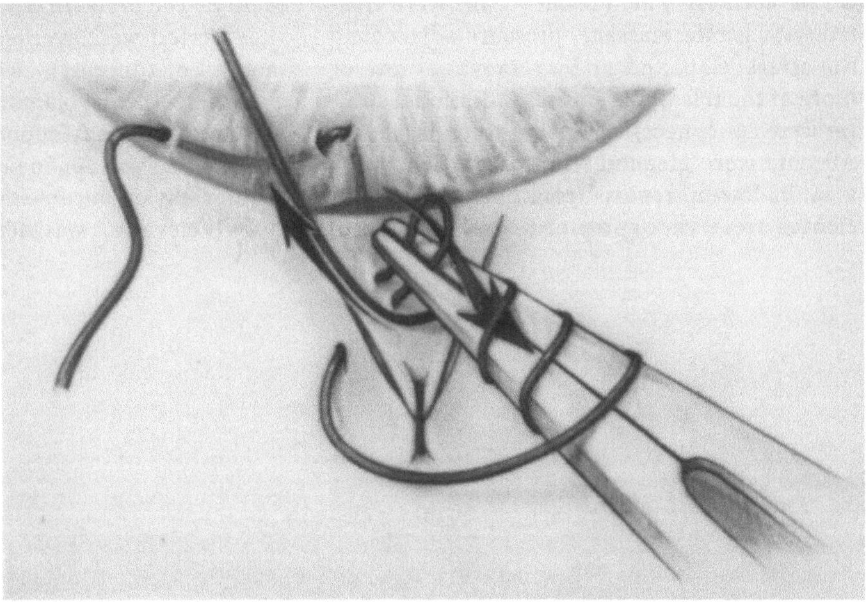

Fig. 5. Tying the proximal suture with a triple throw slip knot

mm Hg or more on the first postoperative day compared to preoperative levels. A change in cup-to-disc ratio > 0.2 was taken to represent a clinically significant progression of optic nerve cupping.
Spherical equivalent was calculated from refraction by adding half the cylinder to the spherical power.
Comparative data were analysed using a paired two-tailed *t* test.

Results

Patient Characteristics

There were a total of 80 eyes included in the study. Patients averaged 76.1 years of age; 52.5% (42 patients) were male and 47.5% (38 patients) were female. The ethnic makeup of the group was 87.5% (70 patients) white, 5% (four patients) black, and 7.5% (six patients) of

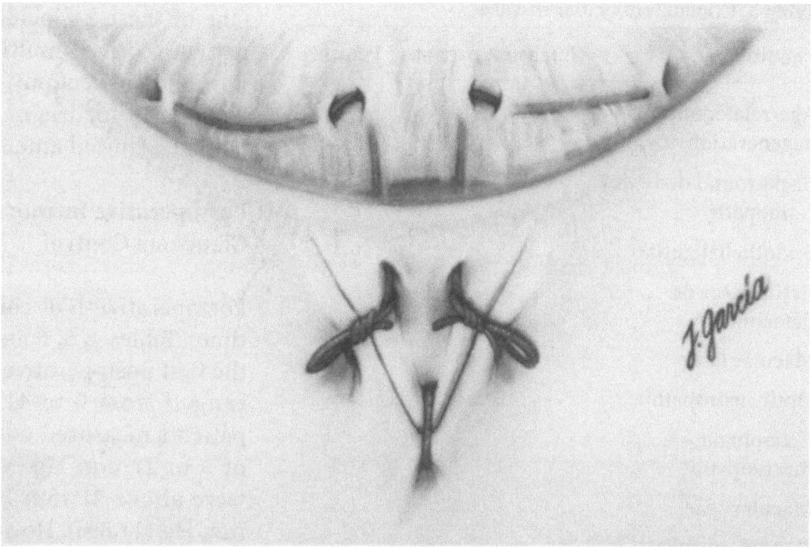

Fig. 6. Final appearance of two releasable sutures used to secure lateral sides of triangular scleral flap

various other backgrounds.

Follow-up time after surgery ranged from 1.5 to 18 months, with an average of 6.9 months. There were 37 patients (46.3%) who were followed for 6 months or longer, and 16 (20%) who were followed for 1 year or more.

Ocular History

Primary open-angle glaucoma was by far the most prevalent condition, involving 61.3% of patients (49 patients); 16.3% (13 patients) had pseudoexfoliation. Low tension and narrow angle glaucoma each occurred in 6.3%. The breakdown on different glaucoma types is listed in Table 1.

Table 1. Glaucoma types

Glaucoma type	Number of patients	Percent
Primary open -angle glaucoma	49	61.3
Pseudoexfoliation	13	16.3
Low tension glaucoma	5	6.3
Narrow-angle glaucoma	5	6.3
Mixed mechanism glaucoma	4	5
Uveitic	2	2.5
Pigmentary dispersion	1	1.3
Postraumatic	1	1.3

Any preoperative procedures or conditions that might predispose to scarring, bleeding, and inflammation were recorded and are listed in Table 2. The most common procedures were laser trabeculoplasty (LTP) and laser peripheral iridotomy (LPI). Table 3 lists other concurrent ocular conditions.

Table 2. Previous surgery and scarring conditions

Procedure or condition	Number of patients	Percent
Laser trabeculoplasty	16	20
Laser peripheral iridotomy	11	13.75
Surgical peripheral iridectomy	1	1.25
Trabeculectomy	2	2.5
Retinal detachment repair	2	2.5
Ruptured globe	1	1.25
Posterior synechiae	3	3.75
Anterior synechiae	1	1.25
Conjunctival scarring	2	2.5
Uveitis	2	2.5

Table 3. Concurrent ocular disease

Condition	Number of patients	Percent
Age-related macular degeneration	9	11.3
Background diabetic retinopathy	7	8.8
Endothelial guttae	5	6.3
Retinal tear or detachment	3	3.8
Macular laser	2	2.5
Optic neuropathy	2	2.5
Cellophane maculopathy	1	1.3
Macular scar	1	1.3
Cystoid macular edema	1	1.3
Myopic degeneration	1	1.3
Central retinal vein occlusion	1	1.3
Strabismus and amblyopia	1	1.3
Corneal scarring	1	1.3

Operative History

All patients underwent combined phacoemulsification, IOL implantation, and trabeculectomy with at least one releasable suture. There were 42 right eyes (52.5%) and 38 left eyes (47.5%). Of 80 trabeculectomies, 26 (32.5%) were designated as small.

In 31 cases (38.75%), sector iridectomy was performed to facilitate cataract extraction, followed later by repair with a 10-0 prolene suture. One of these 31 included sphincterotomy. One patient received multiple sphincterotomies but no sector iridectomy. Two patients underwent iridoplasty for iris or pupil irregularities. One patient required anterior vitrectomy.

Postoperative Intraocular Pressure and Glaucoma Control

Postoperative IOP control was compared over time (Tables 4, 5, 6 and Fig. 7). Average IOP on the first postoperative day was 18.3 mm Hg and ranged from 0 to 41. Nearly half (46.1%) of patients measured outside of the normal range of 9 to 21 mm Hg. More than twice as many were above 21 mm Hg (34.2%) than below 9 mm Hg (11.8%). However, a much smaller proportion of patients were actually considered very elevated (3.9% > 35 mm Hg) or very hypotonous (3.9% < 5 mm Hg). Some 21% (17

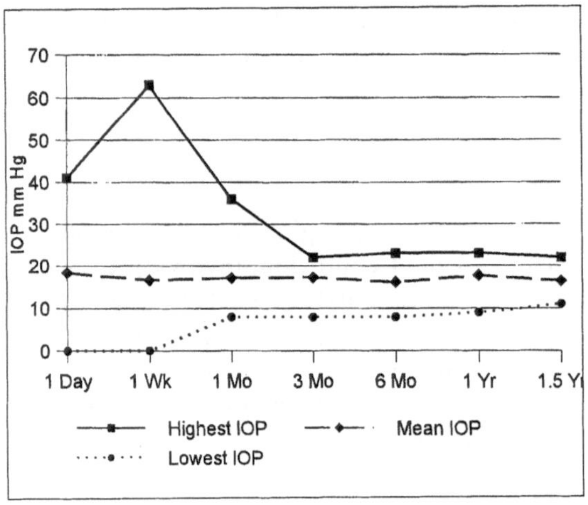

Fig. 7. Postoperative intraocular pressure levels

Table 4. Postoperative pressure control (1 day - 3 months)

Follow-up time	1 Day	1 Week	1 Month	3 Months
N	76	80	68	74
Average IOP (mm Hg)	18.3	16.6	17.1	17.2
Range (mm Hg)	0-41	0-63	8-36	8-22
>35	3 (3.9%)	1 (1.3%)	1 (1.5%)	0
22-35	23 (30.3%)	13 (16.3%)	9 (13.2%)	4 (5.3%)
9-21	40 (51.9%)	55 (68.8%)	57 (83.8%)	69 (93.2%)
5-8	6 (7.9%)	6 (7.5%)	1 (1.5%)	1 (1.4%)
≤4	3 (3.9%)	5 (6.3%)	0	0
0 Medications	76 (100%)	80 (100%)	65 (95.6%)	65 (87.8%)
1 Medication	0	0	2 (2.9%)	9 (12.2%)
2 Medications	0	0	1 (1.5%)	0

Table 5. Postoperative pressure control (6-18 months)

Follow-up time	6 Months	12 Months	18 Months
N=	42	27	8
Average IOP (mm Hg)	16.1	17.7	16.4
Range (mm Hg)	8-23	9-23	11-22
> 35	0	0	0
22-35	1 (2.4%)	1 (3.7%)	1 (12.5%)
9-21	40 (95.2%)	26 (96.3%)	7 (87.5%)
5-8	1 (2.4%)	0	0
≤4	0	0	0
0 Medications	36 (85.7%)	24 (88.9%)	8 (100%)
1 Medication	4 (9 5%)	2 (7.4%)	0
2 Medications	1 (2.4%)	1 (3.7%)	0
3 Medications	1 (2.4%)	0	0

patients) developed immediate IOP elevations (≥ 8mm Hg from preoperative level) on the first postoperative day.

There was a rapid "normalization" of IOP in subsequent follow-up periods: 31.2% outside of 9-21 mm Hg at 1 week, 16.2% at 1 month, 6.8% at 3 months, and 7.5% final. Average IOP also declined from the higher to middle teens. Consistent with other studies [11, 12], a greater proportion of patients were placed on glaucoma medications as follow-up time increased.

A comparison of preoperative and final postoperative pressure control is shown in Table 6 and Fig. 8.

Table 6. Pre- and postoperative glaucoma control

	Preop (%)	Final Postop (%)
N	80	80
Average IOP (mm Hg)	19.5	15.8
Range (mm Hg)	14-29	8-23
> 35	0	0
22-35	19 (23.8)	4 (5)
9-21	61 (76.3)	74 (92.5)
5-8	0	2(2.5)
≤4	0	0
0 Medications	9 (11.3)	65 (81.3)
1 Medication	35 (43.8)	13 (16.3)
2 Medications	22 (27.5)	0
3 Medications	7 (8.8)	2 (2.5)
4 Medications	7 (8.8)	0
CAI use	8 (10)	0
Average number of medications	1.58	0.25

CAI, carbonic anhydrase inhibitor.

Average final postoperative IOP (15.8 mm Hg) was significantly lower ($p < 0.01$) than the preoperative average (19.5 mm Hg) . We observed a greater proportion of postoperative patients (95% vs 76.3% of preoperative patients) under good IOP control (defined as ≤ 21 mm Hg) and using no glaucoma medications (81.3% vs 11.3%). Overall 87.5% of patients were on fewer glaucoma medications postoperatively than preoperatively. Although 13% were on the same number, none were taking a greater number. The average number of medications per patient declined 1.58 to 0.25. Carbonic anhydrase inhibitor usage also dropped from 10% to 0%.

In 78 of the 80 eyes there was some description of bleb appearance postoperatively. The bleb was normal in 61 patients (76.3%), cystic in 2 (2.5%), and flat, absent, or scarred down in 15 (18.8%). Patients with flat and scarred blebs tended to require slightly more glaucoma

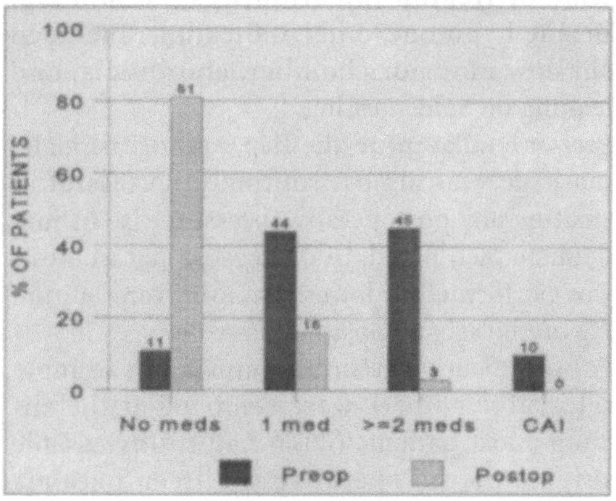

Fig. 8. Comparison of preoperative and postoperative usage of glaucoma medications

medications on average (0.6 medications per patient) for IOP control than the group as a whole (0.25 medications per patient).

No patients had documented progression of glaucoma during their follow-up periods. Of 65 patients with recorded postoperative optic nerve assessments, none were felt subjectively to have any significant increase in cupping; of 29 postoperative visual field tests, none had worsened compared to preoperative perimetry.

Only four of the 80 eyes (5%) had final postoperative pressures more than two points greater than their preoperative levels. However, three of these four were on no medication, while one was using three medications, compared to four preoperatively.

These four patients had slightly more advanced glaucoma, averaging 2.25 anti-glaucoma medications preoperatively, and with two out of the four having undergone LTP. There were no other trends, such as complications or IOL type, that appeared to be factors in these four cases.

Releasable Sutures and Other Postoperative Interventions

Patients were carefully followed up and aggressively treated postoperatively for both hypotony and elevated IOP. Patients were usually seen daily, or even several times in the same day, until pressure was deemed stable and near target range.

Five patients were given viscoelastic (Healon) injections postoperatively. Two of these received Healon on 2 separate postoperative days, and one patient was given Healon on each of his five postoperative days. Average IOP at the time of Healon injection was 2.8 mm Hg. Beside hypotony, other indications included shallow anterior chamber, choroidals, and leaking on Seidel testing.

Pressure adjacent to the flap, and occasionally massage, was almost routinely successful in treating any postoperative pressure rise or inadequate bleb noted. In one case, a paracentesis was performed to lower pressure from 30 mm Hg on the second postoperative day.

For significant pressure elevations, one or more releasable sutures were removed at the slit lamp. Most patients (80%) had two releasable sutures placed operatively. Fifteen patients (18.8%) had only one releasable suture that could be documented. One patient was given three releasable sutures. Releasable suture removal was generally very safe. On only two occasions, out of 134 documented suture releases (1.5%), the suture broke on attempted removal without adverse consequence. After one suture release combined with ocular massage, a postoperative intraocular hemorrhage ensued in a patient with large subconjunctival hemorrhage.

The median removal time of the first releasable suture was postoperative day 5, with a range of 1 day to 11 months postoperatively. Only two out of 80 patients (2.5%) did not have at least one suture removed. The average IOP at the time of the first releasable suture removal was 22.7 mm Hg.

The median removal time of the second releasable suture was postoperative day 19. Where known in 48 patients, the average IOP at the time of second suture removal was 19.6 mm Hg. Five second releasable sutures were left in place, as was apparently the one third releasable suture.

Ten patients (12.5%) required lasering of additional flap sutures after releasable suture removal. Five out of these ten had only one releasable suture placed in surgery. The average time of lasering was 2 weeks postoperative, with an average IOP of 27.4 mm Hg prior to treatment. A trace aqueous leak occurred after one of the laser procedures.

Visual Outcome

The preoperative and postoperative breakdowns of best-corrected visual acuity are compared in Table 7 and Fig. 9. Median visual acuity improved from 20/70 to 20/25. Some 82% of patients saw 20/40 or better at the latest follow-up after combined surgery, compared to 6.3% prior to surgery. Only four patients (5.1%) were 20/200 or worse.

All 14 patients with best-corrected postoperative visual acuities of 20/50 or worse and the nine whose visual acuity improved by less than 2 lines had one of the underlying ocular diseases listed in Table 3. Only three patients (3.82%) declined two or more lines in visual acuity. Their visual impairment was attributable to postoperative retrobulbar neuritis, a postoperative cerebrovascular accident (CVA), and progression of prexisting CME. Only three patients (3.8%) experienced a decrease in visual acuity of two lines or worse.

Table 7. Visual outcome

	Preop (%)	Final Postop (%)
N	80	79
Median VA	20/70	20/25
⩾ 20/20	0	34 (43)
⩾ 20/40	5 (6.3)	65 (82.3)
⩽ 20/50	75 (93.8)	14 (17.7)
⩽ 20/200	15 (18.8)	4 (5.1)
⩾ 2 lines better	—	70 (88.6)
Within 1 line	—	6 (7.6)
⩾ 2 lines worse	—	3 (3 8)

VA, visual acuity.

Refraction and Astigmatism

The average spherical equivalent for the study group preoperatively was -2.43, with a range of-17.25 to +5.75. By contrast, the average final postoperative spherical equivalent was -0.88, with a range from -4.25 to +1.00.

Complications

Table 8 lists the complications encountered after surgery. A patient with more than one complication was counted more than once. The most common complications were hypotony and cystoid macular edema (CME), having seven occurrences (8.75%) each. Most complications resolved in time with proper therapy. Both cases of post-operative diplopia, as well as one case of CME associated with uveitis, had these conditions pre-operatively as well. Retrobulbar neuritis and CVA were acquired after surgery, but unrelated to it.

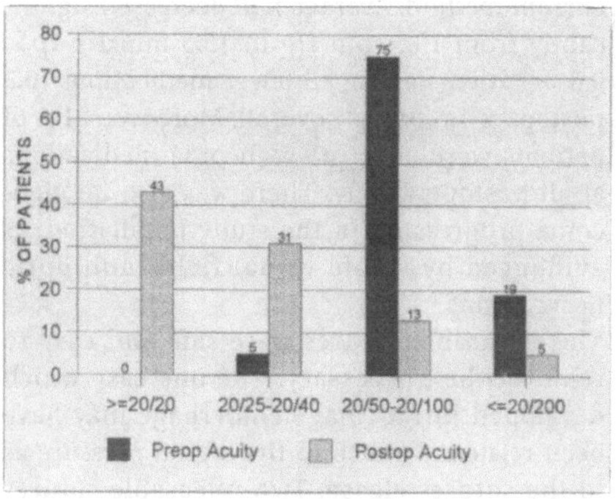

Fig. 9. Comparison of preoperative and postoperative best visual acuity

Table 8. Complications

Complication	Number of patients	Percent
Hypotony	7	8.8
Cystoid macular edema	7	8.8
Bleb leak	6	7.5
Choroidal effusion	6	7.5
Hyphema	6	7.5
Return to surgery for hypotony	4	5
Epithelial abrasion	3	3.8
Filamentary keratitis	2	2.5
Diplopia	2	2.5
Fibrinous iritis	2	2.5
Shallow or flat chamber	2	2.5
High elevation of IOP	2	2.5
Chronic iritis	2	2.5
Opacified posterior capsule	1	1.3
IOL capture	1	1.3
Retinal tear	1	1.3
CVA	1	1.3
Macular ischemia	1	1.3
Unintended myopic refraction	1	1.3
Retrobulbar neuritis	1	1.3
Malignant glaucoma	1	1.3

IOP, intraocular pressure; IOL, intraocular lens; CVA, cerebrovascular accident.

Small Trabeculectomies

Small trabeculectomies were frequently performed when the patient was well controlled preoperatively or had less advanced glaucoma. Small and regular trabeculectomies are compared in Table 9, and have no statistical difference with respect to their final IOPs or prevalence of hypotonous complications.

Table 9. Size of trabeculectomy

	Regular	Small
N	53	27
Preop IOP	19.6	19.3
Final average IOP (mm Hg)	15.7	16.0
IOP postop day 1	19.24	17.8
Hypotony cases	5 (9.1%)	2 (8%)

Intraocular Lens Material

Patients who had foldable lenses implanted had a smaller improvement in pressure than those who received PMMA lenses (Table 10).

Table 10. Comparison of IOL material

	PMMA	Foldable
N	47	33
Median final VA	20/25	20/25
Final postop IOP	15.0	16.9
Preop IOP	19.8	19.2
Number of postop medications patient	0.3	0.2

VA, visual acuity; IOP, intraocular pressure; PMMA, polymethyl methacrylate.

This difference between foldable (silicone except for one acrylic lens) and PMMA lenses was statistically significant ($p = 0.012$). On further analysis, we found that the 12 patients who underwent both small trabeculectomies and foldable lens implantation demonstrated a mean decrease in IOP from 19.4 mm Hg preoperatively to 17.4 mm Hg at final postoperative check. This decrease, however, was not statistically significant ($p > 0.05$). In all other groupings of trabeculectomy and lens type, the patients had significant pressure declines before and after surgery.

Discussion

The theoretical advantages of releasable sutures in the setting of combined phacoemulsification, IOL implantation, and trabeculectomy would include safety and ease of removal, compared to laser suture lysis, and less hypotony, compared to adjunctive anti-metabolites.

Patient history and background did not reveal any obvious trends with respect to complications and results. There were relatively fewer black patients in this series, so a meaningful comparison of their success rates compared to whites cannot be made at this time.

Early in the postoperative period, there were moderate numbers of patients with IOP spikes above 21 mm Hg but relatively fewer patients with hypotony (11.8%), especially severe hypotony (3.9%) which we define as ≤ 4 mm Hg

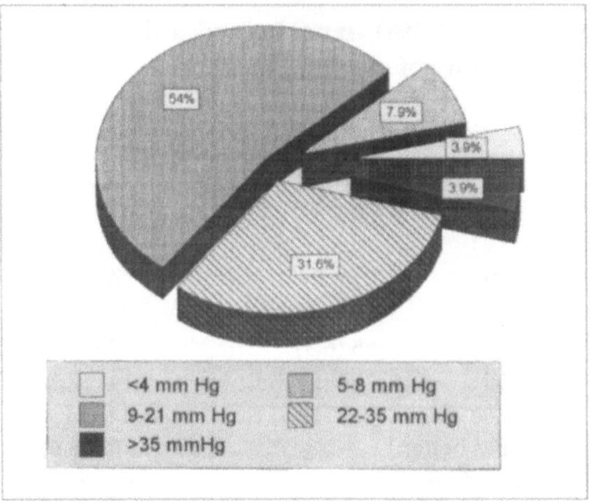

Fig. 10. Intraocular pressure on postoperative day one

(Fig. 10). This is the effect desired with this surgery, as it aims to minimize hypotony and its complications. McGuigan et al. reported on nine of 10 patients with IOPs < 10 mm Hg on the first postoperative day after combined surgery [13].

With an intentionally tighter trabeculectomy flap, the risk of postoperative pressure spiking is probably increased at the same time; however, the releasable sutures facilitate prompt treatment of elevated pressures. Although 21.3% of patients developed immediate postoperative IOP elevations, this number compares to the 62% of nonfiltered glaucomatous eyes that had immediate postoperative spikes after cataract surgery alone in the same study by McGuigan et al. [13].

Comparison of pre- and postoperative glaucoma control demostrates effectiveness in our current method. Average IOP decreased significantly from 19.5 mm Hg to 15.3 mm Hg ($p < 0.01$). Patients averaged fewer medications (0.3 postop. vs 1.6 preop.) overall. Moreover, 81% of patients were using no glaucoma medications at all postoperatively. There was also no glaucoma progression in the study population, as evidenced by stable visual fields and optic nerve exams.

The releasable sutures were safe and easy to remove when necessary. The one case which developed intraocular hemorrhage may have been related as much to the digital pressure as to the suture release. Two releasable sutures appear to be an optimal number of releasable sutures. Patients having only one releasable suture seemed to frequently require subsequent laser suture lysis.

Visual results were generally excellent. Some 82% of patients were seeing better than or equal to 20/40, and 43% had best corrected vision of 20/20 or better. Only four patients (5.1%) had severely decreased vision of ≤ 20/200. All four of these patients had serious underlying optic nerve or macular diseases unrelated to their surgery.

The spherical equivalent data show a tendency toward emmetropia. Only one patient became more myopic than predicted.

Although clinical hypotony was kept at a low incidence, it was not completely prevented by the releasable suture technique. Only four patients (5%), however, had hypotony severe enough to warrant a return to the operating room for treatment. None of the hypotonous eyes ultimately developed corneal decompensation, synechiae, or significant vitreo-retinal sequelae.

CME was identified at some point during the postoperative course of 8.7% of patients, but in general was self-limited or successfully treated without visual sequelae. One case of CME was associated with pars planitis and had been present preoperatively. In another case, the patient had concomitant retrobulbar neuritis, which probably accounted for the majority of the patient's visual loss.

Finally, the small trabeculectomy appears to be equally effective and safe as regular trabeculectomy. PMMA lenses, however, appear to have a slight advantage over foldable lenses with regard to absolute pressure-lowering effect.

In summary, combined phacoemulsification, IOL implantation, and trabeculectomy with releasable sutures is a safe and effective approach to combined cataract and glaucoma surgery. A great majority of patients have excellent visual results, improved control of their IOPs, and less reliance on medical therapy to achieve this control. Complications of hypotony are kept at a low rate. At the same time, postoperative pressure elevations can be treated in a simple and effective manner by selective postoperative suture removal.

Acknowledgement. Appreciation to Jean Chou for performing the statistical analysis.

References

1. McCartney DL, Memmen JE, Stark WJ, et al. (1988) The efficacy and safety of combined trabeculectomy, cataract extraction, and IOL implantation. Ophthalmology 95:754-763
2. Parker JS, Gollamudi S, John G, Stark WJ (1992) Combined trabeculectomy, cataract extraction, and foldable lens implantation. J Cataract Refract Surg 18:582-585
3. Wedrich A, Menapace R, Radax U, Papapanos P (1995) Long term results of combined trabeculectomy and small incision cataract surgery. J Cataract Refract Surg 21:49 54
4. Kriger SH, Tuberville A, Hamilton RS (1989) A review of extracapsular cataract extraction and IOL implantation combined with trabeculectomy. Ann Ophthalmol 21:266-8
5. Wechsler A, Robinson LP (1980) Simultaneous surgical management of cataract and glaucoma. Aust J Ophthalmol 8:151-60
6. Hoskins HD Jr, Migliazzo C (1984) Management of failing filtering blebs with the argon laser. Ophthalmic Surg 15 :731
7. Shin DH (1987) Removable-suture closure of the lamellar scleral flap in trabeculectomy. Ann Ophthalmol 19:51-55
8. Cohen JS, Osher RH (1988) Releasable scleral flap suture. Ophthalmol Clin North Am 1: 187-197
9. Kolker AE, Kass MA, Rait JL (1994) Trabeculectomy with releasable sutures. Arch Ophthalmol 112:62-66
10. McAllister JA, Wilson RP (1986) Glaucoma. Butterworths-Heinemann, Boston, pp 243-250
11. Menezo JL, Maldonado MJ, Munoz G, Cisneros AL (1994) Combined procedure for glaucoma and cataract: a retrospective study. J Cataract Refract Surg 20:498-503
12. Simmons ST (1992) Results: combined cataract extraction and trabeculectomy. CLAO Journal 18:205-208
13. McGuigan LJB, Gottsch J, Stark WJ, et al. (1986) Extracapsular cataract extraction and posterior chamber lens implantation in eyes with preexisting glaucoma. Arch Ophthalmol 104:1301-1308

Surgical Treatment of Hydrodynamic Changes Following Vitrectomy

M. Stirpe, R. Fedeli, A. M. Coppe, and G. Ripandelli

Ophthalmology Foundation G. B. Bietti, Piazza Sassari 5, 00161 Rome

Introduction

Transient or permanent increase of intraocular pressure (IOP) is a frequent post-operative complication of pars plana vitrectomy. Mild to moderate IOP elevation is observed in a high percentage (20%-48%) of vitrectomized eyes within 48 h after surgery [1, 2]; 6%-28% of eyes develop a secondary glaucoma within 1 year [3-7].

Both acute and chronic IOP elevation in vitrectomized eyes is due to an obstruction of the aqueous flow. Hyperproduction of normal or plasmoid aqueous may be hypothesized in selected cases. Open-angle obstruction mechanisms include post-trabecular and trabecular block; closed-angle mechanisms include angle block, pupillary block, and posterior block [8]. Pre-existing obstruction mechanisms represent risk factors for secondary glaucoma [2, 3].

The presence of internal tamponade compounds and postoperative fibrin production are critical factors affecting both genesis and management of ocular hypertension in vitrectomized eyes.

Hydrodynamics

Pars plana vitrectomy is performed by continuous saline infusion. Internal tamponade with water-insoluble compounds (gas, silicone oil) is usually accomplished, when required, at the end of surgery.

Intraocular saline undergoes gradual substitution by aqueous humor in the first post-operative days. IOP still depends on aqueous production and outflow as in the non-operated eye, since the absence of the vitreous body does not influence IOP level.

Intraocular gases (air, SF6, C_2F_6) are replaced by newly formed aqueous at different reabsorption rates, depending upon the physical and chemical properties of the specific gas. As the gas volume expands with absorption of hematic nitrogen, the bubble pushes the retina onto the pigment epithelium. In these conditions, IOP depends on the gas volume and concentration rather than on aqueous production and outflow. Gas pressure and surface tension can also affect the aqueous intraocular flow (pupillary block) inducing iris and/or lens dislocation.

Silicone oil (SO) usually fills 70%-80% of the vitreous cavity, the remainder being filled by aqueous humor inferiorly. In phakic and pseudophakic eyes, the SO bubble is contained by the lens; in aphakic eyes a 6 o'clock basal iridectomy allows circulation of aqueous between posterior and anterior chamber [9, 10] and helps to keep the SO posteriorly.

Sites of Obstruction of Aqueous Flow and Clinical Features

Post-trabecular block implies an increase of episcleral venous pressure following episcleral surgical procedures. Encircling scleral buckle may induce episcleral and/or vortex veins compression; surgical maneuvers can cause rupture of two or more vortex veins; in both cases IOP may increase. The IOP elevation is usually mild (3-6 mm Hg), transient and requires no therapy. In serious choroidal effusion the IOP increase is more severe than in hemorrhagic effusion.

Trabecular block can be induced by inflammatory cells, ghost cells, corticosteroid therapy, neovascularization and SO [2, 11].

Angle-block can follow anterior rotation of the ciliary body due to ciliary edema associated with choroidal detachment. Hypotony of iris musculature, with or without iris retroversion, produces peripheral anterior synechiae. Pressure exerted by intraocular gases and, less frequently, by SO may result in a postero-anterior force directed toward the iris or irido-lenticular diaphragm, which accounts for the higher incidence of angle block in these eyes. The ocular hypertension can become chronic if adhesion between iris and angular structures occurs.

Pupillary block, with or without *iridocorneal adhesion*, may complicate gas or SO tamponade in aphakic eyes; this occurred frequently in the past, before the introduction of peripheral inferior iridectomy [9, 10]. Dislocated lens, IOL and fibrin membrane may also obstruct the flow of aqueous toward the anterior chamber. Clinical features in these cases include anterior chamber shallowing and IOP elevation. Fibrin membrane, blood, inflammatory cells and granulation tissue may close the 6 o'clock iridectomy thus predisposing to pupillary block [12].

Posterior block is an uncommon event determined by SO or gas bubble pushing forward the lens; a circular diaphragm of peripheral vitreous residuals and plasmatic trasudate contribute to the onset of the block, soon complicated by peripheral irido-corneal adhesion and angle block. It is more frequently observed in highly myopic eyes with zonular weakness and gas tamponade, but sometimes follows SO tamponade. Clinical features include early IOP elevation, shallow anterior chamber, absence of pupillary block, peripheral iris adhesion.

Silicone Oil Glaucoma

The pathogenesis of chronic, open-angle SO glaucoma is related to trabecular obstruction and/or inflammation by SO emulsion. Different factors have been proven to elicit emulsification of SO: low viscosity, poor purity of the oil, insufficient filling of the vitreous cavity [13], tensioactive cell membrane constituents, presence of vitreous septa, vitreous residuals and vitreoretinal membranes. The incidence of SO emulsification ranges from 20 to 100% of cases [12, 14], while the incidence of SO glaucoma is 6%-20% [3, 5]. This discrepancy, as well as the high number of normotonic eyes with SO emulsion and angle deposits, may be explained by the fact that the outflow obstruction can be hidden by a reduced production of aqueous.
Prophylaxis of the SO-related glaucoma includes adequate filling of the vitreous cavity, reduction of the inflammation and fibrinogenesis and drainage of the hematic fluid, aimed at washing out of tensioactives.
The first step in treating SO glaucoma is medical therapy (local and systemic). The effectiveness of SO removal is debatable. Different authors report controversial data (9%-75% of IOP normalization following SO removal) [14, 15]. In our series the efficacy of this procedure was poor (31%, personal unpublished data) and unpredictable. Moreover, the risk of retinal complications has to be considered [16]. Other surgical procedures are discussed below.

Surgical Management

Surgical management of glaucoma in vitrectomized eyes offers several difficulties related to the anatomical features of these eyes, to the presence of tamponade, and to the high risk of secondary hypotony. Surgical procedures have three main purposes: to resolve acute postoperative hypertension, to avoid chronicization and to treat established glaucoma.
The first step in surgical treatment of acute post-operative hypertony should be the drainage of any inflammatory substance from the anterior chamber. Fibrine, haematic essudate or blood can be drained through a small inferior limbal incision while the patient is sitting at the slit lamp, under topical anesthesia.
Peripheral anterior synechiae can be prevented by myotics and heparin injection. Aggressive treatment is advised to avoid chronicity. Surgical lysis of the synechiae can be performed through the cornea by means of a thin spatula. A viscoelastic substance is used in more severe cases. In many cases, however, the atony of iris musculature makes the iris return to the initial position. Intraoperative diathermy of the pupillary margin induces tissue contrac-

tion and leads to persistent closure of the pupil. Before performing this procedure, newly formed tissue and vitreous fibers connected with the posterior iris surface must be detected and throughly removed, since their contraction under diathermy would lead to further pupillary dilation.

Both pupil and inferior iridectomy can be closed by fibrin membranes, blood and/or inflammatory tissue. The inferior iridectomy is more often involved because of its position and because the wounded edges of the iridectomy elicit an inflammatory process. Prophylaxis involves accurate intraoperative hemostasis, myotics and heparin. Treatment of this complication includes use of heparin or recombinant tissue plasminogen activator (r-TPA) and surgical dissection of membranes occluding the iridectomy. YAG laser photodisruption of the membranes is generally ineffective.

Posterior block glaucoma usually requires lensectomy and accurate removal of peripheral vitreous residuals. An atypical case of posterior block may occur because of SO slippage through a weak zonular ligament from vitreal cavity to posterior chamber. The SO pushes the iris toward the cornea, simulating an anterior dislocation of the lens. Displacement of the SO from the posterior to the anterior chamber is obtained by gently pushing on the iris by two thin spatulas inserted through the cornea. The SO can be removed from the anterior chamber through a limbal incision by injecting a viscoelastic substance through a second limbar incision on the opposite side. Two basal iridectomies at 6 and 12 o' clock allow the aqueous flow between posterior and anterior chamber in any eye position. Moreover, SO trapped in the anterior chamber can flow posteriorly through the superior iridectomy.

The medical treatment of chronic glaucoma is based on myotics, β-blockers, topic sympathomimetics, and carbonic anhydrase inhibitors.

β-blockers should be used carefully because of the risk of anomalous hypotensive responses in vitrectomized eyes.

Cyclodisruptive treatment (photocoagulation, cryotherapy) should be carefully evaluated for the risk of secondary severe hypotony; these techniques can be used in neovascular glaucoma, when SO cannot be removed due to the high risk of recurrence of the retinal detachment. The treatment should be performed on 90° of the ciliary body each time.

The scarring processes affecting the scleroconjunctival tissues after surgical manipulation and physical treatments make trabeculectomy and other conventional filtering procedures scarcely useful for the therapy of SO-related and other chronic forms of glaucoma. In our series, we found that the best results followed surgical cyclodiastasis, opening the uveoscleral pathway to the aqueous flow. Due to the risk of severe hypotony, cyclodiastasis should not be associated with removal of SO from the posterior chamber. Mechanical devices (Molteno implant, Schocket shunt) represent good surgical alternatives when the anatomical conditions of the eye allow their implantation [17].

References

1. Nguyen QH, Lloyd MA, Heuer DK, Baerveldt G, Minckler DS, Lean JS, Liggett PE (1992) Incidence and management of glaucoma after intravitreal silicone oil injection for complicated retinal detachments. Ophthalmol 99:1520-1524
2. Han DP, Lewis H, Lambrou FH Jr, Mieler WF, Hartz A (1989) Mechanisms of intraocular pressure elevation after pars plana vitrectomy. Ophthalmol 96:1357-1362
3. Lucke K, Strobel B, Foerster M, Laqua H (1990) Sekundarglaukome nach Silikonolchirurgie. Klin Monatsbl Augenheilkd 196:205-209
4. Karel I, Kalvodova B (1994) Long-term results of pars plana vitrectomy and silicone oil for complications of diabetic retinopathy. Eur J Ophthalmol 4:52-58
5. Lucke K (1993) Silikonol in der Chirurgie komplizierter Netzhautablosungen. Ophthalmol 90:215-238
6. Riedel KG, Gabel VP, Neubauer L, Kampik A, Lund OE (1990) Intravitreal silicone oil injection: complications and treatment of 415 consecutive patients. Graefes Arch Clin Exp Ophthalmol 228:19-23
7. Dimopoulos S, Heimann K (1986) Spatkomplikationen nach Silikonolinjektion. Langzeitbeobachtungen an 100 Fallen. Klin Monatsbl Augenheilkd 189:223-227
8. Billington BM, Leaver PK (1986) Vitrectomy and fluid/silicone-oil exchange for giant retinal tears: results at 18 months. Graefes Arch Clin Exp Ophthalmol 224:7-10
9. Ando F (1987) Usefulness and limit of silicone in management of complicated retinal detachment. Jpn J Ophthalmol 31:138-146

10. Beekhuis WH, Ando F, Zivojnovic R, Mertens DA, Peperkamp E (1987) Basal iridectomy at 6 o'clock in the aphakic eye treated with silicone oil: prevention of keratopathy and secondary glaucoma. Br J Ophthalmol 71:197-200
11. Oldendoerp J, Spitznas M (1989) Factors influencing the results of vitreous surgery in diabetic retinopathy. I. Iris rubeosis and/or active neovascularization at the fundus. Graefes Arch Clin Exp Ophthalmol 227:1-8
12. Federman JL, Schubert HD (1988) Complications associated with the use of silicone oil in 150 eyes after retina-vitreous surgery. Ophthalmol 95:870-876
13. Heidenkummer HP, Kampik A, Thierfelder S (1992) Experimental evaluation of in vitro stability of purified polydimethylsiloxanes (silicone oil) in viscosity ranges from 1000 to 5000 centistokes. Retina 12 (Suppl):S28-32
14. Moisseiev J, Barak A, Manaim T, Treister G (1993) Removal of silicone oil in the management of glaucoma in eyes with emulsified silicone. Retina 13:290-295
15. Nowack C, Lucke K, Laqua H (1992) Silikonolentfernung zur Behandlung des sog. Emulsifikationsglaukoms. Ophthalmol 89:462-464
16. Franks WA, Leaver PK (1991) Removal of silicone oil: rewards and penalties. Eye 5:333-337
17. Senn P, Buchi ER, Daicker B, Schipper I (1994) Bubbles in the bleb: troubles in the bleb? Molteno implant and intraocular tamponade with silicone oil in an aphakic patient. Ophthalmic Surg 25:379-382

Discussion

Question: Montanari

My question is to Prof. Brancato. In retreatment, how many spots do you apply? 16 like in the first treatment or less?

Answer: Brancato

Generally in the same number, but it may change according to what we should like to obtain.

Question:

I have some questions. The first question is to Dr. Jampel. Can you compare the difference in outcome between phacoemulsification combined and trabeculectomy with Mitomycin? I have already seen that you have a difference in extracapsular combined and phacocombined, but what's the difference with trabeculectomy alone and phacocombined alone? The second question is to Dr. Stark. Do you use releasable suiters with phacocombined without Mitomycin? I used releasable suiters with trabeculectomy alone, I mean with antimetabolite, but I don't see the need of releasable suiters with phacocombined because there is no hypotony.

Answer: Jampel

The question was a comparison of phacocombined with trabeculectomy and Mitomycin versus trabeculectomy with Mitomycin without cataract surgery. I can only give you my impression because I don't know of any study or how valid a study was done comparing those two. I can tell you that Mitomycin C has been shown to improve the success rate of trabeculectomy in high risk eyes, and up to date there is not a study on that.

Answer: Stark

The success rate in the high pressure patients surgically treated is about 90%. I would like to ask a question to Jampel. I think that the use of an antimetabolite may be very dangerous for the patient. You can wind up with wound leaks and have tremendous post-operative patient management. I see a tremendous variation in the concentration of Mitomycin C and the in time of application on the sclera. Can you give us the range and what is the lowest dose that might have some beneficial effects?

Answer: Jampel

First I will preface my answer by saying that there is a tremendous variation in how glaucoma specialists use Mitomycin C. Even in the small city of Baltimore the variation ranges from glaucoma specialists who hardly ever use Mitomycin C to those who use it in every case. It remains my clinical impression that the concentration of Mitomycin C is more important to determine than the duration of the application. No one has been able to show a regular difference between 0.2 and 0.4 mg; if you go another 10 fold less than 0.2 I don't think you will be able to see any effect. I believe this was the objective of Dr. Kitazawa's study. So I think the most important decision is whether to use it or not, and if one is at all hesitant I would suggest a lower concentration.

Question: Cardia

To Dr. Jampel. Can you tell us a little more about the time of application of mitomycine?

Answer: Jampel

In eyes for which I feel the highest risk of surgical failure I will use a high dose of 0.4 mg for a full 5 minutes. If I think the likelyhood of surgical failure is lower, let's say an eye which simply had uncomplicated phacoemulsification, then I will use a dose of 0.2 for two minutes. I try to make my life easier by only having a certain number of combinations that I use. In summary, my low dose will be 0.2 for 2 minutes, my high dose would be 0.4 for 5 minutes.

Question: Fruscella

To Dr. Jampel or Dr. Stark. In patients who underwent keratoplasty there are more chances of failure of the filtering bleb, and also mitomycine is toxic for the cornea: how do you manage these patients?

Answer: Jampel

In eyes that had previous corneal transplantation I would usually use an antimetabolite, and I usually use Mitomycin C. The discussion on Mitomycin C and the corneal endothelium suggests that if you can keep Mitomycin C out of the eye the damage to the eyegraft wouldn't be so great. I think that one of the golden rules for advocation of Mitomycin C is not to apply it at a time when there is an open hole in the eye. I will supply Mitomycin C before doing the fistula into the anterior chamber and I would never give Mitomycin C post-operatively when there is entrancy to the anterior chamber. I have not been able to attribute too many graft failures to the use of Mitomycin C, although when there is a graft in glaucoma surgery there are so many possible reasons that I couldn't say for certain that it didn't have a major effect.

Answer: Stark

I tend to agree with that, because of the high toxicity of 5FU. If you give it over a period of several days it will go to the corneal epithelium and I think you want to avoid a possible antigraft. I used both, but I prefer Mitomycin C in those graphs that have glaucoma. Post-operatively the management is going to be very difficult then we would prefer it, and we also had previous surgeons who preferred to combine the operation with the use of Mitomycin C.

Question: Gandolfi

I have a question and a comment to Dr. Jampel's presentation. The question is: It is well known that the prognosis for patients undergoing trabeculectomy is worse if they have been treated for a long time with miotics. Do you suggest to use antimetabolites immediately after surgery? My comment is: It is evident from literature that mitomycine is toxic for intraocular tissues and at least three groups have demonstrated that mitomicyne may damage the ciliary body, so I would suggest to be very careful with this drug.

Answer: Jampel

I believe the first part of your question concerns the use of Mitomycin C in eyes that haven't had previous surgery. No, it was not that. The second part was that we should we be more cautious with the use of Mitomycin C, given data suggesting that it has intraocular toxicity not necessarily so much to the cornea but perhaps to the ciliary epithelium or even the retina. I agree with you fully. We should be concerned about that and you are correct in your statement that a growing literature shows that Mitomycin C can not only lower intraocular pressure through making blebs better, but also cause a sort of chemical ciliary destruction. If I hadn't emphasized that enough during my talk, I would emphasize now that I think the use of Mitomycin C in eyes without previous surgery is generally not a good idea, and that if you have any doubt about its use you should not use it in that particular case.

Question:

How do you manage hypotony after Mitomycin C?

Answer: Jampel

It's simply that the pressure is low; then I will do nothing and most of the times it will resolve. However, if the patient has hypotony maculopathy with decreased visual acuity that is an urgent situation, I think the intraocular pressure needs to be restored as soon as possible surgically.
If you think that the flap sutures are tightened, something else should be done either by placing a graft over the trabeculectomy area or by performing criotherapy to the bulb. Something to restore the intraocular pressure. I have a handful of patients who still tell me that they have problems and this hypotony maculopathy has a striking incidence.

Question: Minckler

A couple of questions to Dr. Jampel and Dr. Stark relating to penetrating cheroplasty and filtering surgery. Our impression is that whether you do drain tube installation to control glaucoma associated with penetrating cheroplasty or filtering surgery, the graft rection rate is really much higher and I think that is a consideration that certainly relates to whether or not you add antimetabolites. Another point which hasn't been mentioned.
My presumption is that 5FU given to some kinds of patients away from the surgical side has its benefits if you will use it, because it gets into the eyes diffused through the aqueous or via the aqueous out through the filter. Mitomycin C, presumably because used locally, is more effective in that context. We basically use 5FU almost exclusively now during surgery, applied just like Mitomycin C and supplemented with relatively few injections.

Answer: Jampel

I am sure that drainage device surgery has increased the risk of graft failure, that is why I like to use drainage device surgery when the cornea is cloudy and before penetrating cheroplasty so that my surgery doesn't get blurred because of the graft failure but I think that is a real concern. Secondly, concerning the use of interactive 5FU I used it quite a bit in cases that I feel have a marginal indication for antimetabolites and one can then supplement them with injections that in my opinion hurt rather than help. Science has limited data about how well that works and all studies unfortunately don't show much of an effective 5FU combined surgery which would be nice if it did more.

Answer: Stark

Glaucoma is definitely a risk factor for graft failure. It's a high risk factor and so, in looking at large series in the corneal transplant studies which your institutions took part in, if a patient has pre-operative glaucoma and if nothing is done he has a much higher chance for graft failure rejection. Control studies have not been done to determine either pre-operative glaucoma operations by ciliary destructive procedures or the ouflow tubes or an operation at the time of surgical control glaucoma. All reduces the chances of graft rejection in these high risk cases. I think that of the approximately 80 cases that we did and presented at the Academy last year, about 90% had normal pressure. If you don't do some type of glaucoma operations in people who have a glaucoma, a cornea transplant is needed and pressure becomes very high. After surgery it's difficult to manage and then the success rate goes down. Our overall success rate in those eyes was about 60%. Dr. Jampel has probably done 10 or 20 of my grafting patients and even though the tube is fairly far from the cornea and the pressure is controlled, the graft often begins to thicken several months later.

Question: Rama

Again on Mitomicyne, I have no experience in glaucoma surgery but I saw many complications following pterigyum surgery plus Mitomicyne because of the complete scarring induced by this drug. How do you manage bleb lysis or scleral melting?

Answer: Jampel

Fortunately I have not observed scleral melting after the application of Mitomicyn C, probably because of the amount we give in glaucoma surgery and due to the fact that we give it only interruptively.

Valves and Drainage Implants *

T. Krupin and L. F. Rosenberg

Department of Ophthalmology, Northwestern University Medical School, Tarry 5-715, 300 East Superior Street, Chicago, Illinois 60611, USA

Introduction

Standard filtration surgery creates a limbal sclerostomy which serves to bypass conventional outflow pathways and permits aqueous humor to flow from the anterior chamber to the subconjunctival space with establishment of an external filtration bleb. Adjunctive use of antifibrotic agents, either subconjunctival injections of 5-fluorouracil (5-FU) [1, 2] or intraoperative application of mitomycin-C (MM-C) [3, 4] or 5-FU [5] increases the chance of intraocular pressure (IOP) reduction in eyes at high risk for filtration failure. However, satisfactory filtration may still be difficult to achieve in some of these types of cases. Plastic devices offer a different approach to IOP control. These implants have increased in popularity and are an alternative surgical treatment in eyes with a poor surgical prognosis. Reduction of IOP by modern implants is accomplished by shunting of aqueous through an open tube from the anterior chamber to an area of encapsulation around an explant located 8-12 mm posterior to the limbus. These devices are not "setons" (i.e., use of a foreign material to prevent closure of a surgical wound), a frequently and inaccurately used term to describe these implants. Posterior tube shunt implant more correctly describes these devices which differ in regard to the presence or absence of a flow limiting element and design of the episcleral explant.

Principles of Posterior Tube Shunt Surgery

Early studies by Molteno [6] were directed toward designing an implant which would promote formation of a functioning bleb. His original implant consisted of an acrylic tube connected to a circular (8.5 mm diameter) episcleral plate around which encapsulation occurred. The plate was sutured to the sclera only a few millimeters posterior to the limbus. Since the resulting large area of limbal encapsulation often caused discomfort and formation of corneal dellon, the explant was moved posteriorly toward the equator. This enabled the use of an enlarged (13 mm diameter) episcleral disc which resulted in a large posterior bleb [7]. Molteno's pioneering concept of a posteriorly placed episcleral bleb-promoting implant has been incorporated into devices described by Schocket [8], Baerveldt [9], Krupin [10, 11], Joseph [12], White [13], and Ahmed [14]. All of these implants consist of an open tube which is placed into the anterior chamber to shunt aqueous posteriorly into an area of encapsulation around an episcleral explant. These devices differ in regard to the presence or absence of a flow limiting element and the design of the episcleral explant (Table 1). General concepts common to all of these devices will be presented, with unique attributes of the Molteno, Baerveldt, Krupin and Ahmed devices discussed separately.

* The authors have no proprietary interests in the Krupin Eye Valve with Disk or Hood Laboratories, Inc.

Table 1. Dimensions of episcleral plate: posterior glaucoma implants

	Material	Shape	Surface area[a] (mm²)	Anterior chamber tube (outer/inner diameter mm²)
Nonrestrictive				
Molteno	Polypropylene	Round	134 (single plate)	0.63/0.3
Schocket	Silicone	Rectangle	300 (for 360° band)	0.64/0.3
Baerveldt	Silicone	Curved	250, 350, 425	0.64/0.3
Restrictive				
Krupin	Silastic	Oval	180	0.58/0.3
Joseph	Silicone	Rectangle	765 (for 360° band)	0.64/0.3
White	Silicone	Round	280	0.64/0.3
Ahmed	Polypropylene	Pear	184	0.64/0.3

[a]Two-dimensional surface area based on a circle = πr^2 where r = radius; ellipse = πab where a = shorter radius and b = longer radius; and rectangle = length x width. Surface areas of the Baerveldt and Ahmed implants are published by respective manufacturers.

Anterior Chamber Tube

The opening of the anterior chamber tube functions as the effective sclerostomy for aqueous flow from the anterior chamber to the attached episcleral explant. The tube has the advantage that it can be inserted within the anterior chamber beyond areas of peripheral anterior synechiae. In addition, the tube prevents sclerostomy closure.

Posterior Explant Encapsulation

The posterior episcleral explant stimulates fibrovascular encapsulation of the plate [15]. This process requires at least several weeks for completion. The internal surface of the encapsulation is an open, collagenous meshwork which is not lined by a continuous layer of cells and therefore, is not a true cyst [16, 17].

The area of encapsulation functions as a filtration bleb. Aqueous humor penetrates the bleb capsule (see below) and moves through intercellular spaces and is absorbed by orbital capillaries and lymphatics. The posterior location of the bleb is an advantage in eyes having had prior surgery resulting in conjunctival scarring around the limbus. The outer capsular wall becomes progressively more dense with layers of collagenous bundles. An external vascular layer covers the capsule. The capsule appears to remain separate from Tenon's layer [15] and is unable to form a firm attachment to the plastic plate surface.

Physiology of Posterior Filtration Bleb

Minckler et al. [15] using the Molteno implant in animal eyes, have shown that the main resistance to aqueous flow and IOP reduction, is the capsular wall. These investigators have also demonstrated that latex microspheres as large as 0.2 µm in diameter pass freely through the capsular wall. Moreover, the marker horseradish peroxidase (molecular weight 50 000) moves between the collagenous bundles and reaches the capillaries in the vascular layer. Similar movement of horseradish peroxidase across the encapsulated space surrounding the encircling silicone implant used in the Schocket procedure [18] and the Joseph implant [19] has been demonstrated.

Reduction of IOP is accomplished by passive flow of fluid across the capsular wall [20]. Ultrasonography (Fig. 1) demonstrates that the

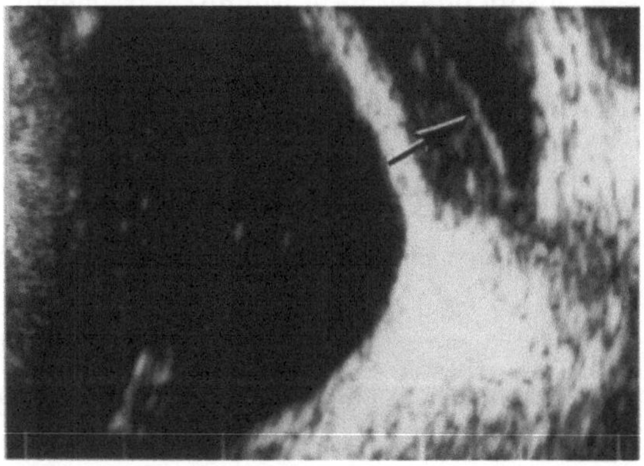

Fig. 1. Ultrasonography of fluid reservoir surrounding the episcleral plate of Krupin disc (arrow)

fluid reservoir surrounding the plate is significantly larger than the plate itself [21]. Pressure reduction is dependent upon the resistance of aqueous flow across the capsular wall (the thinner the capsule, the lower the pressure) and the total surface area of encapsulation (the larger the surface area, the lower the pressure) [22]. It is reasonable to assume that the size of the episcleral explant (see Table 1) determines, at least in part, the size of the encapsulated bleb. However, IOP reduction is not directly related to the size of the explant: IOP is not lower with the 500 mm^2 compared to the 350 mm^2 Baerveldt implant [9]; while pressure reduction is better in eyes that receive a double compared to a single plate Molteno implant, there is no significant difference in IOP control between double and quadruple plate implants [23]; IOP reduction is lower or similar using the double-plate Molteno implant compared to the Schocket encircling device, an implant with a calculated larger surface area [24, 25]. There appears to be an upper limit to explant size beyond which further increases in explant surface area may not improve IOP, and may even be detrimental to the surgical outcome [23-26].

Surgical Indications

Posterior tube shunt implants are indicated in patients with an uncontrolled IOP despite maximum tolerated medical therapy and prior failure of filtration procedures with adjunctive antifibrotic agents. These devices are used in closed-angle, open-angle, and congenital glaucomas, and a variety of glaucomas associated with poor filtration surgery success, such as aphakia, pseudophakia, uveitis, and rubeosis iridis. Primary implantation of a posterior tube shunt implant may be advised in eyes with neovascular glaucoma, closed-angle glaucoma with anteriorly located synechiae which prevent a limbal sclerostomy from communicating with the anterior chamber, or in eyes with extensive perilimbal scarring. In most other eyes, filtration surgery with adjunctive antifibrosis agents should be attempted prior to a posterior tube shunt implant because shunt implant surgery is associated with a higher rate of operative and postoperative complications than trabeculectomy [27-30].

Posterior Tube Shunt Implants

Implant designs fall into one of two categories based on the absence or presence of an element which limits aqueous flow through the anterior chamber tube. Nonrestrictive implants (e.g., Molteno and Baerveldt) permit the free flow of fluid through the anterior chamber tube to the episcleral explant. Restrictive implants (e.g., Krupin and Ahmed) incorporate an element (valve or membrane) designed to impede fluid flow in order to prevent postoperative hypotony and flat anterior chamber. In addition, the size, shape and material used for the episcleral explant differs among the various implants (see Table 1).

Nonrestrictive implants

Molteno Implant

The Molteno implant (IOP Inc., Costa Mesa, Ca) is currently the most frequently used implant for filtration surgery. It consists of a circular, 13 mm diameter, convex, rigid polypropylene episcleral plate. The scleral surface area of the plate is 134 mm^2 (one side). Holes within the rim guide are used to suture the plate to the sclera. A silicone tube (outside diameter 0.63 mm, inside diameter 0.3 mm) which is attached to the plate, passes through the rim and opens onto the convex upper surface of the plate.
Several variations of the Molteno implant are available. A double plate system has two polypropylene plates connected to each other by a 10 mm long silicone tube of similar dimension to the anterior chamber tube. Both right- and left-eyed versions of the double plate Molteno system are available. Molteno has described a quadruple plate system [23]. A pediatric size plate (8 mm diameter) is also available for use. A dual-chamber Molteno implant [31, 32] incorporates a ridge dividing the upper surface of the plate into two separate chambers. This design is intended to reduce postoperative hypotony without tube occlusion.

Baerveldt Implant

The Baerveldt implant [9] (Pharmacia, Inc.

Columbus, OH) is a single-plate, silicone implant which is currently manufactured in three sizes based on presumed collecting reservoir surface areas of 250, 350, and 425 mm^2. It is implanted with the silicone plate underneath two adjacent rectus muscles delimiting one ocular quadrant. The nonrestrictive anterior chamber silicone tube has a 0.30 mm inner and a 0.64 mm outer diameter.

The Baerveldt episcleral plate has been modified to include fenestration holes. The holes allow growth of fibrous tissue through the plate and to the other side of the bleb wall, thereby reducing the height and volume of the bleb. This change was made due to the high incidence of postoperative diplopia associated with this device (see below).

Restrictive Implants

Krupin Eye Valve with Disc Implant

The modified long glaucoma valve implant [10, 11] (Hood Laboratories, Pembroke, MA) consists of a silastic anterior chamber tube with an outside diameter of 0.58 mm and an inside diameter of 0.38 mm. The distal end of the tube is sealed and contains horizontal and vertical slits which function as a unidirectional and pressure sensitive valve. The valve is constructed to open at a pressure of approximately 11 mm Hg and to close at a pressure of approximately 9 mm Hg. The slit-valve design permits one-stage implantation without the need for restrictive ligatures in order to achieve immediate lowering of IOP. The valve end opens on an oval Silastic episcleral plate (13 mm x 18 mm; flat surface area of 183 mm^2) which has a 1.75 mm high side wall. A version with a lower side wall is available. The disc is contoured to approximate the curvature of the globe and has a Silastic platform for fixation of the explant to the sclera (Fig. 2). Design features of this implant maximize the size of the scleral explant to optimize surrounding encapsulation volume in a single quadrant between adjacent rectus muscles, thereby providing a large surface area reservoir for aqueous filtration.

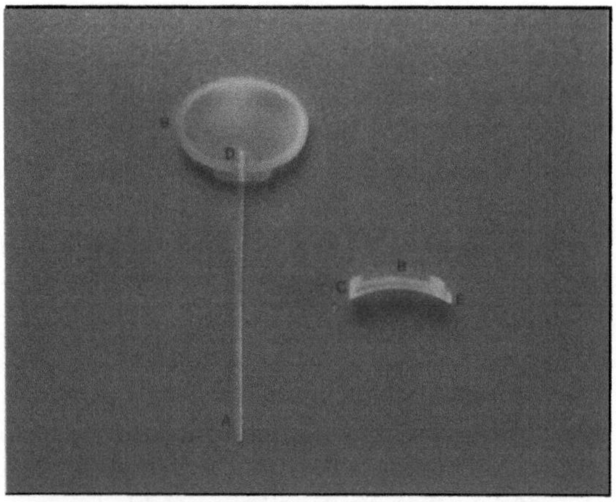

Fig. 2. Krupin eye valve with disc implant. The implant consists of: **A**, an open anterior chamber silastic tube which is trimmed before placement into the chamber; **B**, an oval episcleral silastic disk (13 mm by 18 mm) with a 1.75 mm high side wall; **C**, the disc is contoured to conform to the curvature of the globe (see cross-sectional view); **D**, an unidirectional, pressure-sensitive slit valve; **E**, a silastic platform for fixation of the explant to the sclera. (Courtesy of Hood Laboratories, Pembroke, Massachusetts)

Ahmed Implant

The Ahmed glaucoma valve implant [14] (New World Medical, Rancho Cucamonga, Ca) consists of a pear-shaped polypropylene explant. The rigid plate is 13 mm at widest width, 16 mm long, and 1.9 mm high. The surface area is 184 mm^2. Aqueous passes from the anterior chamber tube between two layers of a thin, silicone elastomer membrane on the upper surface of the plate. This membrane is enclosed within the anterior portion of the implant, creating a Venturi effect on aqueous flow through the device. A force of 8-12 mm Hg is required to separate the layers of the silicone membrane and allow aqueous to pass through the valve, into the reservoir, by Bernoulli's hydrodynamic principle where the velocity of a fluid increases as it travels from the large inlet to the smaller outlet port.

Surgical Implantation

Implantation of the various posterior tube shunt devices is performed using local or general anesthesia and share a number of common surgical techniques (see [33]). Differences relate regarding the need to limit aqueous flow at the time of implantation in the nonrestrictive devices.

Implantation of Nonrestrictive Implants

Two-Stage Insertion

Primary insertion of a nonrestrictive, open anterior chamber tube and the episcleral plate is frequently associated with excessive flow of aqueous humor resulting in hypotony, flat anterior chamber, and choroidal detachment. Because of these complications, Molteno recommended a two-stage implantation [34]. This allows encapsulation to occur around the episcleral plate prior to inserting the tube into the anterior chamber. During the first stage, the plate is attached to the episclera 8-10 mm posterior to the limbus as described above. The open end of the anterior chamber tube is placed under the plate or beneath an adjacent rectus muscle and attached to the episclera using a black silk suture to assist in later identification during the second surgical stage. Since the first stage operation does not reduce IOP, a trabeculectomy is frequently perfomed for interim pressure control. The trabeculectomy is done at a different site from where the tube will later be inserted into the anterior chamber. Medical antiglaucoma therapy is administered postoperatively as required to lower IOP.

The second operative stage, insertion of the tube into the anterior chamber, is performed 2-6 weeks later. The two-stage procedure is recommended in patients at high risk for suprachoroidal hemorrhage or flat anterior chamber, such as aphakic or pseudophakic glaucoma, especially if there has been prior vitreous loss, high myopia, congenital glaucoma, shallow anterior chamber, and closed-angle glaucoma.

Flow of aqueous humor through the tube creates a posterior filtration bleb by dissecting the fibrous encapsulation off the surface of the episcleral plate. During this interval, IOP is frequently elevated to preoperative (or even higher) levels and marked inflammation is observed in the region of the posterior bleb. Antiglaucoma medications and topical corticosteroids are administered during this transient hypertensive phase which may last several weeks [28]. Gradually IOP declines and the bleb inflammation resolves, permitting withdrawal of antiglaucoma medications. Long-term IOP control is usually not affected by this hypertensive phase which may be similar to the bleb remodeling ("high bleb phase") observed after trabeculectomy [35]. The magnitude of the hypertensive phase is reduced with the double-plate Molteno system [36].

One-Stage Insertion

The one-stage operation for nonrestrictive implants consists of attaching the episcleral plate(s) and inserting the anterior chamber tube during the same procedure, thereby eliminating a second operation. Various methods have been used to convert one-stage insertion into a functional two-stage insertion by temporarily occluding the flow of aqueous through the anterior chamber tube of the nonrestrictive implant until the episcleral plate becomes encapsulated. These techniques require intervention to reverse the occlusion. These methods which are not required with restrictive implants, are limited by the difficulty encountered in completely occluding flow through the small bore anterior chamber tube.

1. Buried tube ligature: The tube is occluded with a suture ligature placed around the tube posterior to the scleral flap or donor graft. Various suture materials have been used. We prefer an 8-0 vicryl suture [37] which generally dissolves in 2-4 weeks. If the suture is visible through the conjunctiva, argon laser lysis may be performed if early release is needed or if the vicryl suture dissolves incompletely. Alternately, the suture can be cut via a conjunctival incision.
2. Exposed tube ligature: A releasable nylon or chromic [38] suture is tied around the tube and exposed externally. Care must be taken not to dislodge the tube when this suture is removed. Another releasable suture technique [39] has been described wherein a nylon suture is passed through corneal stroma to emerge from the sclera and beside the tube. A triple-turn of the suture makes a slip knot which, when tied securely, occludes the tube lumen. Infection is an important potential complication with an exposed suture.
3. Anterior chamber tube ligature: Prior to inserting the distal end of the tube into the anterior chamber, a polypropylene suture is

tied to the wall of the tube, and then around the end of the tube and tied [40]. If IOP is elevated, laser lysis is used to cut the suture to release the occlusion while the suture remains attached to the tube wall. In a similar fashion, two interrupted nylon sutures are tied around the anterior end of the tube before insertion into the anterior chamber [41]. However, if laser lysis is indicated, the loose suture will be retained in the inferior anterior chamber angle. Both of these techniques obviate manipulation of the conjunctiva.

4. Internal suture tube occlusion: The internal lumen of the tube is occluded with a 4-0 chromic suture which exits the conjunctiva, and is therefore exposed, over the episcleral plate. The occlusive suture is removed by pulling the externalized suture end [42-44]. This "rip-cord" technique may serve as a conduit for infection. Suture removal can be associated with severe intraocular inflammation, including hypopyon [45]. Alternately, a nonexposed, nondissolvable 5-0 nylon [46] or 3-0 Supramid suture is used to internally block the tube, and the opposite end of suture is placed subconjunctivally 90°-180° away from the tube for removal via a conjunctival incision at a later date. Venting slits in the extrascleral portion of the tube are made and provide early IOP control [47] until the plate is encapsulated. An anterior bleb is noted during this interval.
5. Collagen plug: A collagen lacrimal plug is used to occlude the proximal end of the tube [48]. Unfortunately, the plug may not dissolve and require surgical removal. This may be because of the relative lack of proteolytic enzymes and collagenases in the aqueous humor [49].

Surgical Results

It is difficult to compare accurately the success rates among the current posterior tube shunt implants. Success with respect to control of IOP depends upon the type of glaucoma. The highest success rates (60%-80%) occur in eyes with open- or closed-angle glaucoma, either phakic or aphakic/pseudophakic, and in eyes which previously failed filtration surgery. The lowest success usually occurs in eyes with neovascular glaucoma (25%-67%) [33].

Postoperative Complications of Posterior Tube Implant Surgery

Filtration surgery with posterior tube implant procedures is associated with similar operative and postoperative complications as those occurring following any intraocular procedure in a glaucomatous eye, e.g., anterior chamber hemorrhage, pupillary block, suprachoroidal hemorrhage, retinal detachment, malignant glaucoma, endophthalmitis. However, glaucoma implant surgery is frequently associated with a higher rate of complications due to the underlying ocular disease processes and the numerous prior surgical procedures in the eyes undergoing this type of surgery [27-29, 50-52]. Suprachoroidal hemorrhage occurs in 5%-8% of eyes undergoing implant surgery [28, 53]. Late (> 3 months) postoperative complications which are unique to the posterior tube implant procedure are described below. These complications can occur with any of the implant types described in this paper.

Increased Intraocular Pressure

Late failure with increased IOP can be caused by: (1) blockage of the anterior chamber tube opening, including posterior tube migration out of the anterior chamber; (2) blockage within the tube between the anterior chamber and the episcleral plate; or (3) a nonfunctioning encapsulated bleb. Blockage of aqueous humor egress to the episcleral plate fails to produce a bleb. The overlying conjunctiva is flat against the plate. Visible occlusion of the tube at its opening may be treated by the argon or Nd:YAG laser. If this is not successful or possible, surgical revision is necessary. At surgery, we perform a paracentesis incision and place a 27-gauge blunt-tipped cannula into the tube for injection of balanced salt solution [54]. If the tube is patent, this maneuver may elevate the fibrous encapsulation off of the episcleral explant with formation of a bleb. Failure to irrigate through the tube may indicate a more distal tube obstruction. A wire (e.g., the stylet from a 25-gauge spinal needle) is inserted through the paracentesis tract into the tube and advanced toward the plate. This maneuver may open an obstructed tube. Success is assured by repeat injection of balanced salt into the tube and formation of a bleb over the episcleral explant.

Failure to create a bleb after injection of balanced salt solution through the tube indicates either blockage of the tube on the surface of the episcleral plate or a thickened encapsulation adherent to the plate. This situation is best managed by bleb revision. In our experience, revision by needling of the bleb [27] and withdrawal of aqueous humor followed by 5-FU injections has a low success. Therefore, our preferred method of revision includes dissection of the area of encapsulation over the plate and excision of the fibrous wall. Intraoperative MM-C may be applied to the fibrous capsule overlying the plate [55], although its use is empiric and improved efficacy is not established. Alternatively, a failed procedure can be managed by implantation of additional episcleral devices.

Hypotony

An attempt at reversal of postoperative hypotony resulting from overfiltration by the posterior shunt implant should be considered when there is associated visual loss from hypotony maculopathy, or when there is choroidal detachment, extreme shallowing of the anterior chamber, and/or severe ocular inflammation. Surgical revision would consist of one or more of the techniques described previously for preventing aqueous flow through the anterior chamber tube. Ocular hypotony refractory to these methods would then demand removal of the implant in favor of an alternate method for IOP reduction.

Tube Migration

Posterior migration of the tube out of the anterior chamber requires external dissection to expose the tube. Inadequate anchoring of the tube to the episclera can result in fibrous tissue "pulling" the tube out of the anterior chamber. The tube will be kinked rather than having a straight course from the episcleral plate. In this situation, the tube is isolated and repositioned into the chamber. Episcleral sutures are used to anchor the tube in place.

Migration of the tube either out of or further inside the anterior chamber can occur from slippage of the episcleral plate. This can result from an anchoring suture pulling out of the sclera or following use of an absorbable anchoring suture. In this situation, the tube and anterior encapsulation around the plate are dissected, the plate repositioned so that the tube is in proper position within the anterior chamber, and the plate resutured to the sclera using nonabsorbable sutures.

Implant Erosion

Late erosion of the tube through the conjunctiva can occur, especially if the scleral graft melts. We do not repair this type of defect unless there is leakage of aqueous humor at the site (a positive Seidel test) or ocular irritation due to the exposed tube. Exposed sutures which may incite the erosion, are removed. Repair of an exposed tube requires placement of a donor tissue graft over the site as closure of conjunctiva alone over the tube is inadequate. Dehydrated human dura mater [56] is commercially available and is an alternative to human donor sclera [57] which carries the potential for infectious disease transmission as well as melting. Autologous fascial grafts from either the fascia lata femoris or the temporal fascia [58] may also be considered. A large defect may require a conjunctival graft. Epithelial ingrowth into the fibrous capsule surrounding the episcleral plate has been reported and is associated with persistent aqueous fluid leakage through the conjunctival wound [59].

Late erosion and exposure of the episcleral plate can also occur. Adequate mobilization of the posterior Tenon's space at the time of implantation is essential to prevent this complication. Application of MM-C over the plate may predispose to erosion of the explant. Exposure of the episcleral plate may require removal of the device. Erosion of the episcleral plate into the vitreous cavity is another potential complication.

Cornea

Contact of the tube against the endothelium with migration of the tube out through the entire thickness of the cornea is an unusual complication. More commonly, progressive corneal endothelial cell loss results [60]. Constant tube-corneal touch initially causes reduction in cell count but usually results in a stable fixed corneal attachment without further cell loss. However, intermittent tube touch such as that might be produced when the patient rubs the eye, causes repeated endothelial wounding, endothelial cell migration, and progressive cell loss.

An increased incidence of corneal graft rejection in eyes with previous penetrating keratoplasty may be associated with plastic drainage devices [61, 62]. The causes of corneal decompensation and graft failure are unclear in the majority of eyes. Some probably relate to the eyes having undergone multiple previous surgeries and episodes of inflammation, as well as the effect of uncontrolled glaucoma on graft survival. Others may relate not only to corneal-tube contact, but also to the fact that the anterior chamber is exposed to the extraocular environment. This is further supported by the observation in uveitis patients that leukocytes were deposited from the anterior chamber into the equatorial Molteno filtering bleb [63].

Cataract

Tube-lens touch may be associated with the formation of cataract. Usually the lens opacity is localized to the area of tube contact.

Calcification of Implant

There is one report [64] of calcification noticed on the surface of the distal portion of the silicone tube of a Molteno implant in a childs eye 6 years afler implantation. The source of calcium deposition is left to speculation, but youth, inflammatory eye disease, and presence of the implant for many years are considered risk factors for its development.

Endophthalmitis

Endophthalmitis is a rare complication of drainage devices [65-68]. There are few reports in the literature, and it is unclear whether removal of the implant is indicated. Differentiation from sterile endophthalmitis is imperative since the latter responds to topical corticosteroids.

Diplopia

Many patients experience transient diplopia after posterior tube implant surgery similar to patients undergoing retinal detachment surgery. In most patients, symptoms resolve when postoperative periocular edema subsides. Permanent strabismus is characterized by a nonprogressive limitation of eye movement in the direction of the implant. Possible causes include: (1) a posterior fixation effect induced by scarring between the rectus muscle, the encapsulation surrounding the explant and the sclera [69]; (2) a large bleb resulting in a crowding effect that limits movement of the eye [70, 71]; (3) scarring between the oblique muscle and the explant. A progressive muscle imbalance suggests the possibility of a fat adherence syndrome [72].

Permanent restrictive strabismus is more likely to develop when implants are placed near or under the insertion of a rectus muscle or in eyes which develop a large bleb, particularly in the superonasal quadrant [73-76] or inferonasal quadrant [77]. While strabismus can occur with any of the posterior tube drainage devices, it is more common with the Baerveldt implant [74]. The Baerveldt implant has been modified to reduce the height of the bleb and incidence of diplopia. The plate is fenestrated to allow growth of fibrous tissue through the plate, to the other side of the bleb wall, thereby limiting the size of the bleb.

In cases of intolerable diplopia refractory to treatment with prisms, the implant must be removed. A Baerveldt implant may be replaced by a double plate Molteno [74] or another implant placed in the superotemporal quadrant, if possible.

Summary

The use of aqueous humor drainage implants is an important option in the treatment of refractory glaucoma. The efficacy of these devices has improved and the complications reduced by such modifications as enlarging the surface area of the collecting reservoir, aqueous humor flow reducing techniques, and the use of a donor tissue patches to cover the tube. The clinical outcomes of these implants are most influenced by the type of glaucoma. The variable criteria for success among reported series limits direct comparison of the efficacy of the different types of drainage implants.

The two major problems with implant surgery are the occurrence of hypotony in the early postoperative period and excessive encapsulation around the external implant preventing adequate aqueous humor filtration. The optimal method by which to prevent hypotony still does not exist, but current methods to reduce outflow have decreased the incidence of this complication.

The permeability and surface area of the fibrous capsule surrounding the explant are key factors in final IOP control. There is an optimal explant size for which filtration is most likely achieved. Perhaps the addition of antifibrosis medications at the time of surgery and/or during the postoperative period will further promote bleb formation and long-term IOP control. However, the long-term efficacy of these agents in glaucoma implant surgery has not yet been determined.

References

1. The Fluorouracil Filtering Surgery Study Group (1989) Fluorouracil filtering surgery study one-year follow-up. Am J Ophthalmol 108:625-35
2. Weinreb RN (1987) Adjusting the dose of 5-fluorouracil after filtration surgery to minimize side effects. Ophthalmology 94:564-70
3. Skuta GL, Beeson CC, Higginbotham EJ, Lichter PR, Musch DC, Bergstrom TJ, et al. (1992) Intraoperative mitomycin versus postoperative 5-fluorouracil in high-risk glaucoma filtering surgery. Ophthalmology 99:438-44
4. Chen CW (1983) Enhanced intraocular pressure controlling effectiveness of trabeculectomy by local application of mitomycin C. Trans Asia-Pacific Acad Ophthalmol 9:172-7
5. Smith MF, Sherwood MB, Doyle JW, Khaw PT (1992) Results of intraoperative 5-fluorouracil supplementation on trabeculectomy for open-angle glaucoma. Am J Ophthalmol 114:737-41
6. Molteno ACB (1969) New implant for drainage in glaucoma. Clinical trial. Br J Ophthalmol 53:606-615
7. Molteno ACB, Strachan JL, Ancker E (1976) Long tube implants in the management of glaucoma. S Afr Med J 50:1062-1066
8. Schocket SS, Lakhanpal V, Richards RD (1982) Anterior chamber tube shunt to an encircling band in the treatment of neovascular glaucoma. Ophthalmology 89:1188-1194
9. Lloyd ME, Baerveldt G, Heuer DK, Minckler DS, Martone JF (1994) Initial clinical experience with the Baerveldt implant in complicated glaucomas. Ophthalmology 101:640-650
10. Krupin T, Ritch R, Camras CB, Brucker AJ, Muldoon TO, Serle J, et al. (1988) A long Krupin-Denver valve implant attached to a 1800 scleral explant for glaucoma surgery. Ophthalmology 95:1174-1180
11. Krupin Eye Valve Filtering Surgery Study Group (1994) Krupin eye valve with disk for filtration surgery. Ophthalmology 101:651-658
12. Joseph NJ, Sherwood MB, Trantas G, Hitchings RA (1986) A one piece drainage system for glaucoma surgery. Trans Ophthalmol Soc UK 105:657-664
13. White TC (1992) Clinical results of glaucoma surgery using the White glaucoma pump shunt. Ann Ophthalmol 24:365-373
14. Coleman AL, Hill R, Wilson MR, Choplin N, Kotas-Neumann R, Tam M, et al. (1995) Initial clinical experience with the Ahmed glaucoma valve implant. Am J Ophthalmol 120:23-31
15. Minckler DS, Shammas A, Wilcox M, Ogden TE (1987) Experimental studies of aqueous filtration using the Molteno implant. Trans Am Ophthalmol Soc 85:368-392
16. Rubin B, Chan C, Burnier M, Munion L, Freedman J (1990) Histopathologic study of the Molteno glaucoma implant in three patients. Am J Ophthalmol 110:371-379
17. Philipp W, Klima G, Miller K (1990) Clinicopathological findings 11 months after implantation of a functioning aqueous-drainage silicone implant. Graefe's Arch Clin Exp Ophthalmol 228:481-486
18. Schocket SS (1986) Investigations of the reasons for success and failure in the anterior shunt-to-the-encircling-band procedure in the treatment of refractory glaucoma. Trans Am Ophthalmol Soc 84:743-798
19. Peiffer RL, Popovich KS, Nichols DA (1990) Long-term comparative study of the Schocket and Joseph glaucoma tube shunts in monkeys. Ophthalmic Surg 21:55-59
20. Wilcox MJ, Minckler DS, Ogden TE (1994) Pathophysiology of artificial aqueous drainage in primate eyes with Molteno implants. J Glaucoma 3:140-151
21. Lloyd M, Minckler DS, Heuer DK, Baerveldt G, Green RL (1993) Echographic evaluation of glaucoma shunts. Ophthalmology 100:919-927
22. Prato JA, Santos RCR, LaBree L, Minckler DS (1995) Surface area of glaucoma implants and perfusion flow rates in rabbit eyes. J Glaucoma
23. Molteno ACB (1981) The optimal design of drainage implants for glaucoma. Trans Ophthalmol Soc NZ 33:39-41
24. Wilson RP, Cantor L, Katz LJ, Schmidt CM,

Steinmann WC, Allee S (1992) Aqueous shunts: Molteno versus Schocket. Ophthalmology 99:672-678
25. Smith M, Sherwood MB, McGorray SP (1992) Comparison of the double-plate Molteno drainage implant with the Schocket Procedure. Arch Ophthalmol 110:1246-1250
26. Krupin T (1993) Discussion of paper by MA Lloyd, et al. Intermediate-term results of a randomized clinical trial of the 350- mm² vs the 500-mm² Baerveldt implant. Ophthalmology 101:1463-1464
27. Melamed S, Cahane M, Gutman I, Blumenthal M (1991) Postoperative complications after Molteno implant surgery. Am J Ophthalmol 111: 319-322
28. Minkler DS, Heuer DK, Hasty B, Baerveldt G, Cutting RC, Barlow WE (1988) Clinical experience with the single-plate Molteno implant in complicated glaucomas. Ophthalmology 95: 1181-1188
29. Lloyd MA, Sedlak T, Heuer DK, Minckler DS, Baerveldt G, Lee MB, et al. (1992) Clinical experience with the single-plate Molteno implant in complicated glaucomas. Ophthalmology 99:679-687
30. Bluestein EC, Stewart WC (1993) Trabeculectomy with 5-fluorouracil versus single-plate Molteno implantation. Ophthalmic Surg 24:669-673
31. Freedman J (1992) Clinical experience with the Molteno dual-chamber single-plate implant. Ophthalmic Surg 23:238-241
32. Molteno ACB (1990) The dual chamber single plate implant. Aust NZ J Ophthalmol 18:431-436
33. Rosenberg LF, Krupin T (1996) Implants in glaucoma surgery. In: Ritch R, Shields MB, Krupin T (eds) The glaucomas. 2nd ed CV Mosby, St. Louis, pp 1783-1807
34. Molteno ACB, Van Biljon G, Ancker E(1979) Two-stage insertion of glaucoma drainage implants. Trans Ophthalmol Soc NZ 31:17-26
35. Scott DR, Quigley HA (1988) Medical management of a high bleb phase after trabeculectomies. Ophthalmology 95:1169-1173
36. Heuer DK, Lloyd MA, Abrams DA, Baerveldt G, Minckler DS, Lee MB, et al. (1992) Which is better? One or two? A randomized clinical trial of single-plate versus double-plate Molteno implantation for glaucomas in aphakia and pseudophakia. Ophthalmology 99:1512-1519
37. Molteno ACB, Polkinghorne PJ, Bowbyes JA (1986) The vicryl tie technique for inserting a draining implant in the treatment of secondary glaucoma. Aust NZ J Ophthalmol 14:343-354
38. Hoare Nairne JEA, Sherwood D, Jacob JSH, Rich WJCC (1988) Single stage insertion of the Molteno tube for glaucoma and modifications to reduce postoperative hypotony. Br J Ophthalmol 72:846-851
39. El-Sayad F, El-Maghraby A, Helal M, Amayem A (1991) The use of releasable sutures in Molteno glaucoma implant procedures to reduce postoperative hypotony. Ophthalmic Surg 22:82-84
40. Price FW Jr, Whitson WE (1989) Polypropylene ligatures as a means of controlling intraocular pressure with Molteno implants. Ophthalmic Surg 20:781-783
41. Liebmann JL, Ritch R(1992) Intraocular suture ligature to reduce hypotony following Molteno seton implantation. Ophthalmic Surg 23:51-52
42. Lieberman MF, Egbert PR (1989) Internal suture occlusion of the Molteno glaucoma implant for the prevention of postoperative hypotony. Ophthalmic Surg 20:53-56
43. Latina MA (1990) Single stage Molteno implant with combination internal occlusion and external ligature. Ophthalmic Surg 21:444-446
44. Egbert PR, Lieberman MF (1989) Internal suture occlusion of the Molteno glaucoma implant for the prevention of postoperative hypotony. Ophthalmic Surg 20:53-56
45. Ball SF, Loftfield K, Scharfenberg J (1990) Molteno rip-cord suture hypopyon. Ophthalmic Surg 21:407-412
46. Susanna R (1991) Modifications of the Molteno implant and implant procedure. Ophthalmic Surg 22:611-613
47. Sherwood MB, Smith MF (1993) Prevention of early hypotony associated with Molteno implants by a new occluding stent technique. Ophthalmology 100:85-90
48. Stewart W, Feldman RM, Gross RL (1993) Collagen plug occlusion of Molteno tube shunts. Ophthalmic Surg 24:47-48
49. Ball SF, Herrington RG (1993) Long-term retention of chromic occlusion suture in glaucoma seton tubes. Arch Ophthalmol 111:169
50. Krupin T (1988) Setons in glaucoma surgery. In: Waltman SR, Keates RH, Hoyt CS, et al. (eds) Surgery of the eye. Churchill Livingstone, New York, pp 377-385
51. Lotufo DG (1991) Postoperative complications and visual loss following Molteno implantation. Ophthalmic Surg 22:650-656
52. Waterhouse WJ, Lloyd ME, Dugel PU, Heuer DK, Baerveldt G, Minckler DS, et al. (1994) Rhegmatogenous retinal detachment after Molteno glaucoma implant surgery. Ophthalmology 101:665-671
53. Sherwood MB, Joseph NH, Hitchings RA (1987) Surgery for refractory glaucoma: results and complications with a modified Schocket technique. Arch Ophthalmol 105:562-569
54. Krupin T, Rosenberg LF, Ruderman JM (1994) Drainage implants. In: Kaufman PL, Mittag TW (eds) Glaucoma. Mosby, St. Louis, pp 9.62-9.75
55. Susanna R, Nicolela MT, Takahashi WY (1994)

Mitomycin C as adjunctive therapy with glaucoma implant surgery. Ophthalmic Surg 25:458-462
56. Brandt JD (1993) Patch grafts of dehydrated cadaveric dura mater for tube-shunt glaucoma surgery. Arch Ophthalmol 111:1436-1439
57. Watzke R (1984) Scleral patch graft for exposed episcleral implants. Arch Ophthalmol 102:114-115
58. Dresner DB, Boyer DS, Feinfeld RE (1991) Autogenous fascial grafts for exposed retinal buckles. Arch Ophthalmol 109:288-289
59. Sidoti PA, Minckler DS, Baerveldt G, Lee PP, Heuer DK (1994) Epithelial ingrowth and glaucoma drainage implants. Ophthalmology 101:872-875
60. McDermott ML, Swendris RP, Shin DH, Juzych MS, Cowden JW (1993) Corneal endothelial cell counts after Molteno implantation. Am J Ophthalmol 115:93-96
61. O'Day DG, Stulting RD, Lynch MG, Brown RH (1992) Graft survival and intraocular pressure control after Molteno valve implantation for postkeratoplasty glaucoma. Invest Ophthalmol Vis Sci 33 (Suppl):1273
62. Stewart DH, Swendris RP, Shin DH, Cowden JW, Siegel MJ (1992) Outcome of Molteno implantation for glaucoma associated with penetrating keratoplasty. Invest Ophthalmol Vis Sci 33 (Suppl):1273
63. Hill RA, Nguyen QH, Baerveldt G, Forster DJ, Minckler DS, Rao N, et al (1993) Trabeculectomy and Molteno implantation for glaucomas associated with uveitis. Ophthalmology 100: 903-908
64. Fellenbaum PS, Baerveldt G, Minckler DS (1994) Calcification of a Molteno implant. J Glaucoma 3:81-83
65. Ellis BD, Varley GA, Kalenak JW, Meisler DM, Huang SS (1993) Bacterial endophthalmitis following cataract surgery in an eye with a preexisting Molteno implant. Ophthalmic Surg 24:117-120
66. Krebs DB, Liebmann JM, Ritch R, Speaker M (1992) Late infectious endophthalmitis from exposed glaucoma setons. Arch Ophthalmol 110:174-175
67. Perkins TW (1990) Endophthalmitis after placement of a Molteno implant. Ophthalmic Surg 21:733-734
68. Heher KL, Lim JI, Haller JA, Jampel HD (1992) Late-onset sterile endophthalmitis after Molteno tube implantation. Am J Ophthalmol 114:771-772
69. Christmann LM, Wilson ME (1992) Motility disturbances after Molteno implants. J Pediatr Ophthalmol Strabismus 29:44-48
70. Ball SF, Ellis GS Jr, Herrington RG, Liang K (1992) Brown's superior oblique tendon syndrome after Baerveldt glaucoma implant. Arch Ophthalmol 110:1368
71. Wilson-Holt N, Franks W, Noureddin B, Gregson R, Hitchings RA (1990) Hypertropia following inferiorly sited double plated Molteno tubes. Ophthalmology 9 (Suppl):143
72. Munoz M, Parrish R (1992) Hypertropia after implantation of a Molteno drainage device. Am J Ophthalmol 113:98-100
73. Prata JA, Minkler DS, Green RL (1993) Pseudo-Brown's syndrome as a complication of glaucoma drainage implant surgery. Ophthalmic Surg 24:608-611
74. Smith SL, Starita RJ, Fellman RL, Lynn JR (1993) Early clinical experience with the Baerveldt 350-mm^2 glaucoma implant and associated extraocular muscle imbalance. Ophthalmology 100:914-918
75. Munoz M, Parrish RK II (1993) Strabismus following implantation of Baerveldt drainage devices. Arch Ophthalmol 111:1096-1099
76. Dobler AA, Sondhi N, Cantor LB, Ku S (1993) Acquired Brown's syndrome after a doubleplate Molteno implant. Am J Ophthalmol 116:641-642
77. Çardakli UF, Perkins TW (1994) Recalcitrant diplopia after implantation of a Krupin valve with disc. Ophthalmic Surg 25:256-258

Re-intervention as a Treatment of Glaucoma

D. S. Minckler

Glaucoma Services, Doheny Eye Institute and University of Southern California Medical School, Los Angeles, CA, USA

Introduction

Re-intervention as treatment of glaucoma must be considered whenever previous therapies have failed to achieve desired intraocular pressure (IOP). Surgical interventions in particular, whether initial or repeat procedures, provide challenging complications necessitating re-interventions. This report briefly discusses some practical aspects of surgical re-interventions as therapy for common complications of trabeculectomy and glaucoma drainage device (GDD) installations.

Since important features of any clinical problem can change with time or as a result of previous surgery, it is essential to continually review the pathophysiology of an eye's disorder. The likelihood of management errors must surely increase if we fail to assess ongoing tissue alterations or assume that either the mechanisms or the most appropriate treatment of glaucoma in any specific case will remain static. For example, many eyes initially in the chronic open-angle glaucoma category and responsive to medications develop progressive peripheral anterior synechiae (PAS) after laser or surgical interventions. Over time they transition into a more complex "combined disease" category in which angle closure plays an increasing role, normal outflow pathways become less responsive, and filtering surgery inevitable. Continued age-related lens enlargement in globes with small anterior segments may put a previously "cured" and stable eye at risk for recurrence of angle closure in spite of an open peripheral iridectomy. In such instances, the most rational treatment may be clear lens extraction. Besides continually reviewing the ophthalmological findings, decisions about surgical re-interventions must also consider an eye's vision potential and systemic aspects of the individual patient.

Expectations After Filtering Surgery

Besides the potential for intraoperative or immediate postoperative complications, 30%-50% of primary trabeculectomies performed without antifibrotic agents still fail by 6-10 years after surgery [1, 2]. The failure rate of trabeculectomy in complicated glaucomas with one or more previous surgeries is 50% - 70% at 3 years, even with 5-flurouracil antifibrosis therapy at the time of surgery [3]. The principal reason for failure with or without antifibrotics remains progressive fibrosis at the episcleral surface and closure of the trabeculectomy cleft. Although they clearly improve short-term results, 5-flurouracil (5-FU) and mitomycin-C (MMC) have yet to be demonstrated to improve long-term results of initial or repeat trabeculectomies [4]. Multi-year studies of GDD results also demonstrate failure of IOP control at rates of 10% - 20% per year in non-neovascular glaucomas [5, 6].

Complication Rates

In spite of improvements in technique, trabeculectomy still has a significant likelihood of complications. If we define a complication after trabeculectomy as any minor or major "adverse event," approximately 50% of cases are complicated during the first 12 months postoperatively [4]. The majority of complications are minor, occur shortly after surgery and do not require surgical re-interventions. Minor complications include most shallow and some flat anterior chambers, most choroidal effusions and many choroidal hemorrhages, transient corneal endothelial decompensation and most instances of transient visual loss or delay of visual recovery [4-7]. Major complications including wound dehiscences, many flat chambers, some choroidal hemorrhages and infections may require prompt surgical re-interventions. Acceleration of cataract formation after trabeculectomy accounts for most cases of further visual loss and is best treated by cataract extraction many weeks to months later after inflammation has resolved and IOP has stabilized. Persisting further loss of central vision after trabeculectomy is infrequent, about 7% through 9 months, and most likely in aged eyes with advanced optic nerve injury when surgery is followed by prolonged hypotony [7]. The more advanced the optic nerve and visual field injury, the more likely visual recovery will be delayed.

Anesthesia

Local anesthesia, including facial nerve and retrobulbar blocks, is adequate for most glaucoma surgery and combined procedures. Peribulbar irrigation of local anesthetic into the retrobulbar space directly with a blunt cannula is preferable to retrobulbar needle injection in axially elongated, buphthalmic, or staphylomatous eyes, and can be supplemented more easily to enhance anesthesia during prolonged surgery. Topical applications of anesthetic and a small subconjunctival injection over the trabeculectomy site work well for the initial incision, after which a peribulbar irrigation into the retrobulbar space can be accomplished. The duration of anesthesia after local injection or irrigation will be shortened if the periocular tissues are inflamed.

General anesthesia is best if cooperation by the patient is questionable for the time required.

Sudden, unexpected tensing of the orbit or proptosis and increased IOP during retrobulbar injection suggests retrobulbar hemorrhage. Blood typically dissects around the globe and stops at the insertion of Tenon's fascia 2 mm posterior to the cornea scleral junction. Conjunctival hemorrhage will not respect Tenon's insertion. The appearance of hemorrhage anteriorly after a retrobulbar bleed may be delayed for many minutes depending on its size and how rapidly clotting occurs. Release of the lateral canthal ligament is indicated if IOP is sufficiently high to stop central retinal artery pulsation. Delaying surgery for at least 3 weeks is generally advised after a retrobulbar hemorrhage and general anesthesia may be preferable at the next attempt.

Perforation of the globe during a retrobulbar needle insertion should prompt an immediate retinal exam and determination of need for retinal treatment or vitrectomy to best deal with any intraocular injury. Sudden clouding of the cornea during placement of retrobulbar anesthetic suggests intraocular injection of solution and extremely high IOP.

Location of Initial and Repeat Surgical Interventions

Centering the initial trabeculectomy in the upper nasal quadrant and avoiding the twelve o'clock position provide the most flexibility for subsequent glaucoma or cataract procedures. In eyes with pre-existing filtering blebs superiorly, cataract surgery can perhaps be best done by small incision surgery using phakoemulsification from the temporal or inferior temporal side, avoiding direct trauma to the filtering bleb. Cataract surgery alone in eyes at risk for developing glaucoma may also be done from the temporal side via small incision surgery sparing the superior conjunctiva for later trabeculectomy. Cataract wounds alone, when done from above, should be limited to one quadrant if possible. My present preference for combined cataract and glaucoma procedures is to do a temporal phakoemulsification followed by a separate upper nasal trabeculectomy with intraoperative 5-FU or MMC. All cataract incisions in combined glaucoma and cataract procedures should be securely sutured to enable safe massage of the globe postoperatively if necessary. Clear corneal phakoemulsification may be preferable to scleral tunnel approaches if bleeding is expected or if speed is important because of anesthesia limitations.

If medical treatment is ineffective, repeat trabeculectomy at a new site superiorly is usually the most desirable surgical re-intervention for failed trabeculectomy. Revision of a failed trabeculectomy at the previously used location, even with MMC application before scleral re-dissection or postoperative 5-FU, still has a relatively low success rate. After two or more failed trabeculectomies superiorly, consideration should be given to a GDD installation superiorly or trabeculectomy inferiorly. Inferior trabeculectomy has been associated with a relatively high late infection rate [8]. Inferior trabeculectomy also has the disadvantages of increased exposure and persisting discomfort. GDD installations superior nasally or inferiorly have a higher risk of symptomatic strabismus than when used superior temporally [9].

After scleral buckling procedures in eyes with 180° or larger silicone-rubber encircling elements in position for 3 weeks or more, a "modified" Schocket procedure is an effective treatment for persisting high IOP [10]. This procedure is particularly useful as the glaucoma portion of a combined cataract and glaucoma surgery following scleral buckles in which the conjunctiva has been extensively damaged or when silicone oil remains in the eye. The portion of the tube placed in the buckle capsule should be side-perforated to decrease the risk of obstruction. A permanent (prolene) suture should be used to secure the tube to the episclera to prevent later intraocular migration.

Hypotony

Immediate or delayed hypotony (IOP $\leq$ 4mm Hg) remains the "common denominator" of most complications requiring re-interventions after trabeculectomy. We can speculate that hypotony causes episcleral obstruction (scissoring) of vortex vein outflow with resulting choroidal venous congestion and transudation of fluid and serum into the suprachoroidal space. Other consequences of ocular decompression may include a variation of central vein occlusion with optic disc swelling and hemorrhagic retinopathy [11]. Detachment of the ciliary body by the effusion presumably impairs aqueous production and causes anterior rotation of the lens-iris diaphragm and shallowing of the anterior chamber. A flat anterior chamber with lens or IOL-corneal touch associated with choroidal effusions is a justification for prompt surgical re-intervention to drain choroidal effusion and reform the anterior chamber. In any case, a thorough search for the cause of hypotony must be undertaken including especially the exclusion of wound leaks.

Some shallow anterior chambers will reverse with vigorous cycloplegia alone, or after air, balanced salt solution or viscoelastic installation. Neither air nor balanced salt solution will deepen a flat or shallow anterior chamber if even a modest choroidal effusion is present and will just bubble out along the paracentesis tract during attempted injection. Viscoelastics can be used to forcibly deepen chambers in eyes with choroidal effusions but may result in an intolerable rise in IOP.

Persisting hypotony after GDD installation is rare but may imply that the drainage field established exceeds the eye's ability to produce aqueous. Eyes with iris and anterior segment neovascularization associated with diabetes or vascular occlusions or which have had trauma or multiple previous surgical interventions or cyclodestructive procedures are candidates for persisting hypotony after drain tube installation. Reversal of persisting hypotony with GDDs may require removing or reducing the size of the explant or temporary or permanent ligature of the drain tube. An unusually large response to preoperative aqueous suppressing drugs such as systemic carbonic anhydrase inhibitors in "battered eyes" is reason for caution before using large GDDs.

Titration of Intraocular Pressure Postoperatively

Erring toward tight wound closure, especially when intraoperative antifibrotic agents are used, and employing either removable scleral flap sutures or planned transconjunctival laser suture lysis several days later often permit effective clinical titration of postoperative IOP and avoidance of hypotony. Antifibrotic agents, particularly MMC, extend the time frame during which suture release or suture lysis is effective from a few to many days, permitting conversion to a full-thickness procedure when outflow resistance beyond the scleral flap is sufficient to minimize hypotony. If intraoperative hemorrhage renders the conjunctiva and Tenon's non-transparent, removable sutures may be preferable to planned laser suture lysis. Persisting hypotony may still result after suture release, even many days after surgery, if conjunctival inflammation has been minimal. Also strain-induced sudden circumferential expansion of the filtering bleb may occur even months after surgery when MMC has been used.

Maintaining physical separation of the Tenon's-conjunctival surface from the episclera is desirable to prevent fibrous bridging and obliteration of the bleb. Moderate pressure on the globe 180° away from the fistula may restore a flattened bleb or further elevate a low bleb postoperatively. Vigorous massage in the immediate postoperative period can disrupt the limbal adhesions securing a fornix-based flap or may result in undesirable, sudden expansion of the bleb under a limbus-based flap. Controlled "burping" of the sclera flap by focal pressure along the lateral edges with a cotton swab or smooth instrument is a better controlled manner to re-establish aqueous escape, especially when done under slit lamp view. Any physical distortion of the scleral flap wound during the first few days does have a risk of provoking hemorrhage, sometimes with back bleeding into the eye. Fortunately, most of this type of delayed bleeding will self tamponade and will not completely block the fistula. Small hyphemas are common at the first postoperative visit and generally do not require any intervention. Large postoperative hemorrhages (eight-ball) with high IOP which obstruct the fistula should be irrigated out of the anterior chamber through a second paracentesis.

Tissue Plasminogen Activator for Fibrin Obstruction of Trabeculectomy Clefts or Drain Tubes

Tissue plasminogen activator (tPA) is very effective for dissolving fibrin obstruction of filtering clefts and tubes [12]. Irrigation via a paracentesis of 4-8 μg of tPA into the anterior chamber can effect clearing of fibrin obstructions in minutes and may be preferable to mechanical solutions in some eyes such as massage or suture lysis. It may also be useful to increase aqueous exchange in those occasional cases which have high IOP in spite of large non-hemorrhagic blebs which are apparently filled with serum products and fibrin during the first few days. The obvious hazard of tPA is additional bleeding, presumably triggered by lysis of fibrin clots closing small vessels in or around the scleral flap. This material can be stored in small doses suitable for single use for at least 1 year at -30 °C.

Wound Leaks

Conjunctival bleb leaks recognized at wound closure by Seidel testing with fluorescein should be sutured before leaving the operating room. Brisk leaks recognized postoperatively require suturing if they are large enough to see clearly by slit lamp, especially if antifibrotics were used. Leaks over portions of the scleral cleft (jet stream leaks) frequently require limited closure of the scleral cleft and diversion of aqueous flow elsewhere. Small round (non-cutting) vascular needles mounted on non-braided absorbable suture (9-O polygalactin) work well for routine wound closure and seem ideal for repair of conjunctival leaks if no episcleral suturing is required.

Delayed wound leaks, recognized many days after surgery with antifibrotics, are most common in the avascular conjunctiva overlying the scleral flap. Most of these occur in areas of extremely thin or necrotic conjunctiva and some are impossible to suture. In such instances, debridement of the necrotic conjunctiva and sliding or freehand conjunctival grafts may be necessary.

In extreme cases, especially when the scleral flap has disintegrated, a donor scleral patch graft over the original scleral flap may be necessary. Exposed or eroded hardware (drain tubes or explant materials) must be covered by healthy host Tenon's and conjunctiva or by preserved, sterile donor tissues (sclera, fascia lata, pericardium, dura).

Overfiltration

In the absence of a detectable leak, "overfiltration" due to lack of scleral flap resistance may be proven if compression of the flap at the slit lamp effects immediate deepening of the anterior chamber. Overfiltration is likely as the cause of anterior chamber shallowing if a diffuse 360° bleb has formed. Overnight tamponade by simple patching, patching over a large soft contact lens, or use of a Simmons shell or symblepharon ring which compresses the scleral flap may speed resolution of overfiltration. Chamber shallowing due to overfiltration will resolve as conjunctival inflammation and resistance increase. Deferring or minimizing topical application of steroids and postoperative injections of 5-FU are sensible pending leak closure and normalization of the anterior chamber depth.

Paracentesis during Surgery and Cycloplegia

Routine placement of a paracentesis during surgery and routine use of atropine postoperatively are desirable. Atropine probably decreases the risk of anterior chamber shallowing since some shallow chambers in non-cyclopleged eyes will rapidly normalize with vigorous cycloplegia alone. Pseudophakic eyes, regardless of implant type, are less likely than phakic eyes to become shallow or flat with profound hyptony, probably because the implants haptics act as struts.

Choroidal Effusions, Aqueous Misdirection, and Choroidal Hemorrhage

Expansion of the choroid by serous effusion often accompanies postoperative hypotony. Choroidal effusion may be diffuse and not visible by fundus exam or limited to only the most anterior portions of the suprachoroidal space. Diffuse choroidal effusion can be easily detected with commonly available B-scan units but limited anterior (anular) choroidal effusions require a non-contact (stand-off technique for ultrasound visualization). Anular choroidal effusions may be confused clinically with aqueous misdirection especially if IOP measurements are artifactually high because of anterior chamber shallowing. Expansion of the choroid makes aqueous misdirection very unlikely as the explanation for anterior chamber shallowing.

Aqueous misdirection may respond to vigorous cycloplegia. In cases non responsive to medical treatment, surgical re-interventions may include attempts at vitreous disruption with the Nd:YAG laser, vitreous needle tap via the pars plana, clear lens extraction with anterior vitrectomy, or pars plana vitrectomy without or with lens extraction. Because of the potential confusion between this rare occurrence and annular choroidal effusions, a preoperative ultrasound is wise. In any case, checking for choroidal effusion before penetration of the eye wall for vitrectomy is reasonable.

Surgical re-intervention with drainage of choroidal effusions and reformation of the anterior chamber is indicated if lens-cornea touch occurs or is threatened, in order to protect the corneal endothelium. Many shallow anterior chambers will spontaneously deepen as IOP rises above 4-6 mm Hg typically by 3-6 weeks. IOP often will be noted to be rising just before choroidal effusions suddenly subside. A single drainage with flattening of the choroid and anterior chamber reformation with air or viscoelastic will usually reverse the course, ending the hypotony, particularly if conjunctival resistance is sufficient to keep IOP above 4- 6 mm Hg. Since the use of antifibrotic agents and steroids will slow the development of conjunctival resistance to aqueous escape, delaying choroidal drainage for several weeks after 5-FU or MMC trabeculectomies and minimizing topical steroid use is desirable before surgical intervention. The presence of at least limited inflammation of the conjunctival wound is perhaps the only practical guide as to when resistance to aqueous escape may be adequate to avoid immediate recurrence of choroidal effusion.

A practical technique for choroidal drainage is to utilize a single sclerotomy, placed 4 mm behind the limbus (3 mm in aphakia) over the largest choroidal fluid collection localized preoperatively by ultrasound, usually inferior temporally. The sclerotomy can be left open or a small window of sclera excised. A blunt 23 gauge anterior chamber infusion cannula held by the assistant allows continuous internal tamponade during release of choroidal fluid from the sclerotomy and minimizes trauma to the anterior segment structures. Indirect ophthalmoscopy can be used to confirm flattening of the choroid. A large air bubble injection at closure and topical atropine perhaps aid the reattachment of the ciliary body and resumption of aqueous production.

Choroidal hemorrhage, most likely 24-72 h postoperatively, frequently occurs in hypotonous eyes with pre-existing choroidal effusion. Choroidal hemorrhage may be signaled by intense pain in or around the eye, although some are painless [13, 14]. Many reports have described their occurrence while the patient was straining at stool, justifying the routine use of stool softeners and cautions against vigorous Valsalva maneuvers during the first several days after surgery. Most often, clotting and self-tamponade rapidly occur limiting the elevation and lateral extent of choroidal hemorrhage. Visual consequences obviously depend on the size and location of the choroidal hemorrhage, but are often surprisingly minimal [13, 14]. Only rarely do choroidal hemorrhages recur or continue to extend after the initial bleed. Choroidal hemorrhages associated with break-through vitreous or anterior chamber bleeding have a poor prognosis. Surgical intervention in choroidal hemorrhage is justified only in unusual cases with intractable pain or extremely elevated IOP or when inflammation or adhesions along kissing portions of the retina are noted. Evacuation of choroidal blood is generally impossible until clot lysis occurs, usually best documented by ultrasound 2-3 weeks after the event [14]. Systemic anticoagulants should be stopped before surgery and their resumption delayed for several days postoperatively to minimize the risk of choroidal bleeding.

Hypotony-Maculopathy

Hypotony associated with choroidal folds and macular edema (hypotony-maculopathy) has been most common in young myopic eyes undergoing their first trabeculectomy with antifibrotic agents, either 5-FU or MMC [4]. The majoritv of hypotony maculopathy cases will resolve spontaneously, but may require an agonizingly long period of many weeks to many months. Prolonged hypotony, especially in older patients, may be associated with central retinal vessel decompensation and cystoid macular edema. Fluorescein angiography (FA) has been useful in some cases to distinguish eyes with only choroidal folds from those with choroidal folds and cystoid retinal edema, the latter having greater risk of permanent central vision damage. Retinal vessel leakage, demonstrated by FA, may be a reasonable criteria to use as justification for a re-intervention in cases of prolonged hypotony after trabeculectomy. Autologous blood injection into the filtering bleb has been effective in some cases when blood was retained in the bleb. When indicated for visual rehabilitation, cataract extraction may also provoke inflammation and rise in IOP. Anecdotal reports include eyes with hypotony-maculopathy returning to 20/20 acuity after as long as 18 months of zero IOP following phakoemulsification.

Postoperative Inflammation and Cystic Blebs

Reduction of elevated IOP by aqueous suppressing agents along with continued use of topical steroids probably aids the favorable evolution of cystic blebs, most likely to occur 2-3 weeks after trabeculectomy. High IOP may itself be a stimulus to inflammation and fibrosis of the bleb wall. The degree of optic nerve damage can be used as a guide to the urgency of lowering IOP. Steroid-induced elevation of IOP must be considered when the IOP is high in spite of a clinically favorable bleb appearance. If IOP remains unacceptable and the cystic bleb does not evolve favorable over several weeks, even after resumption of topical antiglaucoma medication, simple needling or surgical revision may be indicated. Injections of 5-FU following these re-interventions probably increase the likelihood of success.

Reports of delayed "scleritis" after MMC trabeculectomies reminds us that previously unknown or rare complications of filtering surgery may appear following every modification of surgical technique [15, 16]. Three recent personal experiences with immediate postoperative clinical "scleritis" in two highly myopic eyes and one eye with congenitally thin sclera suggested that topical application of MMC in thin walled eyes might trigger a chemical uveitis and scleritis. Postoperatively in these three cases, the globes were exquisitely tender, the most severe requiring hospitalization for intravenous pain control! Megadoses of systemic steroids may offer the best option of resolving the more severe of these rare occurrences when topical steroids are ineffective. In rabbits, topical scleral application of MMC can induce significant rectus muscle injury [16]. Minimal concentrations and shortened time applications of MMC are obvious adjustments to consider to minimize chemical irritation.

Late Infection

The most severe problem being reported in alarming numbers after trabeculectomy with antifibrotic agents is late bleb infection with progression to endophthalmitis. Reports have indicated that the risk of late infection approximates 9% at an average of 2 years after surgery with inferior blebs and 3% with superior blebs [8]. These high rates of late infection seem likely to persist or increase with longer follow-up time because of the inevitable rupture or leak of the typical avascular conjunctival blebs resulting from trabeculectomy with antifibrotic agents. Patients should be continually reminded to report immediately any unusual irritation, pain, vision decrease or discharge indefinitely after successful trabeculectomy, particularly when antifibrotic agents have been employed. Patients with chronic lid inflammations or infections of the lids or lacrimal drainage apparatus may be inappropriate candidates for trabeculectomy. GDDs, installed without antifibrotic use, may be preferable in patients with conjunctival, lid or lacrimal disease which renders them infection-prone. In one recent personal case, a second episode of bleb infection and endophthalmitis in the only seeing eye within months of an otherwise successful MMC trabeculectomy prompted surgical revision and closure of the scleral flap combined with installation of a GDD. The second episode in the same eye strongly suggested that the filtration bleb was incompetent to prevent infection and that it was a clinical time-bomb!

Chronic tear deficiency has not been evaluated as a risk factor for delayed infection after trabeculectomy with antifibrotic agents but is an obvious and important potential contributing disorder. The-long term effects of filtering surgery on the tear film, with or without antifibrotic agents, is also a deserving subject for investigation.

Combination Surgical Treatments

A variety of complex re-interventions have been successfully used in eyes with complex glaucomas. For example, neovascular glaucoma presenting with acute pain, elevated IOP, and corneal edema, associated with vitreous hemorrhage and hyphema in diabetes, may require staged re-interventions. If corneal decompensation precludes adequate visualization for panretinal photocoagulation (PRP), a drain tube installation for temporary IOP control may permit resolution of inflammation, media clearing and later vitrectomy, lensectomy and endolaser. Even seemingly hopeless cases with complicated retinal detachments and decompensated corneas may benefit from staged interventions with return to useful vision after sequential cornea, retina and glaucoma surgeries. Planning for post operative IOP control using a first stage GDD at the time of corneal and retina-vitreous procedures may be very helpful to an eventual good outcome.

Cyclodestruction

Traditional cyclodestructive procedures including cyclocryotherapy and newer laser treatments such as transscleral Nd:YAG seem most appropriate when central vision potential is poor because of continued reports of relatively high rates of further decrease in central vision following cyclodestruction [18]. However, in eyes with multiple previous failed procedures, regardless of vision potential, cyclodestructive intervention may be the most reasonable next alternative. Long-term results with Nd:YAG cyclodestruction for intractable glaucoma continue to indicate a relatively high risk of continued vision loss (approximately 40%) whether or not IOP is successfully lowered. Many eyes require multiple (repeat) treatments and the success of IOP control drops from about 70% at 3 years to about 45% at 5 years [17].

Sequence of Glaucoma Interventions and Re-interventions

We should remember that filtering surgery without antifibrotics in the aged eye undergoing its first glaucoma operation is relatively likely to succeed, at least for a few years [1, 2]. Importantly, trabeculectomy without antifibrotics has a low rate of late endophthalmitis. Antifibrotic agents are likely to be utilized currently by most glaucoma specialists in the United States at the first trabeculectomy even in routine cases and certainly in young patients or in repeat filtering surgery and aphakic eyes. GDDs are currently considered appropriate in any eye with multiple previous surgeries, some eyes with congenital anomalies precluding standard surgery, or after previous failed trabeculectomy. Antifibrotic agents have yet to be shown in large, prospective studies as enhancing success rates with GDDs, although short-term results in one report are encouraging [19].

While we all may acknowledge that antifibrotics diminish inflammation and improve short-term results after trabeculectomy, we should remain skeptical about the long-term benefits of these agents until proven by proper clinical studies. It is possible that the effects of these agents are transient, simply delaying the inevitable episcleral fibrosis in many cases and rendering the filtering blebs unusually vulnerable to infection in others. It is possible that late endophthalmitis following trabeculectomy with adjuvant antifibrotics may actually be blinding more eyes from late infection than were previously lost to poorly controlled IOP.

References

1. Araujo SV, Spaeth GL, Roth SM, Starita RJ (1995) A ten-year follow-up on a prospective, randomized trial of postoperative corticosteroids after trabeculectomy. Ophthalmology 102:1753-1759
2. Nouri-Mahdavi K, Brigatti L, Weitzman M, Caprioli J (1995) Outcomes of trabeculectomy for primary open-angle glaucoma. Ophthalmology 102:1760-1769
3. The Fluorouracil Filtering Study Group (1993) Three-year follow-up of the flurouracil filtering surgery study. Am J Ophthalmol 115:82-92
4. Prata JA Jr, Seah SKL, Minckler DS, Lee MB, Baerveldt G, Lee PP, Heuer DK (1995) Postoperative complications and short term outcome after 5-flurouracil or mitomycin-C trabeculectomy. Glaucoma 4:25-31
5. Lloyd MA, Sedlak T, Heuer DK, Minckler DS, Baerveldt G, Lee MB, Martone JF (1992) Clinical experience with the single-plate Molteno implant in complicated glaucomas. Update of a pilot study. Ophthalmology 99:679-687
6. Lloyd MA, Baerveldt G, Fellenbaum PS, Sidoti PA, Minckler DS, Martone FJ, LaBree L, Heuer DK (1994) Intermediate-term results of a randomized clinical trial of the 350 versus the 500-mm² Baerveldt implant. Ophthalmology, 101:1456 1464
7. Seah SKL, Prata JA Jr, Minckler DS, Lee MB, Baerveldt G, Lee PP, Heuer DK (1995) Visual recovery after trabeculectomy. Glaucoma 4:228-234
8. Wolner B, Liebmann JM, Sassani JW, Ritch R. Speaker M, Marmor M (1991) Late bleb-related endophthalmitis after trabeculectomy with adjunctive 5-flurouracil. Ophthalmology 98:1053-1060
9. Prata JA JR, Minckler DS, Green RL (1993) Pseudo-Brown's syndrome as a complication of glaucoma implant surgery. Ophthalmic Surg 24:608-611
10. Sidoti PA, Minckler DS, Baerveldt G, Lee PP, Heuer DK (1994) Aqueous tube shunt to a preexisting episcleral encircling element in the treatment of complicated glaucomas. Ophthalmology 101:1036-1043
11. Fechtner RD, Minckler DS, Weinreb RN, Frangei G and Jampol LM (1992) Complications of glaucoma surgery: Ocular decompression retinopathy. Arch Ophthalmol 110:965-968
12. Lundy D, Sidoti P, Heuer DK, Minckler DS, Lee PP (1996) Intracameral tPA after glaucoma surgery. Ophthalmology 103:274-282
13. Rockwood EJ, Kalenak JW, Plotnik JL, Yoon JS, Sculley L, Medendorp SV (1995) Prospective ultrasonographic evaluation of intraoperative and delayed postoperative suprachoroidal hemorrhage from glaucoma filtering surgery. Glaucoma 4:16-24
14. Chu TC, Cano MR, Green RL, et al. (1991) Massive suprachoroidal hemorrhage with central retinal apposition. A clinical and echographic study. Arch Ophthalmol 109:1575-1581.
15. Fourman S (1995) Scleritis after glaucoma filtering surgery with mitomycin C. Ophthalmology 102:1569-1571

16. Prata JA Jr, Minckler DS, Mermoud A, Baerveldt G (1996) Effects of mitomycin-C on the function of Baerveldt glaucoma drainage implants in rabbits. Glaucoma 5:29-38
17. Fluorouracil Filtering Surgery Study Group (1992) Risk factors for suprachoroidal hemorrhage after filtering surgery. Am J Ophthalmol 113:501-507
18. Dickens CJ, Nguyen Ngoc, Morea JS, Wong PC, Tran H (1995) Long-term results of noncontact transscleral neodymium: YAG cyclophotocoagulation. Ophthalmology 102:1777-1781
19. Perkins TW, Cardakli UF, Eisele JR, et al. (1995) Adjunctive mitomycin-C in Molteno implant surgery. Ophthalmology 102:91-97

Outcomes of Surgical Treatment for Primary Open-Angle Glaucoma*

J. Caprioli, K. Nouri-Mahdavi, L. Brigatti, and M. Weitzman

Glaucoma Section, Department of Ophthalmology and Visual Science, 330 Cedar Street, New Haven, CT 06520-8061, USA

Introduction

Trabeculectomy has become the most commonly performed operation for the surgical treatment of glaucoma since its introduction by Koryllos [1] and Cairns [2]. Recent modifications include the use of antimetabolites [3, 6], laser suture lysis [7], and releasable sutures [8]. Prior studies have described the short- and long-term effects of trabeculectomy on intraocular pressure [9-17]. Few studies have addressed long-term outcomes with respect to optic nerve structure and function [11, 17-19], and have mostly used manual methods of visual field evaluation. We studied the long-term outcomes of patients after trabeculectomy for primary open-angle glaucoma.

Materials and Methods

The charts of all consecutive phakic patients who underwent trabeculectomy between January 1984 and December 1991 were reviewed. Eligibility criteria were: a diagnosis of primary open-angle glaucoma (POAG), age > 30 years, no previous ocular surgery, no intraoperative or postoperative use of antimetabolites, and a minimum follow-up of 2 years after surgery with at least three visual fields available during this period and at least one baseline preoperative field. Coexisting retinal or neurologic disease that may have affected the visual field was a specific criterion for exclusion. In cases in which both eyes of a patient were eligible, the eye with the longer follow-up was included. POAG was defined as the presence of a reproducible visual field defect consistent with glaucoma and the appearance of the optic disc and an open angle with no signs of secondary causes of glaucoma. Indications for surgery were: (1) intraocular pressure (IOP) which, in the opinion of the examiner, placed the patient at high risk of glaucomatous progression while on maximally tolerated medical therapy; (2) worsening of the visual field while on maximally tolerated medical therapy; or (3) deterioration of the optic disc while on maximally tolerated medical therapy. The mean of the last three IOPs recorded during the three months preceding trabeculectomy formed the preoperative IOP. Progressive glaucomatous damage was defined as worsening of the visual field or deterioration of the optic disc according to criteria detailed below. We defined tonometric "success" as postoperative IOP below 21 mm Hg and an IOP reduction of at least 20%. All surgery was performed by one of the authors (J.C.) and employed a limbus-based flap and standard technique [20].

Automated perimetry (G1, 32, or C08 programs of Octopus, Interzeag, Northboro, MA;

*This work was supported in part by grants from the National Institutes of Health (EY07353); The Alcon Research Institute Award, Merck Sharp & Dohme Inc., Research to Prevent Blindness, Inc., and the Connecticut Lions Eye Research Foundation. Dr. Nouri-Mahdavi was supported in part by a grant from the Iranian Ministry of Health and Medical Education

or 24-2 or 10-2 threshold tests of Humphrey Field Analyzer, Allergan Humphrey, San Leandro, CA) was used to monitor visual field status. The same visual field program was used to examine each eye during follow-up.

Nonglaucomatous causes of visual field deterioration were taken into consideration before confirming that progression of the visual field had taken place.

Visual fields were evaluated independently by two experienced observers. The two observers had access to difference-from-normal grids, gray scale plots, visual field indices, visual acuity at the time of each visual field exam and the date of cataract surgery, if any. Data regarding the IOP and optic nerve head were not available to them. In case of disagreement between the two observers, they re-evaluated the visual fields together so that they could reach a consensus on whether or not a glaucomatous change had occurred.

Stereoscopic color optic disc photographs were taken with a Zeiss fundus camera (Karl Zeiss, Oberkochen, Germany). They were evaluated qualitatively with a stereoviewer by three independent trained observers masked with respect to all clinical information. Decisions about change were made by comparison to a set of reference slides that defined change [21]. Agreement between at least two observers was required before change was determined to have occurred. Serial drawings of the optic disc were performed at baseline and at last follow-up in each case by the treating physician (J.C.). In patients for whom baseline and last follow-up disc photographs were not available, the decision about optic disc change made by the treating physician at the time of the final examination on the basis of serial drawings was used as the optic disc outcome for this study.

Life-table analysis was applied to assess different long-term outcomes of the operated eyes [22, 23]. Gehan's test was used to compare survival curves obtained by the two different criteria for IOP control [23]. The χ^2 test was used to compare outcomes in patients with definite preoperative glaucoma progression vs those without such history [23]. Paired Student's *t* test was used to compare mean IOP before and after cataract extraction in patients who had cataract surgery [23].

Results

Preoperative Characteristics

Table 1 shows the preoperative characteristics of our patient population.

Table 1. Preoperative characteristics of the patient population

Number of patients	78
Men	27
Women	51
Number of eyes	78
Right eyes	43
Left eyes	35
Age (yrs)	
Range	33-38
Mean (± SD)	68.4 ± 10.4
Preoperative IOP (mm Hg)	
Range	13-43
Mean (± SD)	24.1 (± 6.1)
Preoperative Visual Acuity	
Range	0.07-1.25
Mean (± SD)	0.67 (± 0.27)
Number of preoperative medications	
Mean (± SD)	2.56 (± 0.86)
Prior ALT (No. of eyes)	
Yes	26
No	52

SD = standard deviation

A total of 78 eyes (43 right eyes, 35 left eyes) from 78 patients (51 women, 27 men) were eligible. There were eight African-American and two Hispanic patients; all other patients were Caucasian. In 13 eyes the indication for surgery was documented evidence of progressive visual field deterioration or optic disc damage in spite of maximally tolerated medical treatment. In the 65 remaining eyes, surgery was performed because of presumed progression or an IOP deemed too high to maintain stability given the existing optic disc and visual field damage, despite maximally tolerated medical treatment.

Surgical Complications

Malignant glaucoma and flat anterior chamber necessitating anterior chamber reformation and drainage of choroidals occurred in one

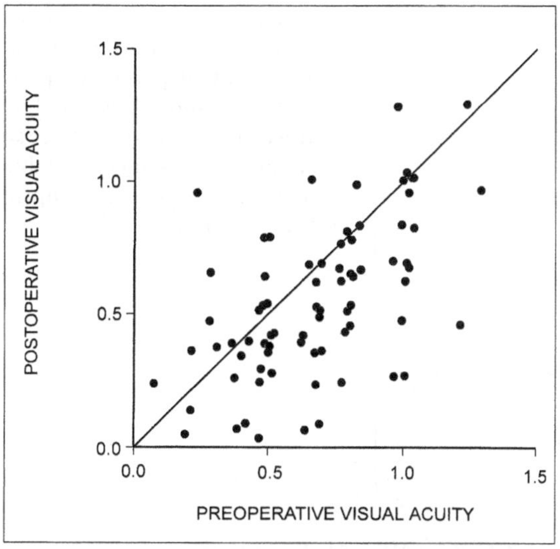

Fig. 1. Long-term changes in visual acuity after trabeculectomy for primary open-angle glaucoma. Points below the line of unity show eyes in which visual acuity decreased postoperatively

eye each. Bleb encapsulation was noted in 13 eyes. In all but one of these cases, IOP normalized after several weeks without surgical intervention.

One late-onset postoperative complication was a bleb leak which appeared 22 months after surgery and resolved after several weeks of conservative management.

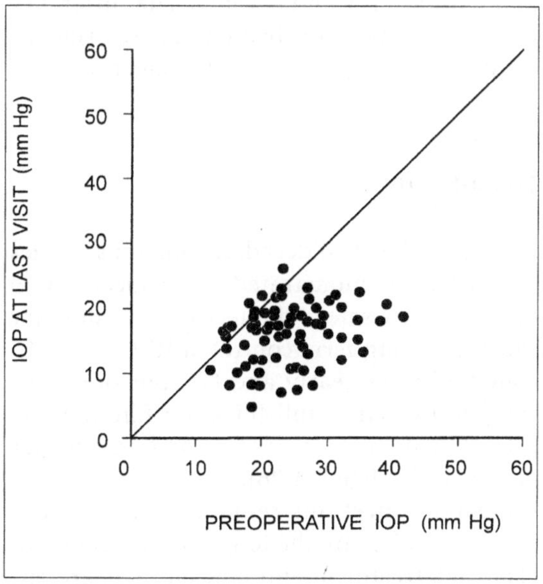

Fig. 2. Long-term tonometric results of trabeculectomy. The points below the line of unity display eyes in which reduction of the intraocular pressure was achieved

Visual Acuity

Figure 1 shows a scatterplot of preoperative visual acuity vs postoperative visual acuity at last follow-up. The mean (±SD) visual acuity decreased from 0.67 (±0.27) preoperatively to 0.54 (±0.29) at the last follow-up visit. In three eyes, significant visual acuity loss was attributed to worsening glaucoma. In three other eyes, visual acuity loss was due to progressive macular degeneration, background diabetic retinopathy, and epiretinal membrane formation, respectively. In all other patients, visual acuity loss could be explained by development or progression of cataract.

Intraocular Pressure

The IOP decreased from a mean (±SD) preoperative value of 24.1 mm Hg (±6.1) to 16.1 mm Hg (±4.2) at the last postoperative visit for all the study eyes. The average (±SD) number of medications used decreased from 2.56 (± 0.86) preoperatively to 0.94 (±1.01) at the last follow-up. Figure 2 displays a scatterplot of preoperative IOP vs postoperative IOP at last follow-up.

Visual Field

Glaucomatous visual field deterioration occurred in 16 out of 78 eyes (21%) during the follow-up period. In five cases, worsening of the visual field occurred before the second surgical intervention. In one eye visual field deterioration occurred despite additional glaucoma surgery. One patient refused additional surgery despite worsening of the visual field. In the remaining cases (9/78), progression occurred at pressures which were deemed unlikely to be lowered by further surgical intervention.

Optic Disc

Twenty-nine eyes had baseline and follow-up stereoscopic optic disc photographs of sufficient quality for evaluation. Progressive glaucomatous damage could be detected in four eyes. In three of these eyes, visual fields did not demonstrate deterioration. In the remaining eye, optic disc was evident 34 months after visual field deterioration. Optic disc deterio-

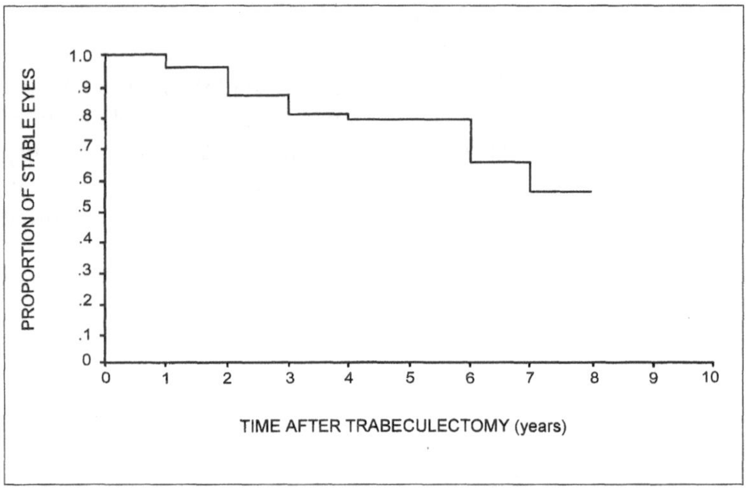

Fig. 3. Proportion of eyes remaining stable after surgical treatment of primary open-angle glaucoma as assessed by life-table analysis. Disease stability was defined as stable visual field and stable optic disc appearance

ration was not detected by the treating physician (J.C.) based on serial drawings of the optic disc in any of the eyes that did not have photographs during the follow-up period.

Other Outcomes

Patients were followed for 25÷112 months (median, 55 months). Fifty-nine eyes did not undergo any further (laser or incisional) surgery. Among those, visual field progression was established in nine eyes. In addition, four eyes showed evidence of deterioration of optic disc, in three of which this was the only evidence of glaucoma progression.

A total of 19 eyes (24%) underwent additional glaucoma surgery because of either evidence of further glaucomatous damage or unacceptably high IOP.

Among these 19 eyes, seven had ALT. Four eyes underwent repeat trabeculectomy combined with extracapsular cataract extraction and posterior chamber lens implantation. Seven remaining eyes had a repeat trabeculectomy with an antimetabolite.

A total of 19 eyes (24%) had cataract extraction during the follow-up period (this does not include the four cases of combined cataract and glaucoma surgery). The mean (± SD) IOP before cataract surgery in this group was 14.1 (± 3.6) mm Hg. It increased to a mean (± SD) of 16.7 (± 4.9) at the last follow-up visit (P = 0.028, paired Student's t test). Two patients required further glaucoma surgery 26 and 45 months after cataract extraction.

To assess the long-term efficacy of surgical treatment of glaucoma in terms of prevention of progressive glaucomatous damage, we analyzed the results of visual field and optic disc evaluation with the life-table method. As shown in Figure 3, the probability of disease stability (i.e., no further visual field deterioration or optic disc damage) was estimated at 81% and 65% at 3 and 6 years, respectively.

The long-term probability of IOP control is shown in Figure 4, and was 48% and 40% at 3 and 5 years, respectively, based on the criteria of IOP < 21 mm Hg and a minimal IOP reduction of 20%.

After redefining "success" as IOP of 20 mm Hg or less, the probability of IOP control was 91% and 81% after 3 and 5 years. The difference between the two survival curves was statistically significant ($P < 0.0001$, Gehan's test).

Discussion

During the last two decades, numerous studies [9-17] have demonstrated trabeculectomy to be a relatively safe and effective procedure for short- and long-term control of IOP. It is associated with less early and late postoperative complications than full-thickness filtering surgery, though at the cost of a somewhat higher postoperative IOP [24-26].

Important questions remain unanswered at this time: what are the long-term outcomes of glaucoma treatment and how effective are our current surgical techniques in preserving visual function? Few studies have addressed these issues. Most published series have dealt with short- and long-term tonometric results

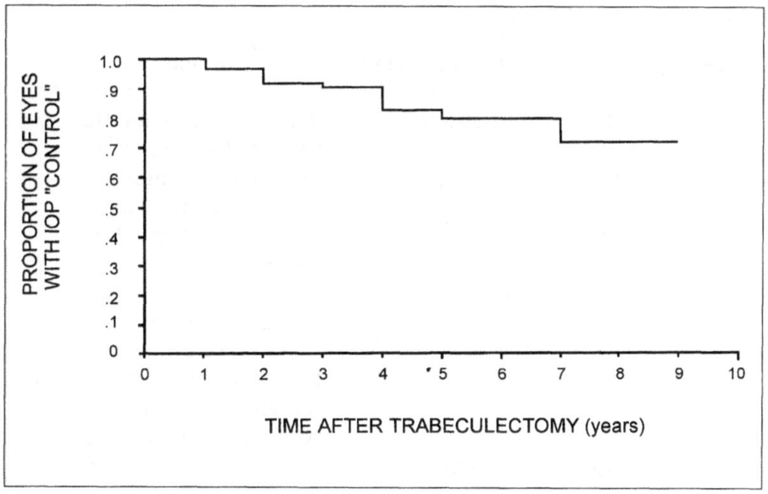

Fig. 4. Proportion of eyes with intraocular pressure (IOP) "control" as assessed by life-table analysis. The curve displays IOP "control" according to the following criteria: postoperative IOP below 21 mm Hg and at least a 20% reduction of IOP

of trabeculectomy. Table 2 lists the published long-term results of trabeculectomy, mostly in terms of IOP control. Long-term tonometric efficacy of trabeculectomy varies from 71% to 98% depending on the duration of follow-up and the criterion used for defining IOP control. Most authors have defined success as maintenance of the IOP below 21 or 22 mm Hg. The unusually high success rate reported by Migdal and colleagues [19] may be explained by the fact that their surgical group included only patients without prior long-term medical treatment. Two recent studies [27, 28] reported from the same center provide evidence that this may actually be the case.

Lamping and colleagues [29] retrospectively studied 252 eyes, within different diagnostic categories, which were followed for 2-14 years. The follow-up time extended from 1967 to 1981. They compared results of initial trabeculectomy (71 eyes) to those of full-thickness procedures (trephine, or posterior lip sclerectomy; 181 eyes). Using rigid criteria to define success (IOP < 19 mm Hg with or without medication, no further visual field loss or disc damage, and no glaucomatous etiology for a decrease in visual acuity) and Kaplan-Meier survival analysis, they reported a success rate of 88% after 6 years (mean follow-up) and 76% after 4 years (mean follow-up) for full-thickness procedures and trabeculectomy, respectively. In the trabeculectomy group, the probability of maintaining success was 85% and 70% at 2 and 5 years. Manual perimetric methods were used in this study and the criteria used to define visual field or optic nerve head deterioration were not detailed.

Roth and colleagues [30] have recently reported the results of a long-term prospective study to evaluate use of corticosteroids after trabeculectomy. Of the 52 eyes that were followed for 5 years, 39 (75%) remained stable. The criteria for success were lower IOP postoperatively and no progressive glaucomatous damage. The study eyes were divided into three groups according to the early postoperative therapeutic protocol (no steroids vs topical steroids vs topical and oral steroids, respectively). Progressive glaucomatous disease was determined by the clinical judgment of the senior author.

The results of two prospective, randomized studies begun in the early 1980s have recently been published [18, 19]. Both were designed to compare primary trabeculectomy to conventional management of POAG (only eyes with a preoperative IOP > 25 mm Hg were included in both studies). Jay and Allan [18] reported a 90% probability of success for preservation of visual function at 3 years in the surgically treated group. Similarly, Migdal and colleagues [19] have shown that visual fields are more likely to progress in the medically treated group. The results reflect those of a selective therapeutic approach (primary surgery) in a selected glaucoma population (eyes with an IOP > 25 mm Hg). The number of the study eyes was relatively small in both studies and older manual methods of perimetry were used during the entire period of the study in one [18]. These results cannot be directly compared to the general population of glaucomatous eyes that generally come to surgery after having received long-term medical treatment.

Table 2. Published long-term results of initial trabeculectomy

Investigators	Number of Eyes	Race	Follow-up Period	Results
David et al.[10]	4	B	6-30 mo	73.4% IOP < 20 mm Hg; 63% needed medications
D'Ermo et al.[13]	90	NA	1 -5 yrs	80% IOP ≤ 21 mm Hg; 9% needed medications
Freedman et al.[9]	51	B	19 mo	82%IOP < 20 mm Hg; 25% needed medications
Inaba[16]	427	A	3 mo to 5 yrs	74% IOP ≤ 21 mm Hg; 49% needed medications
Jerndal and Lundstrom[11]	165	W	18 mo to 3 yrs	71% IOP ≤ 21 mm Hg; 21% needed medications or reoperation; 91.5% had stable Goldmann visual fields
Lavin et al.[28]	43	NA	18 mo	76% IOP, 21 mm Hg*
Migdal and Hitchings[19]	57	NA	4 yrs	98% IOP < 22 mm Hg†
Mills[15]	444	NA	1 - 7 yrs	87.8% IOP < 21 mm Hg; 13.5% needed medications
Roth et al.[36]	52	W	5 yrs	75% had lower IOP postoperatively without disk or field change; 29% needed medications
Thommy and Bhar[14]	111	B	6 - 19 mo	95.4% IOP < 20 mm Hg
Watson and Grierson[17]	424	W	2 - 14 yrs	98% IOP ≤ 21 mm Hg and stable visual fields; 12% needed medications or reoperation
Wilson[12]	309	NA	1 - 7 yrs	75% IOP ≤ 21 mm Hg; 29% needed medications

B = Black; A = Asian; W = White; NA = Not available
*Includes only patients with long-term medical therapy (> 1 year) before surgery.
†Reflects the results in a selected group of patients without long-term prior medical treatment.

In our definition of tonometric success, we required a minimal IOP reduction of 20% relative to the preoperative level in addition to final IOP values below 21 mm Hg. Unfortunately, the problem of how much IOP lowering is required to stabilize disease in an individual eye has not yet been solved. The figure of 20% was chosen as an arbitrary cutoff point because we believed that this criterion (along with an IOP value below 21 mm Hg) was a reasonable amount of reduction that could be expected as a result of surgery. Based on these criteria, the probability of success was 48% and 40% after 3 and 5 years, respectively (Figure 4). These less optimistic results should be judged with a few important points in mind. First, more rigid criteria were used to define success. Second, life-table analysis was used to calculate IOP control at each follow-up interval. Use of life-table analysis (or Kaplan-Meier survival analysis) is a prerequisite for evaluation of any parameter in a group of patients followed over time [22, 23]. Third, the majority of our patients received long-term medical therapy and nearly one third of them had undergone ALT before surgery and may have been at higher risk of failure [31]. Fourth, 24 out of 78 eyes (31%) in our series had a mean preoperative IOP of 20 mm Hg or less. This might have contributed to a less favorable outcome in terms of IOP control. The results obtained by using only the cutoff value of 21 mm Hg were much more optimistic (91% and 81% at 3 and 5 years) and significantly different than those based on the first set of criteria ($P < 0.0001$, Gehan's test). We believe that this significant difference reflects the inadequacy of using a simple cutoff value for defining IOP control.

At the last visit, the mean visual acuity of the entire group had diminished by about one line as compared to the preoperative mean value. Our results are in agreement with other studies [11, 13, 15, 18, 19, 26] in the literature suggesting that reduction of visual acuity, though not very frequent in the short term [32], is a common event after trabeculectomy with longer follow-up, the two most important causes of which are development or progression of cataract, or progressive central field loss. In this study, three eyes developed visual acuity loss due to progressive glaucomatous damage. However, some [18, 19] have suggested that nearly the same amount of visual acuity loss would be observed in a medically treated group of patients followed for a long time. Many of our study eyes (23 eyes, 30%) underwent cataract extraction during the follow-up period.

The long-term probability of disease stability is depicted in Fig. 3. As shown, 81% of the operated eyes remained stable after 3 years. Nearly two thirds (65%) of the eyes remained so at the end of a 6 year period.

The results of this study should be judged with the following caveats in mind. As in any other retrospective study, the possibility of selection bias could not be entirely eliminated. Our clinic is a tertiary care referral center. This could have led to more refractory glaucomas being included in the study, making the final outcomes of trabeculectomy worse than in the general population of glaucoma patients. The same factor could be at work during the postoperative period; that is, patients with a less eventful postoperative course are more likely to be referred back to their primary physicians. By including consecutively operated patients, we tried to reduce this kind of bias. Most of the study eyes had moderate to severe glaucoma. In advanced glaucoma, progressive damage might occur even after significant reduction of the IOP [33, 34]. It should be emphasized that diagnosis of visual field progression remains a difficult task particularly in eyes with moderate to severely advanced field loss. Long-term fluctuation is particularly problematic in such cases [35], making diagnosis of visual field progression more subject to error. Stereoscopic optic disc photographs were not available for all the study eyes. Taking yearly stereoscopic optic disc photographs has been a routine practice in our clinic for many years. The fact that such photographs were available for 29 out of 78 eyes points to the inherent difficulty in obtaining satisfactory photographs in this group of advanced glaucoma patients. Chronic use of miotics, and especially development of posterior synechiae and increasing cataract postoperatively, make successful image acquisition difficult in these eyes. However, in moderate to severe glaucoma, evaluation of the optic disc may be less valuable than in the earlier stages of the disease [20].

In conclusion, two thirds of patients in our study did not suffer progressive glaucomatous damage 6 years after a first trabeculectomy, as measured with automated perimetry and qualitative evaluation of the optic disc. Because of variable and unknown rates of glaucoma progression preoperatively, the issue of efficacy of the surgical treatment of glaucoma in slowing or preventing further deterioration of visual function cannot be addressed quantitatively. These results cannot be directly compared to those of primary surgery in eyes that have not received long-term medical treatment. Standardized prospective data collection from a large number of patients will be important to develop outcome information about surgical treatment of glaucoma.

References

1. Koryllos K (1967) Trabeculectomy: a new glaucoma operation. Bull Soc Hellén Ophtalmol 35:147-57
2. Cairns JE (1968) Trabeculectomy: preliminary report of a new method. Am J Ophthalmol 66:673-9
3. Heuer DK, Parrish RH II, Gressel MG, et al (1984) 5-fluorouracil and glaucoma surgery: II. A pilot study. Ophthalmol 91:384-94
4. The Fluorouracil Filtering Surgery Study Group (1993) Three-year follow-up of the Fluorouracil Filtering Surgery Study. Am J Ophthalmol 115:82-92
5. Chen C-W, Huang H-T, Sheu M-M (1988) Enhancement of IOP control effect of trabeculectomy by local application of anticancer drug. In: Blodi F, Brancato R and Cristini G et

al (eds) Acta XXV Concilium Ophthalmologicum. Proceedings of the 25th International Congress of Ophthalmology; 1986 May 4-10; Rome, Italy. Kugler, Berkeley (CA), vol 2, pp 1487-1491.
6. Palmer SS (1991) Mitomycin as adjunct chemotherapy with trabeculectomy. Ophthalmol 98:317-21
7. Hoskins HD, Jr, Migliazzo C (1984) Management of failing filtering blebs with the argon laser. Ophthalmic Surg 15:731-733
8. McAllister JA, Wilson RP (eds) (1986) Glaucoma. Butterworths, London, pp 243-250
9. Freedman J, Shen E, Ahrens M (1976) Trabeculectomy in a Black American glaucoma population. Br J Ophthalmol 60:573-574
10. David R, Freedman J, Luntz MH (1977) Comparative study of Watson's and Cairns's trabeculectomies in a Black population with open angle glaucoma. Br J Ophthalmol 61:117-119
11. Jerndal T, Lundström M (1977) 330 consecutive trabeculectomies - a follow-up study through 1/2 - 3 years. Acta Ophthalmol 55:52-62
12. Wilson P (1977) Trabeculectomy: long-term follow-up. Br J Ophthalmol 61:535-538
13. D'Ermo F, Bonomi L, Doro D (1979) A critical analysis of the long-term results of trabeculectomy. Am J Ophthalmol 88:829-835
14. Thommy CP, Bhar IS (1979). Trabeculectomy in Nigerian patients with open-angle glaucoma. Br J Ophthalmol 63:636-642
15. Mills KB (1981) Trabeculectomy: a retrospective long-term follow-up of 444 cases. Br J Ophthalmol 65:790-795
16. Inaba Z (1982) Long-term results of trabeculectomy in the Japanese: an analysis by life-table method. Jpn J Ophthalmol 26:361-373
17. Watson PG, Grierson I (1981) The place of trabeculectomy in the treatment of glaucoma. Ophthalmol 88:175-196
18. Jay JL, Allan D (1989) The benefit of early trabeculectomy versus conventional management in primary open-angle glaucoma relative to severity of disease. Eye 3(P+S):528-535
19. Migdal C, Gregory W, Hitchings R (1994) Long-term functional outcome after early surgery compared with laser and medicine in open - angle glaucoma. Ophthalmol 101:1651-1657
20. Spaeth G (ed) (1982) Ophthalmic surgery: Principles and practice. WB Saunders, Philadelphia, pp 270-280
21. Caprioli J (1994) Clinical evaluation of the optic nerve in glaucoma. Trans Am Ophthalmol Soc 92:589-641
22. Feinstein AR (1985) Clinical epidemiology: The architecture of clinical research. 1st ed. WB Saunders, Philadelphia, pp 341-346
23. Dawson-Saunders B, Trapp RG (1994) Basic and clinical biostatistics. 2nd ed., Appleton & Lange, Norwalk, pp 107-110, 149-153, 189-195, 197-199
24. Blondeau P, Phelps CD (1981) Trabeculectomy vs thermosclerostomy: a randomized prospective clinical trial. Arch Ophthalmol 99:810-816
25. Spaeth GL, Poryzees E (1981) A comparison between peripheral iridectomy with thermal sclerostomy and trabeculectomy: a controlled study. Br J Ophthalmol 65:783-789
26. Lewis RA, Phelps CD (1984) Trabeculectomy v thermosclerostomy: A five-year follow-up. Arch Ophthalmol 102:533-536
27. Kidd MN, O'Connor M (1985) Progression of field loss after trabeculectomy: a five-year follow-up. Br J Ophthalmol 69:827-831
28. Lavin MJ, Wormald RP, Migdal CS, Hitchings RA (1990) The influence of prior therapy on the success of trabeculectomy. Arch Ophthalmol 108:1543-1548
29. Lamping KA, Bellows AR, Hutchinson BT, Afran SI (1986) Long-term evaluation of initial filtration surgery. Ophthalmol 93:91-101
30. Roth SM, Spaeth GL, Starita RJ, et al. (1991) The effects of postoperative corticosteroids on trabeculectomy and the clinical course of glaucoma: five-year follow-up study. Ophthalmic Surg 22:724-749
31. Johnson DH, Yoshikawa K, Brubaker RF, Hodge DO (1994) The effect of long-term medical therapy on the outcome of filtration surgery. Am J Ophthalmol 117:139-148
32. Costa VP, Smith M, Spaeth GL, et al. (1993) Loss of visual acuity after trabeculectomy. Ophthalmol 100:599-612
33. Odberg T (1987) Visual field prognosis in advanced glaucoma. Acta Ophthalmol Suppl 182:27-29
34. Grant WM, Burke JF Jr. (1982) Why do some people go blind from glaucoma? Ophthalmol 89:991-898
35. Boeglin RJ, Caprioli J, Zulauf M (1992) Long-term fluctuation of the visual field in glaucoma. Am J Ophthalmol 113:396-400
36. Roth SM, Spaeth GL, Starita RJ, et al. (1991) The effects of post-operative corticosteroids on trabeculectomy and the clinical course of glaucoma: A five-year follow-up Study. Ophthalmic Surg 22:724-729

Discussion

Question: Montanari

I would like to ask Dr. Caprioli which are his criteria to evaluate the visual field.

Answer: Caprioli

This unfortunately was a qualitative evaluation by experts who evaluated all the visual fields. Their task was trying to estimate in patients with an advanced damage the magnitude of altered fluctuation that these fields show.
We required at least 4 visual fields, which I think is an absolute minimum to try to evaluate progression. Any change in the visual field that was considered progression was necessarily larger than the magnitude of long-term fluctuation from test to test. It was a clinical evaluation and not a quantitative one.

Question: Greve

Two questions for Dr. Krupin: Do you really believe that there are more complications in glaucoma implants than in trabeculectomy with Mitomycin C given that you are probably putting the implants where several surgeries have already failed?
If one would compare the same sorts of patients, would the complication be more important?

Answer: Krupin

Even starting at a better level with eyes that have not gone to some previous surgery and using this foreign device as far as earlier or more initial surgery, you still have a hard complication. You have a formal theory giving more chances of having some blockage of that tube within the anterior chamber that you won't have with trabeculectomy. There's more chance of having some sort of erosion posteriorly that you won't have with trabeculectomy and any foreign device still has some limited and extra complications.
The sensible way to think about complications with drainage implants is to simply add those unique to those that you get with regular trabeculectomy. I do have one possible exception, which is endophtalmitis. Our experience has been that it's very rare with drainage implants. Late infection is very rare even when there is erosion.

Question: Caprioli

I agree with that. I think that even with erosion I have not seen problems. I think that incidence of endophtalmitis may be too high or too frequent for using fibrotics agents.

Question: Greve

Could you show the progression pre and post operatively? I know that you don't have the data pre. However, in terms of quality of life it may very well be that you are still showing progression. In our 10 year perspective study published long ago, in ten years half of the patients have died and they died seeing. So in terms of quality of life you may have a 20% progression after the intervention. You may have considerably improved the patients' quality of life, otherwise you may have them blind.

Answer: Caprioli

I certainly agree and I think that is why we do these procedures even in absence of scientific evidence that it does slow the progression as we don't have an appropriate control group. I think that we all believe that this certainly slows the progression so that such a study would not be useful.

Question:

It's a question for Dr. Minckler. I'd like you to elaborate the fact that you said, maybe I didn't get you well, but you said that the outcome of trabeculectomy with 5FU and Mitomycin C is the same. Is it so?

Answer: Minckler

My understanding from literature and from my own short studies is that the complication rates and short term outcome are about the same. My concern relates really to long term problems with Mitomycin C. I think there's probably going to be a much higher rate of late infections. I am actually not aware of long term studies with these agents. These last two studies that I mentioned, in one of which Dr. Caprioli was co-author, are among the few that have looked at survival or failure rates. After any trabeculectomy we certainly need long term data with 5FU and Mitomycin C.

Question: Jampel

Two questions: only 1/3 of your patients have had ALT pre-operatively. Was there any effect of pre-operative ALT upon the surgical outcome?
And secondly, there seems to be a lot of progression in your study at lower pressure and I am wondering if you can make any comment about whether getting the pressure lower was more beneficial than not having the pressure low.

Answer: Caprioli

About the first question with respect to ALT, we were unable to find any correlation in our population between pre-operative ALT and any surgery failure; since we only had 25 patients who had ALT we may not have sufficient statistical data to get in that question, but we didn't find an association.

Secondly we did have a lot of patients who progressed despite low pressures and I think they may have been a "functional eastern" part of the kinds of patients we usually see and operate on. We often get patients who are progressing in the disease despite low pressure with medical therapy; we then operate on.

Question: Pernini

To Dr. Krupin. If I understood well your valve does not need any tube-closing suture while in recent Baerveldt technology for unresponsive or juvenile glaucoma the tube is closed off with prolene or nylon sutures: what is the difference in terms of filtration between a closed and an opened tube?

Question: Balestrazzi

We have experience with double plates Molteno valve. Originally it was suggested to close the tube in order to regulate filtration in the postoperative period. We tried to close the connecting tube between the plates but not the one that goes directly into the anterior chamber. We had good results: at the beginning filtration involves only the first plate, immediately followed by the second one.

Answer: Krupin

First of all, it's probably better not to use the word valve; the word valve is used very commonly by people describing this sort of devices and we have talked here about the Molteno valve. The major concept you should think about is that there are two groups of devices. There are devices that have an open tube in the anterior chamber with no restrictions in the tube at all, and those devices you have to tie off. You do that by using the suture externally or some type of suture within the tube occluding the lumen. If you put open tube in the anterior chamber outside the eye without any kind of restriction device you risk to have free flow of aqueous. In the first group there are no restrictions, that is Molteno, the valve, they are open tools. The second major group includes devices that have some type of element. The only one able to be swipped out is the valve implant, but these devices have some types of elements within the device that limit flow and you don't have to tie off and occlude. It doesn't mean that you get low pressure, but they will have some kind of resistance within the tube to prevent flow.

Question: S. Miglior

My question is to Dr. Caprioli. I understand that in your study almost 30% of patients who underwent glaucoma surgery had their IOP below 21 mmHg with maximal treatment. Did you find any differences between these patients and those with an IOP over 21 mmHg following surgery?

Answer: Caprioli

That's a very good question; unfortunately in our population we were unable to find any correlation between a number of variables we have looked at. One was pre-operated pressure and the second was post-operated pressure and success in terms of further damage. One can conclude two things, either the population was not large enough to detect the relatively small differences, or there is no difference; but I can tell you that there is a considerable evidence from other studies in the literature that there is an association between level of pressure and preservation of visual function, and quite honestly I don't know why we didn't find this correlation in our study.

Question: Falcinelli

When we perform osteo-odonto-keratoprothesis in our patients, we insert a very small tube of approx. 0.20 mm (instead of 3-4 cm) into the anterior chamber and we never had a marked hypotension.

Answer: Minckler

I don't know how many cases Jampel had an experience with. There is an enormous literature which describes simple tools not necessarily taking back to the vicinity of the optic nerve, but basically under the conjunctiva. The problem with those in general has been that they have been kept close to the Molteno and similar devices that basically guarantee that after there is a capsule form and an aqueous flow. There's a physical separation between the inside of the capsule and the orifice, the posterior opening of the tube. We think that mechanical separation has a lot to do with preserving the flow, preventing a closure if one could put it to endospace in such a position that it didn't provoke fiber incapsulation. The problem is with that device which has a very small surface area and restricts the amount of fluid that is diffused through the capsule.

Question:

Since with time there is a loss of the effect of trabeculectomy with and without antimetabolites, do you feel that patients should have long term topical steroids or antimetabolites or even a bit of radiation?

Answer: Minckler

I have no experience with radiation. One of the papers Caprioli mentioned from Philadelphia did look at the issue of steroids versus non-steroids, and the steroid treated patients did significantly better. Based on that and on our own experience, topical steroids in the pre-operative period make sense, I have no reason to believe that long term steroids administration would affect the long term outcome.

Answer: Krupin

Just to come onto the related issue, we do have a lot of papers coming out in general glaucoma relating the surface area of a bulb to the ability to perfuse fluid. I am sure that a general concept is applicable to filtration surgery, trabeculectomy.
The size is a factor in the surface area, is a factor in the functioning of the bulb, and steroids might have something to do with preserving that at least through the period of time. A few years ago we published our results on 5FU after initial trabeculectomy and we had but 50 eyes in each group that were randomizing, 5FU or no 5FU. After the first paper we published we had a much higher success rate with this 3 to 5 5FU injections and lower pressure. We have a 5 year follow-up in a number of patients, as far as visual field we are analyzing their pressure. We have a discontinuing decrease in our failure rate in the eyes that didn't receive 5FU. But in the eyes that got 5FU we didn't have failures and this is over 5 years follow-up. So I think that 5FU in initial surgery may have a benefit as far as long term survival.

Question:

One of the complications that we are seeing more frequently now because of the nature of our surgery is delayed superchoroidal hemorrhages. I was wondering what is your experience with this and if you have any tips on how we can reduce this incidence.

Answer: Minckler

I don't believe there is an incidence of superchoroidal hemorrhages either with filtering surgery or glaucoma draining plant, but we had a continuing very bad experience. Our experience is that usually these things occur after a delay time of 24-72 hours. We have had choroidal hemorrhages occurring even after 2 stage glaucoma draining plants, for example where you are waiting weeks between the initial device and the insertion of the 2 chambers. We have choroidal hemorrhages that occur even after days of stable, well controlled intraocular pressure; sometimes there is a clear history of patients draining, sometimes not. I think choroidal hemorrhages are much less frequent because of our concerns for controlling pressure; that by the way is one of the principal advantages, I think, in small incision cataract surgery where you have a controlled self-sealing wound compared to the extracapsular much larger incision. We have almost no experience with intra-operating choroidal hemorrhages in glaucoma surgery. I don't know how to prevent them. We have tried viscoelastics, we have tried gas, SFX, 2 stage procedures. I don't know what the answer is.

Answer: Greve

An answer to that question is that we have been using gas in a consecutive series of, I believe, 40 high-risk patients, high myopia, high phakics, and we have not seen hemorrhages yet. So we believe that the injection of SFX in the vitreous cavity has a very high potential in preventing these hemorrhages.

Answer: Minckler

We have had a large collective experience with choroidal hemorrhages. In fact, overall they don't do too badly; a relatively small percentage of them are massive in destroying the eye. Most of them occur particularly if it is 2 or 3 days after filtering surgery, and in fact the nasal doesn't involve the macula. Relatively few in my opinion need surgical intervention and the summary of that in my view is that there is no reason to even contemplate that in most cases unless you have uncontrollable pressure, pain that you can't manage in any other way. There is a logic contrast in draining them unless you can demonstrate by ultrasound that there is liquid. If the retinal surfaces are kissing, if there is obvious inflammation along them, if there is intermetrial hemorrhage associated with them, or if you see fiber organization occurring; then I think you do have reason to advice intervention, but fortunately most of them are not so bad.

UP-DATING ON HYPOTENSIVE AND NON HYPOTENSIVE GLAUCOMA THERAPY

Blood Flow: a Target for Ocular Therapy in Glaucoma?

E. P. O'Donoghue

Royal Eye Hospital, Oxford Road, Manchester M13 9WH, UK

Introduction

The pressure/mechanical hypothesis for glaucoma progression is increasingly challenged. Epidemiological studies reveal that, for up to 50% of glaucomas, intraocular pressure (IOP) does not exceed so-called normal values [1]. Moreover, as many as 70% of ocular hypertensives do not develop glaucoma in studies with follow-up as long as 20 years [2]. A proportion of high pressure glaucoma patients who maintain consistent 'target pressures' in the low teens range following treatment continue a relentless visual decline. We are more aware of racial differences; for the same IOP the prevalence of glaucoma in blacks can be as much as four times that of whites. In Japan, prevalence of glaucoma increases despite gradual fall of IOP with age. Clearly other factors are at play.

A growing body of evidence implicates vascular factors. Systemic hypertension and its treatment may influence the course of the disease. Systemic hypotension, and particularly nocturnal hypotension, may be important risk factors for glaucomatous progression [3, 4]. Vasospasm, immune disorder, and a variety of diseases of the arteries, veins and capillaries may be important associations. Haemorheological abnormalities are associated with some glaucomas. Krakau, reviewing the evidence for a vascular aetiology of glaucoma [5], states that disc haemorrhage-frequently unnoticed-may often precede glaucoma and suggests that its "common provenance" with retinal vein occlusions is due to an endothelial vascular abnormality. Release of vasoactive factors following disc haemorrhage may alter local capillary perfusion. As further evidence for the vascular theory of normal pressure glaucoma, Hendryckx [6] has shown that treatment has no effect on the incidence of haemorrhage in normal pressure glaucoma.

Regulation of Ocular Blood Flow

The capacity of the optic nerve head vasculature to autoregulate [7] allows the normal eye to maintain ocular blood flow despite alterations in IOP and other factors [8]. We have better definition of the complex interaction of metabolic, myogenic and neurogenic mechanisms in autoregulation. Much has been learned about the complex role of the vascular endothelium in ocular circulatory regulation and the complex balance between relaxing factors (nitric oxide, prostacyclin, putative hyperpolarising factor, etc.) and constricting factors (endothelins and cyclo-oxygenase pathway products such as thromboxane A2 and prostaglandin H2) [9, 10, 17].

However, there is much to be learned about autoregulatory function and dysfunction in individual glaucomatous states, the relative significance of reduced blood flow vs autoregulatory abnormality, and the impact of factors such as choriocapillaris watershed variation, peripapillary atrophy and changes in the blood-retinal barrier. In terms of future therapy, we must bear in mind that in disease states the autoregulatory reserve may already be maximally utilised and therefore limit therapeutic intervention. Most exploratory journeys into vasoactive therapy have looked at the impact of acute therapy in highly selected groups. Much less is known about the impact of long-term therapy in a general glaucomatous population. Some recent developments in possible vasoactive therapies for glaucoma will be briefly discussed.

Potential Therapeutic Approaches

The Calcium Channel

Much has been learned about the complex labyrinth of the calcium channel in recent years. As intracellular calcium depletion leads to rapid relaxation of vascular smooth muscle, calcium channel blocking agents might be expected to improve ocular blood flow. It is worth noting that only long-acting, voltage -operated channels are sensitive to calcium channel blockers. There are very different rates of activation and inactivation of calcium channels in different vascular beds, in each of which there may be different 'gating' states at any one time.

In terms of treating vasospasm associated with some glaucomas, blocking agents might be expected to be useful if vasospasm is due to calcium channel flux anomaly; however, a positive benefit is less certain if vasospasm is due to abnormal sympathetic hyperactivity or responsiveness, the presence of high levels of circulating sympathetic amines, capillary wall disease, or optic nerve hyponutrition due to large vessel disease. Calcium channel blocking agents such as nifedipine have been shown by Kitazawa to improve visual field performance in some normal pressure glaucomas; this effect was greater in subjects with peripheral vasospasm [11]. Nimodopine has recently been shown by Bose and co-workers [12] to improve contrast sensitivity function in controls and in subjects with normal pressure glaucoma. However this was a short-term study on a relatively small population using relatively basic CSF test measures. As nimodopine is considered safer than nifedipine in terms of risk of hypotension and other adverse drug reactions, it is worth noting in Bose's study that a third of all subjects had a blood pressure decrease of more than 10%.

The mechanism of action of calcium channel blockers in the eye remains unclear and the long-term effects of such therapy are unknown. What is clear is that these are potentially dangerous drugs. Nifedipine is commonly associated with symptoms of headache, flushing, dizziness and lethargy which can have significant implications for quality of life. Treatment may also be associated with cardiac dysrhythmia and hypotension and great care is necessary to exclude patients with postural hypotension (especially those on β-blockers), poor cardiac reserve, hypotension and diabetes. Nifedipine has been implicated in 'steal' phenomena, leading to local ischemia. Overdosage can cause profound hypotension and bradycardia, heart block, and death from myocardial infarction, asystole and cardiogenic shock. Nimodopine, with its preferential effect on cerebral vessels, may be safer but can be associated with hypotension, heart rate changes and symptoms of flushing and headache.

Alternative agents such as the physiological calcium channel blocker magnesium may be safer and existing agents such as ß-blockers may have useful calcium channel blocking activity [30].

The Endothelins

Endothelins are amongst the most potent vasoconstrictors known, with activity up to ten times that of angiotensin-2 [13], and may be implicated in a variety of disease processes including diabetes, hypertension, migraine and Raynaud's disease [14, 15]. Endothelin-1 specifically interacts with the ETA receptor which is predominant in vascular smooth muscle and is also present in pericytes. The endothelin-B receptor is also a potent mediator of vasoconstriction but it has additionally been shown that its stimulation by endothelin-3 is linked to nitric oxide production; it has been suggested that this apparently contradictory activity may function to buffer the effects of endothelin-1, particularly when the levels are highly elevated [16].

Endothelin production is inhibited by nitric oxide, prostacyclin and a putative smooth muscle inhibitory factor [17], which may be useful in devising future modulating strategies. Furthermore, specific antagonists to endothelial A and B receptors have recently been developed. The ETA antagonist FR139137 markedly inhibits endothelin-1 vasoconstriction in the perfused porcine eye [18]. A selective endothelin-B agonist sarafotoxine Stx-S6c, derived from the venom of a middle eastern snake, has been shown to be highly selective for endothelin-3 and to more than double outflow facility in the rabbit [19] but with a potential for undesirable posterior segment vasoactivity as yet to be explored.

Dopaminergic Mechanisms

Two families of dopamine receptor have been defined, D-1 and D-2. D-1 agonists, such as fenoldepam, increase IOP but D-2 agonists (such as bromocriptine) have been shown to significantly reduce IOP [20]. A variety of dopamine antagonists have been investigated, some of which lower IOP in association with evidence of improved ocular blood flow [21]. Chiou also presents evidence to suggest improved retinal function after ischemia. The mechanism of action is via a combination of decreased aqueous production and increased aqueous outflow. A common feature of most dopamine antagonists is potential for conjunctival irritation, and Chiou reports that this is least with droperidol, loxapine and metoclopramide.

Prunte and Flammer have found an additive effect by combining D-1 antagonist with a D-2 agonist (SDZ JLC-756) with a mean intraocular decrease of more than 25% in control and glaucoma subjects; they further report evidence of improved blood flow in rat optic nerve [22].

Such agents may have considerable potential for adverse drug reactions in vulnerable patients on long-term therapy. Dopaminergic agonists may be associated with nausea, drowsiness and confusion, in addition to postural hypotension, Raynaud's syndrome and exacerbation of cardiovascular disease. Dopaminergic antagonists have been associated with Parkinson's disease, tardive dyskinesia, exacerbation of chronic obstructive airways disease, and neuroleptic malignant syndrome, in addition to more common adverse effects such as hypotension and tachycardia.

The Angiotensin System

The potent vasoconstrictor angiotensin II can be an important contributor to regulation of the ophthalmic microcirculation when elevated above baseline levels [17, 23, 24]. Angiotension converting enzyme (ACE) inhibitors have been shown by a variety of authors to inhibit the formation of angiotensin II, to prevent brady-kinin inactivation and to augment endothelial dependent relaxation to bradykinin (with increased nitric oxide production) in isolated arteries, thus improving flow in the ophthalmic microcirculation [17, 24, 25]. Angiotensin II is inhibited by valsartan and the vasodilatory activation of the endothelial L-arginine ni-trous oxide pathway by ACE inhibitors is me-diated by D-2 receptor activation with agents such as enalapril.

The use of such agents may be associated with a malaise complex (dizziness, headache, nausea, fatigue) in addition to confusion and decreased cerebration. Hypotension, myocardial infarction and cerebrovascular accident have been implicated as adverse events of some ACE inhibitors. Other effects include renal dysfunction, angioneurotic oedema, immune disturbance and impotence. The risk of such adverse effect increases in patients over 70 years of age and in those with a history of cardiovascular disease or systemic hypotension. The therapeutic effect may be decreased in Afro-caribbean subjects.

Glaucoma Medications in Current Use

Topical β-blockers have been the mainstay of medical therapy for glaucoma for more than two decades. As effective hypotensive agents, an improvement in ocular perfusion might be anticipated; however, there is some suggestion that the visual benefit of such therapy is less than expected [26]. β-blocker therapy may interfere with endogenous vasodilation [27], and cause optic nerve head arteriolar vasoconstriction [28, 29]. Corrosion casting studies have shown significant differences between individual β-blockers in terms of vasoconstrictive effect of long term therapy. By contrast, the vasorelaxant action of a β-blocker on isolated bovine retinal microarteries, described by Hoste [30], suggests a potential beneficial effect on ocular blood flow. Further clarification is clearly desirable.

The recently available α-adrenergic agent apraclonidine has potent anterior segment vasoconstrictory effects, raising concerns about a possible adverse vasomotor effect on optic nerve head microcirculation that might theoretically negate the benefits of IOP lowering. A recent study has shown no significant effect on optic nerve head blood flow [31]. However this study of impact of chronic therapy was confined to a 3-week treatment period on five rabbits using corrosion casting techniques which remain subject to some controversy regarding the theoretical vasoreactive effect of the technique itself. Other α-adrenergic agents such as phenylephrine and clonidine clearly reduce optic nerve head flow [32]. The long-term safety of apraclonidine in glaucoma treatment is unknown and therefore combination therapy with β-blockers - as recently suggested - should be subject to careful study.

Haemorheological Therapy in Glaucoma

A growing number of studies have found associations between haemorheological abnormalities and glaucoma such as increased viscosity [33-36], altered haematocrit [33, 37] and reduced deformability of erythrocytes and leucocytes. Other factors such as increased platelet activation, erythrocyte hyperaggregatability and shear rate abnormalities have been suggested as possible associated factors with glaucoma progression.

The potential for possible future rheological therapy may be illustrated by looking briefly at one of these factors: reduced red blood cell deformability (increased rigidity) has been associated with some glaucomas and it is of interest that this association is also apparent in diabetes, sickle cell disease, Raynaud's phenomenon, chronic infection and impaired microvascular flow. The trisubstituted xanthine derivative, pentoxyfylline may increase cyclic AMP in erythrocytes, reduce viscosity and improve erythrocyte deformability leading to enhanced oxygenation of ischemic tissues.

Measurement of Ocular Blood Flow

Studies to explore vasoactive therapy for glaucoma will be dependent on accurate, reproducible, noninvasive methods of blood flow measurement. In recent years there have been important developments in both the variety and sophistication of techniques available for such study, a number of which will be briefly reviewed.

Blue field entoptic phenomena have been utilised to estimate leucocyte velocity and density and have been shown to be reliable measures of perimacular haemodynamics in suitable subjects [38]. However one must be cautious about extrapolating such data to conditions in which the primary abnormality lies in the optic nerve head microcirculation.

Laser Doppler velocimetry studies have revealed decreased optic nerve head blood flow velocity in high and normal pressure glaucomas in both treated and untreated states [36, 39]. A limitation of this technique is that it will only offer global information on capillary velocity and it is noteworthy that improved velocity will equate to improved flow only if capillaries are not constricted or the number of capillaries per unit tissue volume is not decreased.

Colour Doppler Imaging (CDI) of ophthalmic circulation has received considerable recent attention. Evidence from CDI have been used to suggest that timolol does not affect blood flow in ophthalmic arteries [40] and that glaucoma therapy does not appear to alter ophthalmic artery blood flow in a normal pressure glaucoma population [41]. Yamazaki and co-workers found no difference between high pressure and normal pressure glaucoma in terms of resistivity index, peak systolic, and diastolic and mean envelope velocities in the ophthalmic artery. Whether this revealed the true situation or a hidden effect of glaucomatous therapy remains uncertain. However, most studies focus on the ophthalmic or central retinal artery; the short posterior ciliary arteries which supply most of optic nerve head circulation are of greatest interest, but results are much more variable.

In a recent study, Harris and colleagues went to considerable lengths to look at test/re-test reproducibility for CDI [42]. This study has shown that blood flow velocity and resistivity parameters in the short posterior ciliary circulation cannot be reliably determined by CDI with the present technology. Angle-induced error remains a major limiting factor; as the angle between ultrasound beam and flow direction increases in perpendicularity, velocities are increasingly underestimated. The observer has to make a subjective estimate of this error and apply an appropriate correction. Lower velocity is associated with larger variability in small vessels. Longitudinal studies may be limited by the impossibility of recreating probe position from one test to the next. CDI is dependent on a highly skilled operator and there is significant potential for inter-observer and inter-centre errors. The effect of globe compression is a further potential confounding factor and there is much to be learned about the normal physiological variation of this technique. Future technological refinements are likely to improve sensitivity, perhaps by using higher insonation frequencies but caution is necessary to avoid drawing inappropriate conclusions from such data particularly with reference to the posterior ciliary vessels.

Fluorescein angiography has revealed filling defects and leakage in the glaucomatous optic nerve head and the extent of such findings has been related to disease progression [43]. In one study, filling defects were found in 100% of primary open angle glaucoma subjects and in approximately 33% of ocular hypertensives [44]. Geijssen also found a high prevalence (85%) of filling defects associated with glaucoma but no differences between normal and high pressure glaucomas [45]. A limitation of fluorescein angiography is that the deeper vessels remain obscured. This may be overcome in part by indocyanine green angiography, with its potential for imaging the peripapillary choroidal circulation. Video-angiography allows estimation of blood velocity and arterio-venous passage time. However, in terms of necessary longitudinal studies, angiography remains invasive with a small but definite risk of severe allergy and accurate quantification is difficult.

Pulsatile ocular blood flowmetry (POFB) has received considerable renewed attention due to the development of a new, rapid, user friendly machine which has been shown to be consistent and reliable [46]. POBF measures the pulsatile component of flow. The nonpulsatile contribution is unknown. The technique assumes standard ocular rigidity and venous outflow and many uncertainties remain regarding what precisely is being measured. Nonetheless, POBF is reduced in normal pressure glaucoma [47, 49] and is significantly improved in some high pressure glaucomas following glaucoma filtration surgery [48]. Quaranta has shown a marked decrease in POBF with increase of IOP in a normal pressure glaucoma population and suggests that the results may be consistent with poor myogenic autoregulation [49]. Boles-Carenini and colleagues found differences in the long-term effect of timolol vs betaxolol therapy but caution about the possibility of inappropriately correlating a choroidal blood flow effect with the pathogenesis of optic nerve head disease.

Scanning Laser Doppler Flowmetry (SLDF) has brought us closer to the elusive goal of rapid noninvasive measurement of blood flow in the optic nerve head and retinal microcirculation. How close remains uncertain. Nonetheless, SLDF, using Heidelberg retinal flowmetry, provides high resolution, two-dimensional maps of perfused capillaries. It has a rapid acquisition time of just over 2 s, and Michelson's work suggests that this is a reliable and valid index of papillary blood flow [50]. At a recent Heidelburg users group in San Antonio, Texas, Michelson presented data revealing reduced optic nerve head and retinal blood flow associated with artificial elevation of IOP. At the same meeting, Harrison and colleagues observed that increased optic nerve head blood flow was induced by 10 Hertz flicker. The effectiveness of this technology in detection of glaucomatous change remains to be determined.

In one Manchester ocular blood flow laboratory we have recently shown a high degree of repeatability for SLDF in both normal and glaucoma subjects for whom volume, flow and velocity parameters all had coefficients of repeatability of approximately 10% [51]. Coefficient of repeatability was expressed as percentage of mean effect of two visits using seven consecutive perfusion measurements per visit (repeated at one week interval) with similar coefficients of repeatability for retina and optic nerve head

[51]. A reproducible, significant decrease in normal parameters was noted in a group of subjects breathing 60% oxygen. An acute decrease in retinal capillary volume is apparent as an acute effect of smoking. An improved strategy for successive image alignment is necessary for accurate longitudinal studies.

Conclusions

Further research is necessary to understand the nature and individual variation of autoregulatory dysfunction in glaucoma subjects before large scale studies of vasoactive therapy can be justified. Many glaucoma patients are relatively frail, elderly subjects, who will be particularly vulnerable to the adverse reactions of many proposed vasoactive drugs. The potential for such adverse responses may be concealed in initial studies which will tend to use highly selected younger, and relatively healthier volunteers. Vasoactive agents which improve overall ocular blood flow may not necessarily usefully improve local optic nerve head perfusion and considerable care will be necessary to avoid secondary hypotension and steal phenomena which may have an undesirable impact for glaucoma progression. We have yet to learn whether useful improvements in ocular blood flow can be achieved in advanced glaucomatous disease. Considerable research is also necessary to eliminate limitations of currently available blood flow measurement techniques. Blood flow measurement strategies must be highly reproducible and valid, with a proven ability to detect subtle physiological change.

Future vasoactive therapy must be shown to be safe, effective, and improve quality of life, and must be subject to rigorous prospective randomised study.

References

1. Sommer A, Tielsch J, Katz J, et al. (1991) Relationship between intraocular pressure and primary open angle glaucoma among black and white Americans. Baltimore Eye Survey. Arch Ophthalmol 109:1090-5
2. Lundberg L, Wettrell K, Linner E. (1985) Ocular Hypertension. A 20 year follow-up at Skovde. Acta Ophthalmol 63 (Suppl.):473
3. Graham, Drance SM, Wijsmank K et al. (1995) Ambulatory blood pressure monitoring in glaucoma: the nocturnal dip. Ophthalmol 102: 61-69
4. Hayreh SS, Zimmerman MB, Podhajsky P, Alward WL (1994) Nocturnal arterial hypotension: Role in optic nerve head and ocular ischemic disorders. Am J Ophthalmol 117: 603-24
5. Krakau, CET (1994) Disc haemorrhages and retinal vein occlusions in glaucoma. Surv Ophthalmol 38:S18-S22.
6. Hendrickx KH, van den Enden A, Rosker MT, Hoyng, PFJ (1994) Cumulative incidence of patients with disc haemorrhages in glaucoma and effect of therapy. Ophthalmol 101:1165-1172
7. Bill A (1985) Some aspects of the ocular circulation. Friedenwald Lecture. Invest Ophthalmol Vis Sci 26:410-424
8. Riva CE, Grunwald JE, Petrig BL (1988) Autoregulation of human retinal blood flow: an investigation with laser doppler velocimetry. Invest Ophthalmol Vis Sci 27:1706-1715
9. Zetlan SR, Sponsel WE, Stodtmeister R (1992)Retinal capillary haemodynamics, visual-evoked potentials and pressure tolerance in normal human eyes. Invest Ophthalmol Vis. Sci 33:1857-63
10. Orgul S, Meyer P, Cioffi GA, et al. (1995) Physiology of blood flow regulation and mechanisms involved in optic nerve perfusion. J Glaucoma 4: 427-443
11. Kitazawa Y, Shirai H, Go FJ (1989) The effect of Ca^{2+}-antagonist on visual field in low-tension glaucoma. Graefes Arch Clin Exp Ophthalmol 227:408-12
12. Bose S, Piltz JR, Breton ME (1995) Nimodipine, a centrally active calcium antagonist, exerts a beneficial effect on contrast sensitivity in patients with normal-tension glaucoma and in control subjects. Ophthalmol 102:1236-1241
13. Yanagisawa M, Kurihara H, Kimura S, et al. (1988) A novel potent vasoconstrictor peptide produced by vascular endothelial cells. Nature 332:411-5.
14. Luscher TF, Boulanger CM, Dohi Y, et al. (1992) Endothelium-derived contracting factors. Hypertension, vol 19, 117-130
15. Luscher TF, Boulanger CM, Yang ZH et al. (1993) Interactions between endothelium-derived relaxing and contraction factors in health and cardiovascular disease. Circulation 87:V36-44
16. McDonald JR, Bailie JR, Archer DB, et al. (1995) Characterisation of endothelin A (ET_A) and endothelin B (ET_B) receptors in cultured bovine retinal pericytes. Invest Ophthalmol Vis Sci 36:1088-1094

17. Haefliger IO, Meyer P, Flammer J et al. (1994) The vascular endothelium as a regulator of the ocular circulation: A new concept in ophthalmology? Surv Ophthal 39:123-132
18. Meyer P, Flammer J, Luscher TF (1993) L-arginine/nitric oxide and endothelin as regulators of flow in the perfused porcine eye. Invest Ophthalmol Vis Sci 34:3614-3621
19. Haque MSR, Taniguchi T, Sugiyama K, et al. (1995) The ocular hypotensive effect of the ETB receptor selective agonist, Sarafotoxin S6c, in rabbits. Invest Ophthalmol Vis Sci 36: 804-808
20. Costagliola C, Carella C, Amato G, et al. (1995) Effect of oral bromocriptine administration in intraocular pressure in normotensive and glaucomatous human subjects. J Glaucoma 4:386-390
21. Chiou JCY (1994) Treatment of open angle glaucoma and ischemic retinopathy with Dopamine antagonists. J Oc Pharmacol 10:371-377
22. Prunte C, Flammer J (1995) The novel dopamine D-1 antagonist and D-2 agonist, SDZ GLC-756, lowers intraocular pressure in healthy human volunteers and in patients with glaucoma. Ophthalmol 102: 1291-1297
23. Ferrari-Dileo G (1988) $ß_1$ and $ß_2$ adrenergic binding sites in bovine retina and retinal blood vessels. Invest Ophthalmol Vis Sci 29: 695-699
24. Meyer P, Flammer J, Luscher TF (1995) Local action of the renin angiotensin systems in the porcine ophthalmic circulation: Effects of ACE-Inhibitors and angiotensin receptor antagonists. Invest Ophthalmol Vis Sci 36:555-562
25. Sramek SJ, Wallow IHL, Tewksbury DA, et al. (1992) An ocular renin-angiotensin system. Immunohistochemistry of angiotensinogen. Invest Ophthalmol Vis Sci 33: 627-1632
26. Rossetti L, Marchetti I, Orzalesi N, et al. (1993) Randomised clinical trials on medical treatment of glaucoma. Arch Ophthalmol 111:96-103
27. Collignon-Brach J (1994) Long term effect of topical betablockers on intraocular pressure and visual field sensitivity in ocular hypertension and chronic open angle glaucoma. Surv Ophthalmol 38:149-155
28. Van Buskirk EM, Bacon DR, Fahrenbach WH (1990) Ciliary vasoconstriction after topical adrenergic drugs. Am J Ophthalmol 109:511-517
29. Martin XD, Ramineau PA (1989) Vasoconstrictive effect of topical timolol on human retinal arteries. Graefes Arch Clin Exp Ophthalmol 227:526-30
30. Hoste AM, Stanislas US (1994) The relaxant action of betaxolol on isolated bovine retinal microarteries. Curr Eye Res 13:483-487
31. Orgul S, Bacon DR, Van Buskirk EM, et al. (1996) Optic nerve vasomotor effects of topical apraclonidine hydrochloride. Br J Ophthalmol 80:82-84
32. Sugiyama K, Cioffi GA, Bacon DR et al. (1994) Optic nerve and peripapillary choroidal microvasculature in the primate. Glaucoma 3:S45-54
33. Klaver JH, Greve EL, Goslinga H et al. (1985) Blood and plasma viscosity measurements in patients with glaucoma. Br J Ophthalmol 69: 765-770
34. Trope GE, Salinas RG, Glynn M (1987) Blood viscosity in primary open angle glaucoma. Can J Ophthalmol 22:202-4
35. Foulds WS (1987) 50th Bowman Lecture. "Blood is thicker than water." Some haemorheological aspects of ocular disease. Eye 1:343-63
36. Wolf S, Arend O, Sponsel WE, et al. (1993) Retinal hemodynamics using scanning laser ophthalmoscopy and haemorheology in chronic open angle glaucoma. Ophthalmol100: 1561-6
37. Garcia-Salinas P, Trope GE, Glynn M (1988) Blood viscosity in ocular hypertension. Can J Ophthalmol 23:305-307
38. Harris A, Shoemaker JA, Burgoyne J, et al. (1995) Acute effect of topical ß-adrenergic antagonists on normal perimacular hemodynamics. J Glaucoma 4:36-40
39. Hamard P, Hamard H, Dufaux J, et al. (1994) Optic nerve head blood flow using a laser Doppler velocimeter and haemorheology in primary open-angle glaucoma and normal pressure glaucoma. Br J Ophthalmol 78:449-453
40. Baxter GM, Williamson TH, McKillop G, et al. (1992) Colour Doppler ultrasound of orbital and optic nerve blood flow: Effects of posture and Timolol 0.5%. Invest Ophthalmol Vis Sci 33:604-10
41. Rojanapongpun P, Drance SN, Morrison B (1993) Ophthalmic artery flow velocity in glaucomatous and normal subjects. Brit J Ophthalmol 77:25-29
42. Harris A, Williamson TH, Martin B, et al. (1995) Test/retest reproducibility of color doppler imaging assessment of blood flow velocity in orbital vessels. J Glaucoma 4:281-286
43. Schwartz B (1994) Circulatory defects of the optic disk and retina in ocular hypertension and high pressure open-angle glaucoma. Surv Ophthalmol 38 (Suppl.):S23-34
44. Nanba K, Schwartz B (1988) Nerve fibre layer and optic disc fluorescence defect in glaucoma and ocular hypertension. Ophthalmol 95: 1227-33
45. Geijssen HC (1991) Studies on normal pressu-

re glaucoma. Kugler Amstelveen, The Nederlands pp168-194

46. Butt Z, O'Brien C (1995) Reproducibility of Pulsatile ocular blood flow measurements. J Glaucoma 4:214-218
47. Ravalico G, Pastori G, Toffoli G, Croce M (1994) Visual and blood flow responses in low tension glaucoma. Surv Ophthalmol 38:S173-176
48. James CB, Smith SE (1991) Pulsatile ocular blood flow in patients with low tension glaucoma. Br J Ophthalmol 75:466-470
49. Quaranta L, Manni G, Donato F et al. (1994) The effect of increased intraocular pressure on pulsatile ocular blood flow in low tension glaucoma. Surv Ophthalmol 38:177-182
50. Michelson G, Schmauss B (1995) Two dimensional mapping of the perfusion of the retina and optic nerve head. Brit J Ophthalmol 79: 1126-1132
51. Ataullah S, Hudson C, Chen H, O'Donoghue E (1996) Repeatability of capillary blood flow measurements assessed with Heidelburg retinal flowmeter in normal subjects and in glaucomatous patients. Invest Ophthalmol Vis Sci 37: 134-138

The Ca^{2+} Channel Blocking Action of β-Blockers in Bovine Retinal Microartery

A. M. Hoste, L. J. Andries, and S. U. Sys

Department of Human Physiology, University of Antwerp, Groenenborgerlaan 171, 2020 Antwerp, Belgium

Introduction

Vascular disorders in the posterior pole of the eye may have a role in the pathogenesis of open-angle glaucoma [1-4]. One should therefore be aware of the vascular effects of antiglaucoma medication. We studied the effects of β-blockers on retinal microarteries in the cow.

Materials and Methods

We described our technique in detail previously [5]. Microarterial segments located between the optic disc and the first intraretinal arterial branching were dissected free. The mean diameter of the segments was 221 μm. Subsequently, the microarterial segments were threaded on two stainless steel wires of 40 μm diameter and the whole preparation was transported to an organ bath containing a physiological salt solution. The top view of the organ bath (Fig. 1) shows how the microarteries were mounted with the stainless steel wires and connected to a force-transducer that could measure the force generated by the microarteries. This experimental set-up yields highly precise measurements of microarterial tone. In addition, we have control of the environment of the preparation under study.

To allow studies of relaxation, the preparations were precontracted (or activated) by: (1) a depolarizing solution containing K^+ 125 m*M* (equimolar replacement of Na^+) or (2) the agonist prostaglandin $F_{2\alpha}$ ($PGF_{2\alpha}$). When we immerse the microartery in the K^+-containing solution, or when we add $PGF_{2\alpha}$ to the physiological salt solution in the organ bath, the microartery starts to contract or develop force. The contraction typically shows a rapid phasic part and subsequent stabilization at a tonic part. When the K^+- or $PGF_{2\alpha}$-containing solution is replaced by the normal physiological salt solution, the artery ceases to develop force or relaxes. During the stable tonic part of the contraction we can perform pharmacological interventions.

Results and Discussion

Absence of Functional ß-Adrenoceptors

In most vessels, stimulation of ß-adrenoceptors causes relaxation or vasodilatation, while stimulation of α-adrenoceptors causes contraction or vasoconstriction. Theoretically, β-blockers might induce vasoconstriction in the retina, since during β-adrenoceptor blockade, α-mediated effects of circulating adrenaline would no longer be opposed. However, this is only a theory, based on the assumption that retinal arteries have functional β-adrenoceptors.

We studied the effects of isoproterenol, a β-adrenergic agonist, to assess whether retinal arteries actually have such receptors. Increasing doses of isoproterenol (10^{-7}-3.10^{-6}*M*) were added to K^+-activated microarteries. Isoproterenol was unable to induce relaxation (Fig. 2). High doses of isoproterenol (3.10^{-6} *M*) were also without effect during $PGF_{2\alpha}$-induced contractions.

Since the β-adrenergic agonist isoproterenol fails to relax bovine retinal microarteries,

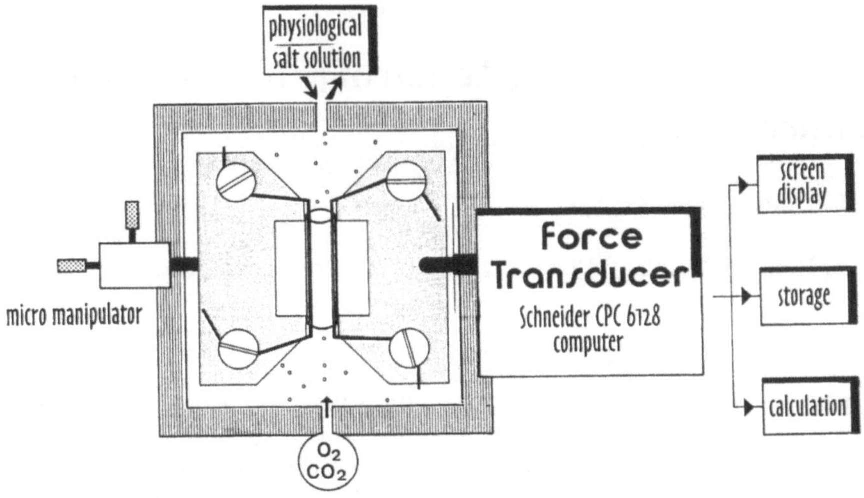

Fig. 1. Top view of the organ bath with mounted microarterial segment

these microarteries do not possess functional ß-adrenoceptors. Hence, β-blockers probably have no adverse constricting effects in retinal microarteries through their β-adrenoceptor blocking capacities. However, β-blockers could affect retinal arterial tone through other mechanisms. Therefore we studied the effects of propranolol.

Relaxant Effects of β-Blockers

Propranolol is the standard β-blocker in pharmacology, and it was the first β-blocker, shown in 1967, to have ocular hypotensive effects [6]. Propranolol (10^{-6}-$3.10^{-5}M$) relaxes K^+-induced contractions dose-dependently (Fig. 2). Racemic *dl*-propranolol, and both stereoisomers *l*- and *d*-propranolol are equieffective in producing relaxation, indicating that the relaxation shows no stereospecificity.

Betaxolol, a well-known β-blocker in ophthalmology, resembles propranolol in relaxing K^+-induced contractions (Fig. 2). The ED_{50} value, which is the mean dose resulting in 50% relaxation, is $10^{-5}M$ for both drugs. Timolol, the standard β-blocker in ophthalmology, only has a slight relaxant action (Fig. 2).

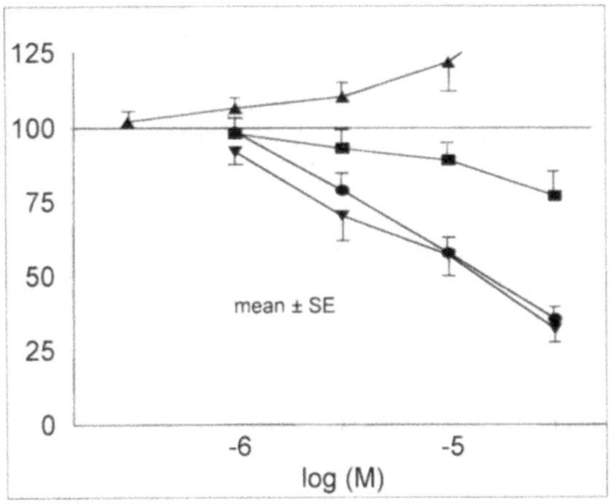

Fig. 2. Mean developed K^+-induced tonic force during increasing doses of isoproterenol (▲, n = 6), propranolol (●, n = 17), betaxolol (▼, n = 7) and timolol (■, n = 9). Control was K^+-induced tonic force prior to drug application

Possible Mechanism of the Relaxant Action of β-Blockers

Which Cell Type Within the Microarterial Wall Mediates the Relaxation by the ß-Blockers?

The β-blockers might relax the K^+-induced contractions through presynaptic effects on the adrenergic nerves: they are known to inhibit the noradrenaline release from depolarized nerve endings [7]. However, the bovine retinal artery, like the retinal artery of other animal species [8], has no adrenergic nerves [9].

The endothelium (lining the internal microarterial surface) is another important determinant of smooth muscle cell tone and might therefore mediate the relaxation by the β-blockers. We can selectively remove the

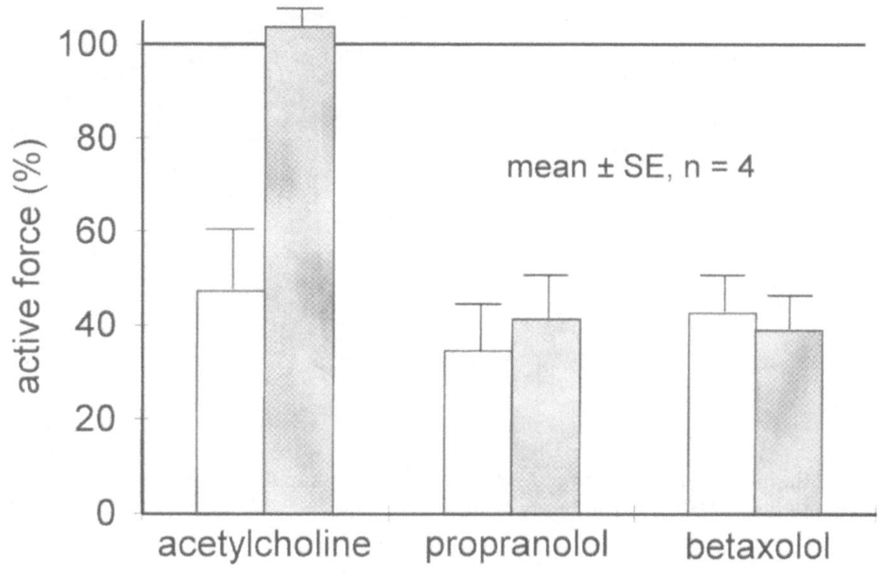

Fig. 3. Mean developed force after adding acetylcholine $3.10^{-6}M$ to $PGF_{2\alpha}$-induced contractions, or after adding betaxolol or propranolol $3.10^{-5}M$ to K^+-induced contractions, (❑) before and (■)after endothelium removal. Control was force prior to drug application. Self-pairing experimental design

endothelium from mounted preparations by blowing gas (95% O_2 - 5% CO_2) through the arterial lumen [10]. Removal of the endothelium blocks endothelium-dependent relaxations, such as the relaxation induced by acetylcholine [10]: acetylcholine markedly relaxes the intact retinal microartery, but fails to do so after the endothelium is removed (Fig. 3). By contrast, removal of the endothelium does not result in a weaker relaxant effect of betaxolol or propranolol (Fig. 3): betaxolol or propranolol induces the same amount of relaxation before and after endothelium removal.

As the relaxing action of betaxolol and propranolol is not mediated by interaction with adrenergic nerves or with the endothelium, the β-blockers act directly on the smooth muscle cells.

Where in the Process of Smooth Muscle Cell Contraction Do the β-Blockers Interact to Produce a Relaxation?

Basically, smooth muscle cell contraction is initiated by an increase of intracellular Ca^{2+} (Fig. 4). This activates the contractile proteins through myosin light chain kinase. Ca^{2+} comes from either intracellular Ca^{2+} stores or from the extracellular space. This Ca^{2+} influx occurs mainly through voltage-operated Ca^{2+} channels. Drugs that block these voltage-operated Ca^{2+} channels are called Ca^{2+} channel blockers. Removal of Ca^{2+} from the extracellular space quickly abolishes the K^+-induced contraction in retinal microartery, indicating that this type of contraction is mainly supported by Ca^{2+} influx from the extracellular space. High concentrations of K^+ are indeed known to open the voltage-operated Ca^{2+} channels through depolarization of the cell membrane [11]. Unlike K^+, $PGF_{2\alpha}$ is still able to induce a contraction in Ca^{2+} free medium. This indicates that prostaglandin-induced contractions are less dependent on Ca^{2+} influx than are the K^+ -induced contractions, the prostaglandin being able to release Ca^{2+} from intracellular stores. As a consequence, prostaglandin-induced contractions are less sensitive to verapamil, a standard Ca^{2+} channel blocker, than are K^+-induced contractions (Fig. 5).

β-blockers probably have Ca^{2+} channel blocking activity, since they relax K^+ -induced contractions that are mainly supported by Ca^{2+} influx through the voltage-operated Ca^{2+} channels. If β-blockers have this activity, one would expect the drugs to induce a weaker relaxation in the prostaglandin-induced contractions than in the K^+ -induced contractions (similar

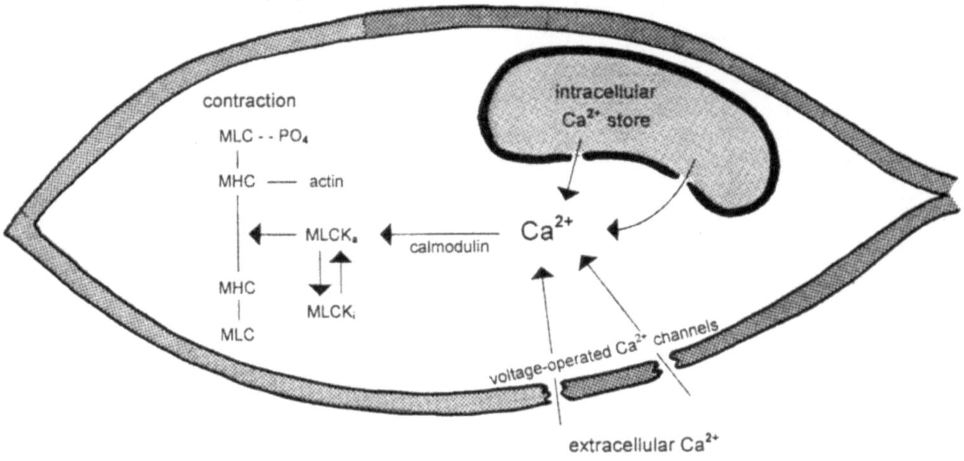

Fig. 4. Vascular smooth muscle cell contraction. *MLC*, myosin light chain, *MLCKi*, inactive- and *MLCKa*, active- myosin light chain kinase, *MHC*, myosin heavy chain

to the standard Ca^{2+} channel blocker verapamil). And this is indeed the case: while a high dose of betaxolol or propranolol is able to relax the K^+-induced contraction markedly, the β-blockers only slightly relax the prostaglandin-induced contraction (Fig. 5). The slight relaxation by betaxolol is significant, the effect of propranolol however is not. Furthermore, what is left of the prostaglandin-induced contraction after removal of Ca^{2+} from the extracellular space must be mainly supported by Ca^{2+} released from intracellular stores. If betaxolol acts as a Ca^{2+} channel blocker, it should be without effects on this intracellular component of the contraction. Indeed, the small relaxation that betaxolol induces during normal conditions, is abolished in Ca^{2+} free medium.

Previous studies of other types of contraction, such as contractions induced by serotonin and stretch, were also in agreement with propranolol and betaxolol having Ca^{2+} channel blocking

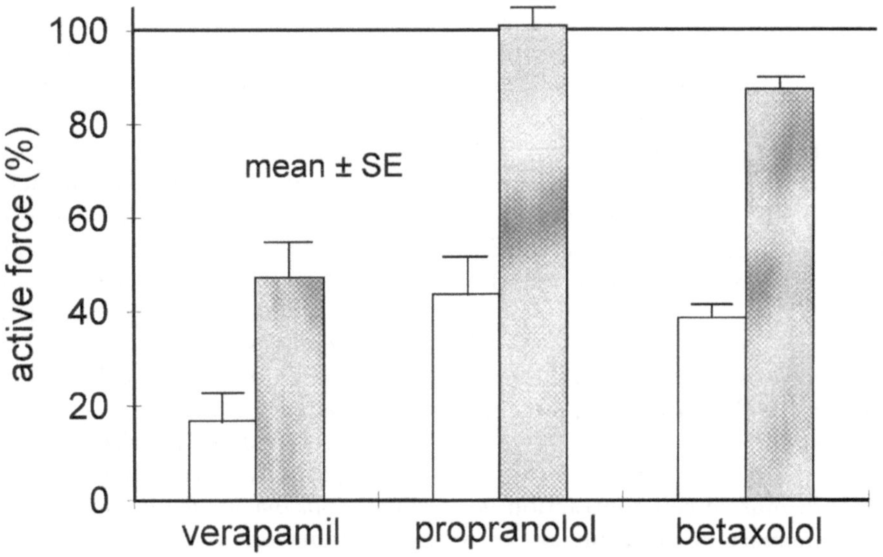

Fig. 5. Mean developed force after adding verapamil $3.10^{-6}M$ ($n = 5$), propranolol 3.10^{-5} M ($n = 6$) or betaxolol $3.10^{-5}M$ ($n = 7$) to (❑) K^+- and (■) $PGF_{2\alpha}$-induced contractions. Control was force prior to drug application. Self-pairing experimental design

activity: the effects of both β-blockers were similar to the effects of verapamil during both types of precontraction [9, 12].

Other studies have demonstrated relaxant effects of betaxolol in porcine long posterior ciliary artery [13], and rat renal, mesenteric and femoral arteries [14]. These relaxant effects were also thought to result from Ca^{2+} channel blocking effects. Recently the Ca^{2+} channel blocking action of betaxolol has been confirmed by an electrophysiological study of guinea-pig mesenteric artery [15].

Possible Clinical Significance of the Ca^{2+}-Channel Blocking Action of ß-Blockers

Propranolol (the standard β-blocker in pharmacology) is not used in the management of glaucoma because the drug also has Na^{+} channel blocking activity that is responsible for its local anesthetic activity [16]. Consequently, application of propranolol to the eye produces marked corneal anesthesia, which after chronic application would lead to corneal disease. However, at least one of the β-blockers used in ophthalmology (namely betaxolol) has a similar relaxant action. Betaxolol could therefore dilate retinal arteries during antiglaucoma therapy, if the drug reaches the retina after topical application. At present, we certainly cannot exclude this possibility. The concentrations of β-blockers in ophthalmic solutions are very high. The betaxolol 0.5% ophthalmic solution contains 1.45 10^{-2} *M* betaxolol, this concentration being 1000 times higher than the concentration required to relax retinal microarteries by 50% in this study. Furthermore, as discussed previously [12], β-blockers could reach the retina by a very short conjunctival-scleral route. Finally, drugs may accumulate in the ocular tissues when they are chronically administered.

At this time the vascular hypothesis in glaucoma focuses on the circulation of the optic nerve head. In this respect, it is interesting to know that the Ca^{2+} channel blocking action of betaxolol has also been demonstrated in ciliary artery [13]. Still, the retinal circulation may be at least as important. None of the papers in which a correlation is shown between impaired ocular perfusion and glaucoma [1, 4] actually measure blood flow in the eye. The exact location of the vascular disorder in the eye still has to be determined [17]. The axons within the optic nerve head originate from the retinal ganglion cells. The retinal circulation maintains the perfusion of these cells (and of all the inner retina as far externally as the outer plexiform layer [18]). Moreover, in the retina the necessity to ensure a good quality optical image has taken priority over the provision of abundant blood supply. The retinal circulation: (1) is sparse; (2) is endarterial in nature; (3) operates with a high arteriovenous oxygen difference; and (4) has a perfusion pressure that is opposed by the relatively high intraocular pressure [19]. This makes the retinal circulation one of the most precarious vascular beds in the entire body, and therefore an interesting research target.

References

1. Phelps CD, Corbett JJ (1985) Migraine and low-tension glaucoma. Invest Ophthalmol Vis Sci 26: 1105-1108
2. Schulzer M, Drance SM, Carter CJ, Brooks DE, Douglas GR, Lau W (1990) Biostatistical evidence for two distinct chronic open-angle glaucoma populations. Br J Ophthalmol 74: 196-200
3. Gasser P, Flammer J (1991) Blood-cell velocity in the nailfold capillaries of patients with normal-tension and high-tension glaucoma. Am J Ophthalmol 111:585-588
4. Graham SL, Drance SM, Wijsman K, Douglas G R, Mikelberg FS (1995) Ambulatory blood pressure monitoring in glaucoma. The nocturnal dip. Ophthalmol 102:61-69
5. Hoste AM, Boels PJ, Brutsaert DL, De Laey JJ (1989) Effect of alpha-1 and beta agonists on contraction of bovine retinal resistance arteries in vitro. Invest Ophthalmol Vis Sci 30: 44-50
6. Philips CI, Howitt G, Rowlands DJ (1967) Propranolol as ocular hypotensive agent. Br J Ophthalmol 51:222-226
7. Weinstock M (1976) The presynaptic effect of β-adrenoceptor antagonists on noradrenergic neurons. Life Sci 19:1453-1466
8. Laties AM (1967) Central retinal artery innervation: Absence of adrenergic innervation to the intraocular branches. Arch Ophthalmol 77:405-409
9. Hoste AM, Boels PJ, Andries LJ, Brutsaert DL, De Laey JJ (1990) Effects of beta-antagonists on contraction of bovine retinal microarteries in vitro. Invest Ophthalmol Vis Sci 31: 1231-1237

10. Hoste AM, Andries LJ (1991) Contractile responses of isolated bovine retinal arteries to acetylcholine. Invest Ophthalmol Vis Sci 32:1996-2005
11. Droogmans G, Raeymaekers L, Casteels R (1977) Electro- and pharmacomechanical coupling in the smooth muscle cells of the rabbit ear artery. J Gen Physiol 70:129-148
12. Hoste AM, Sys SU (1994) The relaxant action of betaxolol on isolated bovine retinal microarteries. Curr Eye Res 13:483-487
13. Hester RK, Chen Z, Becker EJ, McLaughlin M, DeSantis L (1994) The direct relaxing action of betaxolol, carteolol and timolol in porcine long posterior ciliary artery. Surv Ophthalmol (Suppl) 38:S125-S134.
14. Bessho H, Suzuki J, Tobe A (1991) Vascular effects of betaxolol, a cardioselective β-adrenoceptor antagonist, in isolated rat arteries. Jpn J Pharmacol 55:351-358
15. Setoguchi M, Ohya Y, Abe I, Fujishima M (1995) Inhibitory action of betaxolol, a β_1 -selective adrenoceptor antagonist, on voltage-dependent calcium channels in guinea-pig artery and vein. Br J Parmacol 115:198-202
16. Matthews JC, Baker JK (1982) Effects of propranolol and a number of its analogues on sodium channels. Biochem Pharmacol 31:1681-1685
17. Geijssen HC, Greve EL (1995) Vascular concepts in glaucoma. Curr Opinion in Ophthalmol 6:71-77
18. Hogan MJ, Feeney L (1963) The ultrastructure of the retinal blood vessels. J Ultrastruct Res 9:10-28
19. Wise GN, Dollery CT, Henkind P (eds) (1971): The Retinal Circulation: Chapter 6 Physiologic Principles. Harper and Row, New York

Antioxidant Drugs and Glaucoma

R.A. Meduri[1], E. Martini[1], D. Bozza[2], G. Grossi[2], P. Preda[3], C. Sprovieri[1], L. Scorolli[1], and G. Piccinni Leopardi[1]

Department of Ophthalmology, S. Orsola-Malpighi Policlinic, Via Massarenti 9, 40100 Bologna, Italy
[1] Optic Pathophisiology Service; [2] Centralized Laboratory Service; [3] Ultrastructural Biology and Pathology Service

Introduction

The goal of our research was to better understand the role of trabecular meshwork antioxidant activities in chronic open-angle glaucoma.
The basis of our work may be summarized as follows: the trabecular cells are the most active component regarding trabecular structure and function. They actively control aqueous humor outflow and removal of pigment and cellular debris. They ensure the synthesis and turnover of trabecular fibrillar elements in that they synthesize and degrade proteoglycans and glycosaminoglycans [1-3]. In doing so they modify the steric and anionic resistance to aqueous humor outflow, responding to mechanical, humoral and probably even neuronal stimuli.
This intense cellular activity can be seen in the abundance of mitochondria, endoplasmic reticulum and lysosomes and requires extensive activation of cellular energetic oxidative reactions.
The trabecular meshwork is continuously exposed to the action of oxidizing agents which are generated by an intrinsic trabecular metabolism and are also transported from other anterior chamber stuctures, carried by aqueous flow. Remarkable concentrations of hydrogen peroxide (25 μm) were detected in normal aqueous humor as a likely effect of light reaction whit ascorbic acid [4]. The normal trabecular meshwork has an effective antioxidant system which acts against free oxygen radicals [5].
High concentrations of reduced glutathione (and no trace of oxidized glutathione) were found in the trabecular tissue [6]. Components of the main antioxidant enzymatic systems were also detected: superoxide dismutase and catalase [7], glutathione peroxidase [8], glutathione reductase [9]. Cultured trabecular cells are able to actively defend themselves against oxidative stress [10, 11].
Glaucomatous trabecular alterations include a constant and relevant reduction of trabecular cell number [12]. Other quite constant features are a progressive increase of extracellular material, especially "long spacing" (100 nm) and "curly" collagen and plaques derived from collagen and pseudo-elastic fiber sheaths. Both the structural and resistance-type proteoglycans are often altered in quantity and quality [1-3].
The trabeculocyte's metabolic and enzymatic crisis, which underlies the cellular depletion and structural modifications observed in glaucoma, may be caused - or, in any case, may be worsened - by the damaging action of oxygen free radicals, to which trabecular cells have an increased sensitivity and/or a reduced neutralizing capacity [13, 14]. Babizhayev and Bunin [15] detected increased lipid peroxidation in glaucomatous trabecular meshwork as compared to normal. The depletion of glutathione [6] or catalase [16] makes the trabecular tissue more susceptible to hydrogen peroxid's toxic action [17], resulting in a reduction of outflow. Di Staso and co-workers [18] showed that cultured glaucomatous cells have significantly less important enzymatic activities than normal ones. These include glucose-6-phosphate-dehydrogenase, an essential step in the phosphate-pentose shunt upon which production of reduced glutathione depends.
To better understand the role of antioxidant systems in primary glaucoma, we decided to measure and compare the amount of vitamin

E in the serum and aqueous humor of glaucomatous and normal subjects.

Vitamin E [19] is a tocopherol: eight varieties of tocopherol have been identified, but the most abundant and biologically active one is α-tocopherol, which structurally is highly similar to coenzyme Q4 [20], whose activity it shares. Vitamin E is absorbed in the gastroenteric tract by a mechanism similar to that of other liposoluble vitamins. It enters the hematic flow via the lymphatics, associated with chylomicrons and successively to β-lipoproteins. Inside the cell, vitamin E is concentrated at sites where there is considerable production of free radicals (mitochondria and endoplasmic reticulum) and acts as a direct scavenger, seizing the free radicals and decomposing the hydro-peroxides [21]; it also has an indirect role as part of the mitochondrial Q coenzyme system.

Besides, we decided to evaluate a possible correlation between seric or aqueous vitamin E levels and ultrastructural alterations of trabecular meshwork of glaucomatous eyes undergoing trabeculectomy.

Materials and Methods

Our group included 20 patients, 12 male and 8 females (between 41 and 85 years; mean 70.3 ± 10.0) (Table 1). All of the patients had chronic open-angle glaucoma that did not respond to maximal medical therapy (mean IOP 30.0 ± 5.7 mm Hg) as well as worsening visual field damage and were therefore recommended for filtrating surgery. The day before surgery a venous blood sample was taken to measure serum vitamin E. During the trabeculectomy we obtained an aqueous humor sample (0.2 ml) by an anterior chamber puncture with a 30-gauge needle, to measure aqueous humor levels of vitamin E. The trabecular specimen removed during surgery was fixed and examined by transmission electron microscopy (TEM) to detect ultrastructural trabecular alterations. As a control group we selected 15 patients, similar in sex and age distribution, who were completely free of glaucomatous alterations (normal visual field and optic nerve head, IOP<18 mm Hg without any therapy, absence of familial glaucoma and who underwent cataract surgery). Venous blood and aqueous humor samples were obtained from these patients using the same technique.

Vitamin E in serum and aqueous humor was measured by high performance liquid chromatography, using an electrochemical detector with high sensibility and selectivity. The syringers with the sample were immediately frozen at -30°C and thawed later by shaking and inversion at room temperature. The liquid sample was then transferred to an Eppendorf 1.5 ml test tube. A total of 50 μl of the sample plus 1.5 ml of 5% ascorbic acid in 0.1 HCI were put in a glass 16 x 115 mm conical test tube with a screw plug and teflon under seal. The test tube was vortexed; 2 ml of ethanol were then added and again vortexed; 4 ml of n-esane were added and the test tube plugged, controlling that the under-seal was well placed. Thereafter we stirred by constant inversion for 15 min and then centrifuged for 15 min at 4°C and 3500 rpm. A total of 3.5 ml of supernatant were then transferred to a glass test tube and allowed to evaporate under nitrogen at 37°C for 20-30 min. The dry residual is collected with 2 ml of ethanol and put in vials for injection into an HPLC apparatus.

For TEM, the surgical specimens were immediately fixed in 2.5% glutaraldehyde, with cacodylate buffer (0.1M pH 7.4) and postfixated in 1% osmium tetroxide with the same buffer and dehydrated with increasing concentrations of ethanol. After a further dehydration in propylene oxide, the specimens are embedded in araldite. Ultrathin sections (700 Å) were obtained using an OMV 3 Richter ultramicrotome, collected on copper/rhodium grids, covered with formvar and contrasted with uranyl acetate and lead citrate. A Philips 400 T transmission electron miscroscope was used.

Results

The mean serum level of vitamin E was 24 992 ± 7243 μm/l in glaucomatous subjects vs 25 393 ± 5 516 μM/l in normal (cataract) subjects; the difference between the two groups was not statistically significant (Student's *t* test for unpaired data: $p = 0.86$) (Table 1).

The vitamin E level in aqueous humor had a mean value of 0.014 ± 0.006 μM/l in glaucomatous eyes vs 0.026 ± 0.038 μM/l in control eyes;

Table 1. Results of vitamin E level (μM/l) in blood serum and aqueous humor in glaucomatous and normal subjects

Patient number	Age	IOP	Aqueous vitamin E	Blood vitamin E	Control number	Age	Aqueous vitamin E	Blood vitamin E
1	64	21	0.0127	42.20	1	73	0.0220	39.10
2	75	24	0.0234	38.30	2	59	0.0060	25.00
3	41	28	0.0064	27.20	3	80	0.0021	25.90
4	72	25	0.0149	29.00	4	57	0.1555	30.80
5	68	30	0.0192	27.70	5	64	0.0053	27.40
6	67	35	0.0099	10.20	6	72	0.0042	22.50
7	66	27	0.0122	35.25	7	73	0.0260	19.30
8	72	37	0.0167	23.00	8	65	0.0380	26.20
9	73	20	0.0099	22.50	9	76	0.0350	26.20
10	85	38	0.0129	20.00	10	66	0.0100	30.70
11	72	27	0.0144	17.80	11	63	0.0035	17.80
12	74	32	0.0153	26.70	12	75	0.0275	24.60
13	76	34	0.0150	20.90	13	81	0.0187	20.90
14	83	35	0.0040	21.80	14	74	0.0204	26.20
15	56	33	0.0170	21.20	15	67	0.0122	18.30
16	63	35	0.0010	26.00				
17	65	35	0.0060	22.40				
18	74	26	0.0135	20.70				
19	77	36	0.0208	25.70				
20	83	22	0.0262	21.30				

the difference between the two groups is quite evident but is not statistically significant (p = 0.187) (Table 1).

The ultrastructural examination showed in all cases definite alterations of the trabecular meshwork:

- Increased extracellular matrix and the presence of long spacing (100 nm) collagen in 100% of cases; strands of thickened and curly collagen in 60% of cases.
- Nearly constant thickening of basal membranes and lamellar core with a reduction of intertrabecular spaces.
- Significant reduction of trabecular cells that in nine patients (45%) left uncoated areas of trabecular tissue.

In all patients the trabecular cells appeared rich in pigment granules and in 11 patients (55%) showed features of cytoplasmic organelle damage and vacuoles presumably of lysosomal derivation. In three patients (15%), intertrabecular spaces were almost completely obliterated and the rare cells were almost smothered in abundant extracellular matrix. In six patients (30%) there were focal deposits (plaques) in the juxtacanalicular tissue derived from collagen and pseudoelastic fiber sheaths. In four patients (20%), after prolonged contrast with uranyl acetate, we detected a great abundance of proteoglycans. In one patient (5%) the trabecular structure was completely upset and there were calcific degeneration areas.

We attempted to stage trabecular alterations, defining grade 0 as having a normal histologic structure. Grade 1 was defined as thickening of basal membranes, increased extracellular matrix with long spacing and curly collagen, cell number reduction and cellular damage without 'baring' of trabeculae. Grade 2 was assigned to cases with greater cellular loss, leaving uncovered trabeculae, thickened and partially fused. Grade 3 was used to describe complete perturbation of trabecular tissue and the few remaining cells smothered in anomalous extracellular matrix.

According to this staging scheme, 11 of our patients (55%) were assigned to stage 1, six (30%) were classified as having stage 2 disease and three (15%) had stage 3 (Table 2).

Table 2. Stage of trabecular meshwork alterations in 20 trabeculectomy specimens examined by TEM (see text for description)

Stage	Number of cases(%)	
0	0	(0)
1	11	(55)
2	6	(30)
3	3	(15)

The regression analysis between the different variables showed a weak negative correlation between the stage of trabecular alterations and aqueous vitamin E levels x: the patients with lower vitamin E levels in aqueous humor tended to have more severe alterations (Fig. 1). This correlation (r = 0.118) was not statistically significant. A similar negative correlation stands out between IOP and aqueous level of vitamin E: patients with higher IOP have tendentially lower levels of vitamin E (Fig. 2). Again this correlation did not attain statistical significance (r = 0.282).

A good correlation (r = 0.415) appeared between IOP level and trabecular alteration stage. The correlation between age and trabecular alterations showed more severe lesions in younger patient (r = 0.425) (Fig. 3). Age and aqueous vitamin E levels were directly correlated, with the latter increasing with age (r = 0.367) (Fig. 4).

Discussion

Serum vitamin E levels were absolutely similar in normal and glaucomatous patients (24.99 vs 25.39 µm/l; P = 0.86). By contrast, the level of vitamin E in the aqueous humor was lower in glaucomatous eyes (0.014 µM/l) than in normal eyes (0.026 µM/l). The difference did not attain statistical significance due to a wide distribution of values and a wide overlap of distribution curves between the two groups. These data tend to exclude the finding that in glaucomatous patients there is a systemic deficiency of antioxidant system, but suggest the possibility that oxidative damage plays an exacerbating role, perhaps by lowering scavenger activity in the aqueous humor of these patients. Ultrastructural examination of trabecular tissue confirmed a profound tissue rearrangement: particularly important was the reduction of trabecular cell number and the presence of abnormal material, with increased proteoglycans and focal (plaque) deposits derived from collagen and pseudoelastic fiber sheaths.

As we expected there was a good correlation between IOP and trabecular alterations, while the correlation between such alterations and vitamin E level in aqueous humor was quite weak. Surprisingly, the older patients had fewer alterations. One possible explanation is that we dealt with a group of patients undergoing glaucoma surgery and that younger patients needing surgery have more pronounced ultrastructural alterations of trabecular meshwork. It may be interesting to underline that these younger patients also tend to have lower levels of vitamin E in aqueous humor.

We conclude from our work that oxidative damage does not play a primary role in the pathogenesis of glaucomatous trabecular alterations. Nevertheless the reduced level of vitamin E in the aqueous humor of younger patients with more advanced trabecular alterations suggests that oxidative agents have a worsening effect on glaucomatous eyes.

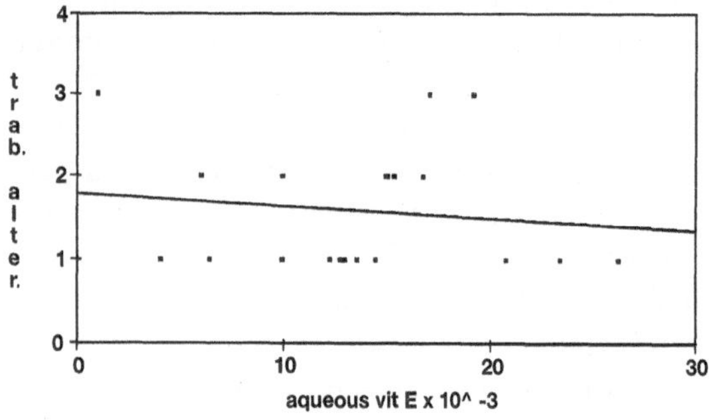

Fig. 1. Weak negative correlation between trabecular alterations and aqueous vitamin E levels (r = -0.118)

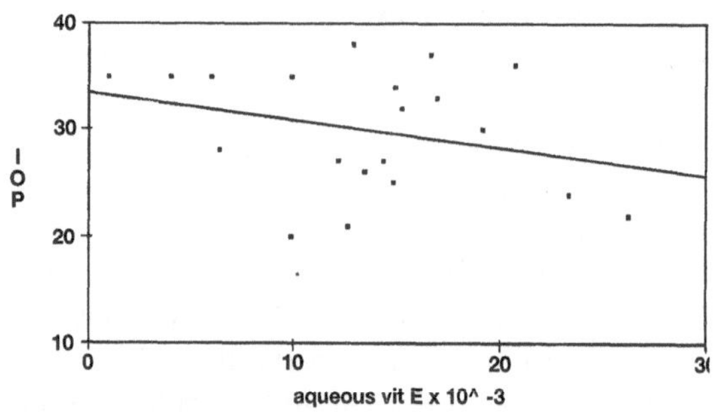

Fig. 2. Negative correlation between the intraocular pressure and aqueous vitamin E levels in glaucomatous eyes (r = 0.282)

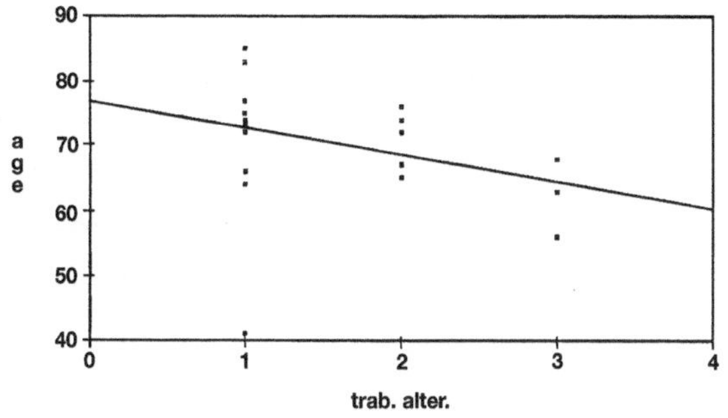

Fig. 3. Negative correlation between age and trabecular alterations: younger patients have more advanced damage (r = 0.425)

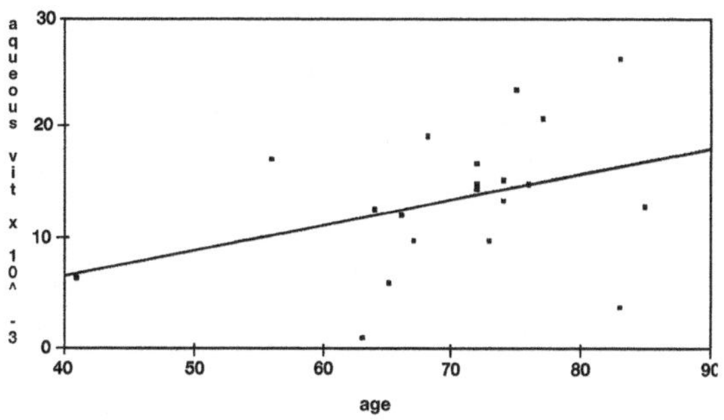

Fig. 4. Direct correlation between age and aqueous vitamin E levels: older patients have higher vitamin E levels (r = 0.367)

References

1. Rohen JW, Lutjen-Drecoll E (1989) Morphology of aqueous outflow pathways in normal and glaucomatous eye. In: Ritch R, Shields MB, Krupin T, (eds) The Glaucomas Mosby, St. Louis pp 41-65
2. Plane C (1992) Voies d'excretion de l'humeur aqueuse. In: Sole P, Dalens H, Gentou C (eds) Biophtalmologie, Masson, Paris, pp III/23-30
3. Bechetoille A. La résistance à l'écoulement de l'humeur aqueuse. In: Demailly P (ed) Traitement actuel du glaucome primitif à angle ouvert, Masson, Paris, pp 11-47
4. Spector A, Garner WH (1981) Hydrogen peroxide and human cataract Exp, Eye Res 33:673-681
5. Bron A, Maupoil V, Garcher C et al. (1991) Le pouvoir antiradicalaire de l'humeur aqueuse chez l'homme. Ophthalmol 5:107-109
6. Kahn MC, Giblin FD, Epstein DL (1983) Glutathione in calf trabecular meshwork and its relation to aqueous humor outflow facility. Inv Ophthalmol Vis Sci 24:1283-1287
7. Freedman SF, Anderson PJ, Epstein DL (1985) Superoxide dismutase and catalase of calf trabecular meshwork. Inv Ophthalmol Vis Sci 26:1330-1335
8. Scott DR, Karagenzian LN, Anderson PJ, Epstein DL (1984) Glutathione peroxidase of calf trabecular meshwork. Inv Ophthalmol Vis Sci 25:599-602
9. Nguyen KPV, Weiss H, Karagenzian LN et al. (1985) Glutathione reductase of calf trabecular meshwork. Inv Ophthalmol Vis Sci 26:887-890
10. Bloom E, Maglio MT, Polanski JL et al. (1990) Effects of oxidative injury on phagocytosis in human trabecular meshwork cells. Inv Ophthalmol Vis Sci, ARVO abstracts 31 (Suppl): 337
11. Anderson PJ, Karagenzian LN, Juzuki R et al. (1988) Effects of oxidative stress on calf trabecular meshwork and pulmonary aortic endothelial cells in culture. Inv Ophthalmol Vis Sci, ARVO abstracts 29 (Suppl): 229
12. Alvarado J, Murphy C, Juster R (1984 Trabecular meshwork cellularity in primary open-angle glaucoma and non-glaucomatous normals. Ophthalmol 91:564-579
13. Mata Flores F (1994) Multiple causes of glaucoma: a role for oxygen free radicals. Chibret Int J Ophthalmol 10/2:24-27
14. Spinelli D (1994) Vitamine e antiossidanti: aspetti clinici. Communication at IV Congresso Nazionale di Farmacologia Oculare, Capri (I), 13-15 October 1994
15. Babizhayev MA, Bunin AY (1989) Lipid peroxidation in open-angle glaucoma. Acta Ophthalmol 67:337-371
16. Polansky JR, Wood I, Maglio MT et al. (1984) Peroxide damage to human trabecular cells: a possible model for morphological alterations in aging and glaucoma. Inv Ophthalmol Vis Sci, ARVO abstracts 25 (Suppl): 122
17. Padgaomkar V, Hiblin FJ, Leverene V et al. (1994) Studies of H_2O_2 induced effects on cultured bovine trabecular meshwork cells. J Glaucoma 3:123-131
18. Di Staso S, Visconti U, Balestrazzi E (1994) Lactate dehydrogenase, malae dehydrogenase and glucose-6-phosphate dehydrogenase activities in normal and glaucomatous human trabecular meshwork cells. Inv Ophthalmol Vis Sci, ARVO abstracts 35 (Suppl): 2748
19. Bieri JG, Farrel PM (1976) Vitamin E. Vitam Horm 34:31-75
20. Symposium (various Authors) (1965) Interrelationships among vitamin E, coenzyme Q and selenium. Fed Proc 24:55-92
21. Molenaar I, Vos J, Hommes FA (1972) Effects of vitamin E deficiency on cellular membranes. Vitam Horm 30:45-82

Clinical Experience with Brimonidine Tartrate, an α-2 Agonist

J.T. Wilensky

Department of Ophthalmology and Visual Sciences, University of Illinois at Chicago College of Medicine, Chicago, IL 60612, USA

More than two decades ago, it was recognized that clonidine, an α-2 adrenergic agonist that was being used to treat elevated blood pressure, also caused a reduction in intraocular pressure [1]. This drug was explored extensively as a topical ocular hypotensive agent, but, because of its effect on systemic blood pressure, it never received widespread application as an anti-glaucoma medication. A derivative of clonidine, paraminoclonidine, which had much less effect on blood pressure, was developed and tested [2]. It was also found to have significant ocular hypotensive activity. Initially, it was used primarily in acute situations such as after laser trabeculoplasty but more recently has been recommended for extended use as an addition to maximum therapy to delay surgery. In this report, I would like to discuss the results that have been obtained from testing with a third agent in this class–brimonidine tartrate.

Brimonidine differs from apraclonidine by having a quinoxaline ring on the molecule (Fig. 1). Brimonidine has a much higher selectivity for α-2 receptors than α-1 receptors. The ratio for brimonidine is 1,781:1 vs 146:1 for clonidine and 76:1 for apraclonidine [3]. This means

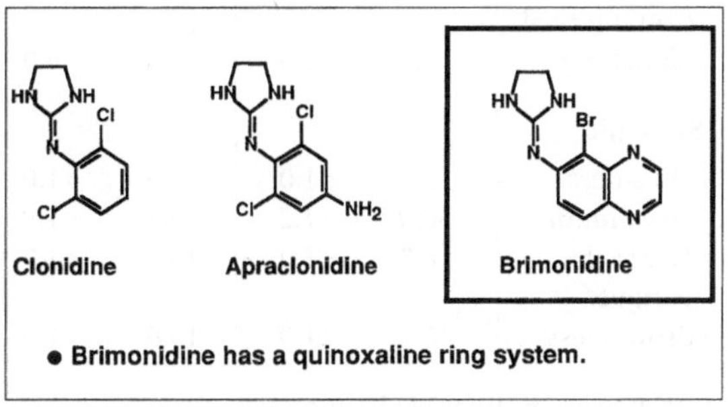

Fig. 1. Chemical structure of α adrenergic agonists

that brimonidine will cause much less α-1 stimulation at a dose that is sufficient to achieve the α-2 stimulation that is necessary for the intraocular pressure reduction.

There have been two major multicenter, 1-year, clinical trials that have been conducted with brimonidine. I participated in the first of these studies along with 24 other test centers. The second study involved 29 test centers. Both studies were double-masked, 1-year studies in which brimonidine (0.2%) was compared with timolol (0.5%). In the first study, randomization was performed on a one-to-one basis. In the second study, it was on a three-to-two basis, with three patients being started on brimonidine for every two on timolol.

The entry criteria for both studies were the same. The patients had either primary open angle glaucoma or ocular hypertension, elevated untreated intraocular pressure with a range between 23 and 34 mm Hg and no greater than a 5 mm asymmetry between the two eyes. The patients could not have been on more than two anti-glaucoma medications prior to washout.

The major outcome variable for the study was intraocular pressure control, while cup-to-disc ratios and visual fields were the secondary outcome variables. Drug safety was assessed. Adverse events, heart rate, blood pressure, and blood chemistry were also recorded in all patients.

A total of 926 patients were enrolled in the study. When they were analyzed, it was found that only 837 of these patients actually met the entry criteria for the study, and these patients were the ones that were analyzed for efficacy of the drug. An approximately equal number of subjects were found ineligible in each study group. Since some of the other patients also did receive treatment prior to determination that they were not eligible, these patients were included in the safety analysis, although not in the efficacy analysis. Within the study population, 58% had open angle glaucoma, 39% ocular hypertension, and, in 3%, there was an overlap between the two diagnoses. Approximately 60% of the patients had been on treatment for glaucoma prior to the study and underwent washout. They were evenly distributed between the study groups. A total of 466 of the patients were started on brimonidine, 371 on timolol. Analysis of the study population showed no significant difference between the two groups for age, race, sex, iris color, or glaucoma diagnosis.

Data analysis has been completed on all of the patients in the first study but has only been completed out to 6 months in the second study. So, the results that I will be presenting include all 837 patients for 6 months but only 374 after 12 months. As can be seen in Fig. 2, the mean intraocular pressure on entry into the study was a little over 24 mm Hg in both study groups. The intraocular pressure dropped significantly in both groups, and, at 2 h after instillation, the mean decrease in intraocular pressure from baseline ranged from 6.0 to 7.2 mm Hg in the brimonidine group and from 5.6 to 6.2 mm Hg in the timolol group. This reduction in intraocular pressure remained fairly stable over the 12-month follow-up period. At the 2-week and 3-month visits, brimonidine actually showed a significantly greater IOP decrease than did timolol ($p < 0.045$). The intraocular pressure reducing effect of the two drugs was also analyzed at the 12-h trough in the morning prior to the instillation of the medication.

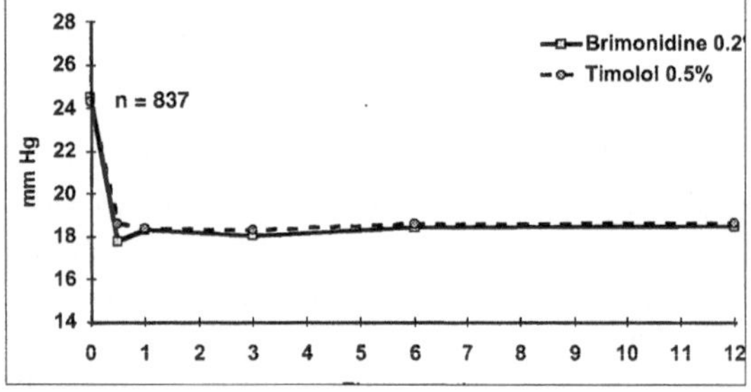

Fig. 2. Mean IOP at study entry and 2 h after treatment with brimonidine or timolol

At this point, the mean reduction from baseline was 3.7-5.0 mm Hg in the brimonidine group over the 12-month period and 6.1-6.6 mm Hg in the timolol group. Again, the mean decreases in intraocular pressures from baseline were statistically significant in both treatment groups at all periods, but timolol did lower the intraocular pressure at trough more than brimonidine over the entire study period.

No difference in changes in cup-to-disc ratio or visual fields were seen between the two groups during the follow-up period. However, really little change in either of these perimeters was seen in any of the patients. So, it is not surprising that there was no difference between the two study groups. No mydriasis was seen in either group.

Table 1 shows the adverse events that occurred during the study. The results were fairly similar between the two study groups with three exceptions.

Table 1. Adverse events[a]

	BRIM 0.2% (*n*=513)		TIM 0.5% (*n*=413)	
	Overall (%)	Exited study (%)	Overall (%)	Exited study (%)
Ocular				
Burning/ stinging	***24.0***	***<1.0***	***40.7***	***<1.0***
Hyperemia	26.3	1.4	23.0	0.0
Foreign body sensation	17.0	<1.0	15.0	0.0
Blurring	17.5	<1.0	20.1	<1.0
Conjunctival follicles	7.8	<1.0	2.9	<1.0
Lid erythema	6.4	0.0	4.6	0.0
Allergy[b]	***9.6***	***7.4***	***0.2***	***<1.0***
Conjunctival blanching	3.3	0.0	3.6	0.0
Systemic				
Dizziness	5.3	<1.0	3.6	<1.0
Dry mouth	***30.0***	***1.2***	***15.5***	***<1.0***
Headache	18.7	<1.0	18.9	<1.0
Fatigue/ drowsiness	15.8	<1.0	13.6	<1.0

BRIM, brimonidine; TIM, timolol.

[a]In both groups, >50% had been treated pre-study with a topical β-blocker.

[b]Allergic conjunctivitis, allergic blepharoconjunctivitis, follicular conjunctivitis, allergic reaction.

Burning and stinging were more common in the timolol group, while allergic reactions and complaints of dry mouth were more common in the brimonidine group. Overall, 9.6% of the patients in the brimonidine group did develop an allergic reaction and 6% of them dropped out of the study because of this. I found it very interesting, however, that no patient was discontinued from the study during the first month of treatment. This is in contrast to what has been seen with iopidine, for which we have found that 10%-15% of patients will develop an acute allergic reaction requiring termination of treatment during the first month [4]. This suggests to me that there is some difference in the nature of these allergic responses.

Systemically, very little difference was seen between these two treatment groups. There was virtually no change in systolic or diastolic blood pressures. There was no change in heart rate with brimonidine, while there was a small but statistically significant decrease in heart rate with timolol; this was expected. There were no changes in any of the blood chemistry studies in either patient group.

In summary, these two studies with over 800 patients have shown that brimonidine appears to be an effective ocular hypotensive agent. It is generally well tolerated, although there was a less than 10% incidence of a mild to moderate allergic response that developed over the course of treatment anywhere from about 2 months up to almost 12 months. The ocular hypotensive response was sustained over 1 year with no suggestion of the development of tachyphylaxis. We believe that these data suggest that brimonidine can be a useful addition to our anti-glaucoma armamentarium.

References

1. Hodapp E, Kolker A, Kass M, et al. (1981) The effect of topical clonidine on intraocular pressure. Arch Ophthalmol 99:1208-1211
2. Stewart WC, Ritch R, Shin DH, et al. (1995) The efficacy of apraclonidine as an adjunct to timolol therapy. Arch Ophthalmol 113:287-292
3. Burke J, Manlapaz C, Kharlamb A, et al. (1995) Alpha-adrenoceptor and ocular pharmacology of brimonidine, p-aminoclonidine and clonidine. Proceedings of the XX Pan-american Congress of Ophthalmology, p 110
4. Kaplan B, Wilensky JT, Hillman DS (1994) Clinical experience with chronic use of iopidine (0.5%). Scientific Poster, American Academy of Ophthalmology, San Francisco, October 1994

Avenues Toward Neuroprotection of the Optic Nerve in Glaucoma*

J. Caprioli

Department of Ophthalmology and Visual Science, Yale University School of Medicine, 330 Cedar Street, New Haven, CT 06520 USA

The Susceptible Optic Nerve

Perhaps the greatest challenge that faces physicians who treat glaucoma patients is the preservation of visual function in patients who continue to worsen despite low intraocular pressures. Such patients generally fall into one of three categories:

1. Relatively young patients (in their 50s or 60s) with normal tension glaucoma associated with a generalized vasospastic disorder; vasospasm is often manifested by migraine headache or Raynaud's phenomenon.
2. Older patients (in their 70s or older) with normal tension glaucoma; in at least some of these patients intraocular pressure lowering appears to be beneficial.
3. Patients with far advanced damage, incurred at high or low pressure, who continue to lose vision despite surgical intervention to lower intraocular pressure to subnormal levels.

Patients in the first two categories often have visual fields with dense localized scotomas, sometimes with sudden and episodic progression, and focal abnormalities of the optic nerve head and nerve fiber layer (Fig. 1). Those in the third category, of course, have far advanced visual field loss with only small central or temporal visual islands.

Treatment Outcomes

It is widely agreed that lowering intraocular pressure benefits most glaucoma patients, particularly those who have suffered damage at high intraocular pressure. The data which support this statement are too numerous to all be cited here. The extent to which intraocular pressure should be lowered in an individual to prevent or slow additional damage and the identification of those who benefit most are questions without satisfactory answers. A retrospective report showed that glaucoma patients with mean intraocular pressure higher than 21 mm Hg during the follow-up period had progressive glaucomatous changes, those with mean pressures lower than 17 mm Hg remained stable, and approximately half of the eyes with mean pressures between 17 and 21 mm Hg had progressive glaucomatous changes [1]. A recent 10 year follow-up study of corticosteroid treatment in trabeculectomy patients showed a direct correlation between level of IOP and stabilization of disc and field [2]. Still, 10% of patients with a mean final IOP of 13 mm Hg continued to show progression despite low intraocular pressures during this period. Another recently published outcome study of trabeculectomy (performed without antimetabolites) showed that progressive glaucomatous damage, by either disc or field, occurred in about one third of patients 6 years after trabeculectomy [3]. In 12% (9/78), pro-

*Supported in part by Alcon Research Institute Award, Connecticut Lions Eye Research Foundation, and the National Eye Institute RO1EY07353

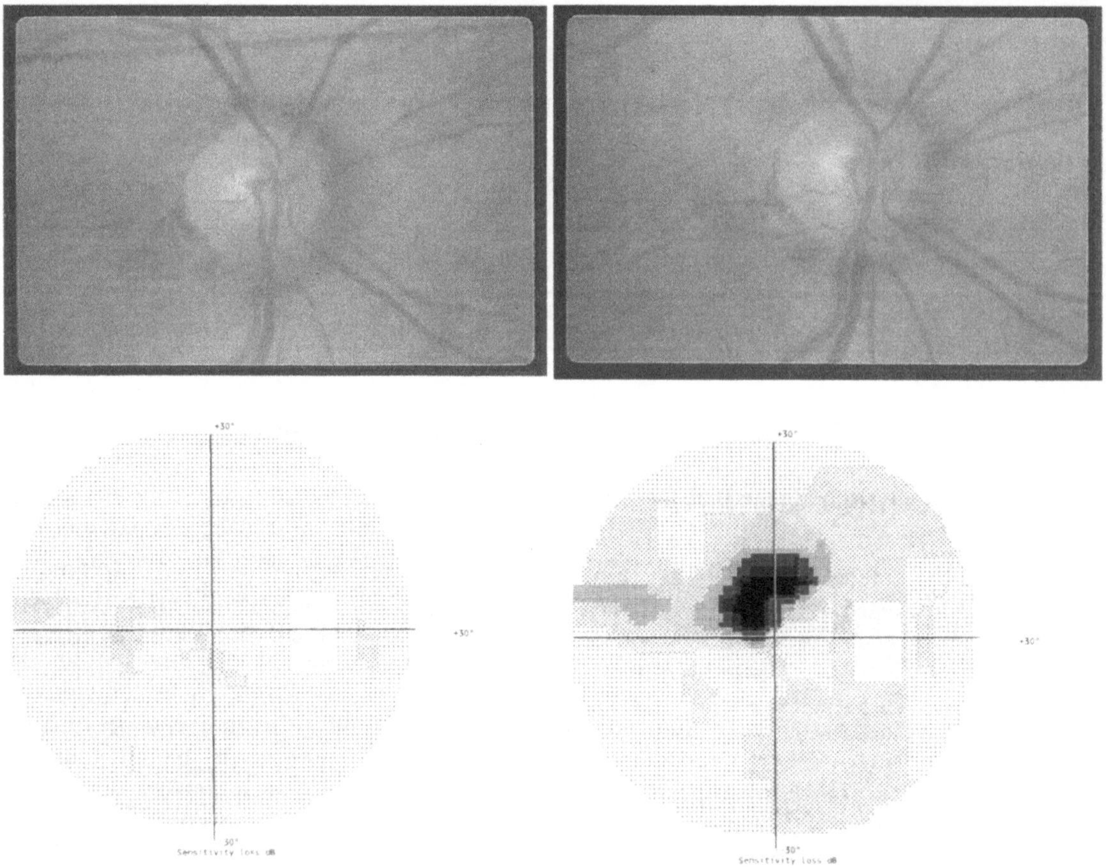

Fig. 1. Optic disc photographs and visual fields of the right eye of a patient with progressive normal pressure glaucoma. *Top*, the right optic disc at baseline (*left*) and 6 years later (*right*). Bottom, the visual field of the right eye at baseline (*left*) and after 6 years follow-up (*right*). Multiple intraocular pressure measurements, including diurnal curve measurements, never revealed pressures greater than 13 mm Hg in this eye

gression occurred at pressures which were deemed unlikely to be lowered by further surgical intervention. In a study of initial trabeculectomy for primary open-angle glaucoma, 40% of patients with advanced field loss continued to progress despite either maximal medical or surgical treatment [4].

Mechanisms of Damage

There is overwhelming clinical evidence that intraocular pressure is an important risk factor for glaucomatous optic nerve damage [5]. Even in normal tension glaucoma, data suggest that intraocular pressure is still a risk factor [6-8]. However, there are ample clinical indications that there are pressure-dependent and pressure-independent causes of glaucomatous optic neuropathy [9]. Such mechanisms might operate over a wide range of intraocular pressure and would contribute to damage both at low and high pressures (Fig. 2). Different patterns of damage, as evidenced by visual field loss and pattern of optic nerve cupping, have been shown in subgroups of patients with low and higher pressures [10-12]. These data hint at the possibility of different predominant mechanisms in these subgroups.

Neuroprotection: New Avenues for Glaucoma Treatment

The search for neuroprotective agents for glaucoma treatment is grounded in desperation: the desperation of continuing visual loss in some patients despite intraocular pressure reduction to quite low levels. Some cases continue to progress despite dramatic intraocular

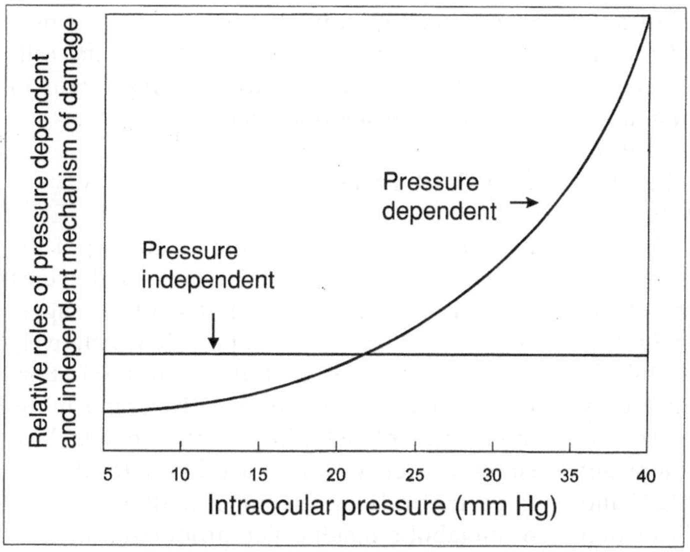

Fig. 2. An hypothesis regarding the relative roles of pressure-dependent and -independent mechanisms of damage. Intraocular pressure is an important risk factor and may operate in patients even with low pressures. Pressure-independent components of damage may operate across a whole range of intraocular pressures in patients with high pressures and low pressures alike

pressure lowering to 5/10 mm Hg (Fig. 1). This is not meant to imply that pressure-independent mechanisms of damage operate solely in the absence of pressure; pressure-dependent mechanisms (we don't know what those are yet) may facilitate the induction of pressure -independent processes, and vice versa. The attack on pressure-independent mechanisms is, of course, impeded by the lack of elucidation of such mechanisms. What we present are possible avenues for neuroprotection, given the likely players in the damage process (Fig. 2). This topic is the subject of a recent review [13].

Calcium Channel Blockade

Calcium channel blockers have been used empirically to treat low tension glaucoma for some years. Those patients with vasospastic conditions and normal pressure glaucoma have been particularly targeted [14, 15]. Nifedipine and nimodipine have both been used for the treatment of normal tension glaucoma. However, blockade of calcium channels at the neuronal cellular level, by interrupting the cascade of events which lead to death from ischemia, is also a reasonable rationale. The systemic lowering of blood pressure by calcium channel blockers should be considered, since this could reduce perfusion pressure to the anterior optic nerve head and potentiate ischemia.

A retrospective clinical study compared 56 patients with glaucoma who were concurrently taking calcium channel blockers to a control group not taking such medications for a mean follow-up period of 3.4 years [16]. In patients with normal tension glaucoma, there was a significant difference in the progression of visual field defects, with 11% (2/18) of patients taking calcium channel blockers, compared to 56% (10/18) of controls showing new visual field defects. The authors concluded that calcium channel blockers may be useful in the management of low-tension glaucoma. A short-term (6 months) prospective study of nifedipine in normal tension glaucoma patients suggested visual improvement in 24% (12/50), with the younger patients with the lowest pressures responding the best [17]. The long-term efficacy of this approach requires the scrutiny of a long-term clinical trial.

Glutamate Blockade

Neuronal injury from glutamate receptor-mediated neurotoxicity has been implicated as a central mechanism in a wide variety of central nervous system diseases, including ischemia, trauma, and some chronic neurodegenerative diseases. Excitotoxicity may also interact with other pathophysiologic processes to enhance or facilitate neuronal damage; this topic has recently been reviewed [18]. The possibility that excitotoxicity may play a role in the chronic neurodegeneration of glaucomatous damage has been suggested [14, 19]. Considerable progress has been made in our understanding of the mechanisms of neuronal death in the central nervous system, but only recently has attention been focused on the importance of these mechanisms in the retina. In the central nervous system, endogenous excitatory amino acids are important agents of neuronal cell death [20], and early studies suggested that they also act in the retina [21]. Hypoxia certainly plays a central role in retinal disease from diabetes and retinal vascular occlusion; its role in the damage of retinal ganglion cells in glaucoma is less certain. It is an important cause of central neuronal damage and its effects appear to be mediated by excitatory amino acids [22]. These excitotoxins, most notably glutamate, are important neurotransmitters in the inner retina [23] and are present in high concentration in retinal ganglion cells, enabling their potential role in pathologic retinal ganglion cell death [24, 25]. Recent reports of elevated levels of glutamate in the vitreous of glaucomatous monkeys and humans have provided additional fuel for this hypothesis [26, 27]. Whether the high vitreous levels of glutamate are a cause or result of damage is undetermined, but high concentrations of this neurotoxin would certainly be toxic to the inner retina.

The effects of hypoxia on retinal ganglion cell survival using an in vitro retinal ganglion cell culture model in the rat have been studied, and compared to the effects of excitatory amino acid administration and the protective effect of an *N*-methyl-*DL*-aspartate (NMDA) antagonist [28]. Ganglion cells were labeled retrogradely by injection of the fluorescent dye Di I into the superior colliculus 2 days prior to dissociation. Exposure of cultured ganglion cells to glutamate and NMDA showed a time- and concentration-dependent survival rate. Exposure of cells to hypoxia demonstrated a survival rate that was dependent on time and O_2 concentration. Excitotoxic and hypoxic damage was entirely blocked by the noncompetitive NMDA blocker MK-801. Retinal ganglion cells cultured on Müller glia showed significantly better survival rates ($p < 0.01$) than those cultured on cortical astrocytes under hypoxia and exposure to 200 μM glutamate. The results demonstrated that excitotoxic and hypoxic damage to cultured retinal ganglion cells is moderated by NMDA receptor blockade and by the presence of glial cells, especially retinal Müller cells. The importance of neuronal-glial interactions cannot be over estimated and a primary defect in Müller cells cannot be ruled as a contributing factor in glaucomatous neuronal damage.

Heat Shock Proteins

Recent advances in the understanding of the biochemical and molecular biological events which lead to neuronal cell death have suggested novel therapeutic approaches. Relatively little attention has been drawn to the importance of intrinsic neuroprotective events in the modulation of cell injury. In this context, heat shock proteins (HSPs) are likely to play an important role in cell survival after a variety of metabolic insults. The production of heat shock proteins (HSP) increases neuronal tolerance to ischemic insults in the cerebral cortex and hippocampus [29]. A protective role for HSPs has also been demonstrated in the rabbit retina against light induced retinal injury [30]. Antibodies that bind HSP can increase the rates of cell death after certain noxious insults, suggesting that these molecules may play an important role in cellular protection [31].

A recent study showed that retinal ganglion cells express the 72 kDa HSP after hyperthermia, sublethal hypoxia, and glutamate exposure in vitro [32]. Furthermore, retinal ganglion cells in culture treated with hyperthermia or sublethal hypoxia were much less susceptible to subsequent damage from excitotoxicity and anoxia. Inhibition of HSP synthesis by the addition of quercetin abolished the protective effect [33]. The neuroprotective effect of the induction of HSP synthesis by hyperthermia and sublethal hypoxia suggests a role for HSP as a protective mechanism against ischemic and excitotoxic retinal ganglion cell death.

Nitric Oxide Synthase Inhibition

Nitric oxide is a rapidly diffusing gas with a very short half-life in vivo. It has a vasodilatory action and may act as a nonconventional neurotransmitter in the brain. Calcium entry into the cell increases nitric oxide synthesis, which is generated from *L*-arginine through the action of nitric oxide synthase. The presence of nitric oxide activates cyclic GMP, whose effects are mediated through protein phosphorylation. Nitric oxide in sufficient concentrations is a potent neurotoxin. The exact place of nitric oxide in the cascade of events associated with ischemic central nervous system damage is not known, but it is almost certainly an important player. Inhibitors of nitric oxide synthase can protect neurons from nitric oxide toxicity [34]. Cultured retinal ganglion cells are significantly less susceptible to damage from anoxia and excitotoxicity in the presence of nitric oxide synthase inhibitors [35].

Antioxidants

The reperfusion phase after ischemic injury produces highly reactive compounds called free radicals. These oxygen containing molecules have unpaired electrons and react with lipids, nucleic acids, and proteins. They are thought to be important mediators of reperfusion injury. Free radicals may also facilitate the release of excitotoxins, and both may work together to bring about cellular death from ischemia [36]. Free radicals have been recently implicated in the slow chronic neurodegeneration of amyotrophic lateral sclerosis [37] so their role in a chronic neural degeneration like glaucoma is entirely feasible. Free radical scavengers include endogenous enzymes, like catalase and superoxide dismutase, and the antioxidant vitamins, especially C and E. Therapy could take the form of turning on the synthesis of endogenous compounds, or providing exogenous ones. Some level of antioxidation can be achieved through vitamin therapy, but requires well controlled clinical studies to determine efficacy.

Optic Nerve Regeneration

Impressive results reported by Aguayo and coworkers demonstrate the feasibility of central nervous system regeneration. Implantation of peripheral nerve sheath grafts into the eyes of rats promotes the regrowth of axotomized retinal ganglion cells into the graft [38]. These regenerated axons also have the ability to establish synaptic connections at target cells [39]. The peripheral nerve sheath appears to confer on the central neurons the ability to regenerate by providing a suitable environment and growth factors. This approach may yield important molecular insights into neuroprotection or neuroregeneration, although we are unlikely to see any clinically applicable therapies in the near future.

Clinical Perspectives

Calcium channel blockers are already in clinical use for the treatment of normal tension glaucoma, but not on an evidential basis; clinical trials are required to demonstrate their efficacy. The use of all the other approaches here are even more experimental and require significant animal study to demonstrate safety and a potential for efficacy. Non-reversible glutamate blockers (e.g., MK-801) are problematic because of central nervous system side effects, and nonselective blockers are also likely to have serious side effects on the inner retina. However, compounds with sufficient selectivity for the desired effects could become available to make this form of treatment feasible. If ischemia is an important process in some glaucoma patients, then inhibition of the potent neurotoxin nitric oxide may be helpful. Compounds for clinical use have not yet been developed, but the approach is being intensively studied for the central nervous system. Heat shock protein therapy will probably require the ability to therapeutically turn on gene translation and transcription selectively. Treatments such as these, while exciting, seem a long way off but within our reach. Approaches to facilitate neuroregeneration are feasible, but again will not be available any time soon. The use of free radical scavengers is still in the realm of animal experimentation, but the antioxidant approach can be achieved immediately through vitamin therapy and requires well controlled clinical studies to determine efficacy.

There should be a great deal of optimism, as well as caution, with respect to the future of neuroprotective treatment to prevent glaucomatous optic neuropathy. Intensive research must be directed to this area if we are to realize any of the potential benefits.

References

1. Mao LK, Stewart WC, Shields MB (1991) Correlation between intraocular pressure control and progressive glaucomatous damage in primary open-angle glaucoma. Am J Ophthalmol 111:51-55
2. Araujo SV, Spaeth GL, Roth SM, Starita RJ (1995) A ten-year follow-up on a prospective, randomized trial of postoperative corticosteroids after trabeculectomy. Ophthalmol 102: 1753-1759
3. Nouri-Mahdavi K, Brigatti L, Weitzman M, Caprioli J (1995) Outcomes of trabeculectomy for primary open-angle glaucoma. Ophthalmol 102:1760-1769
4. Jay JL, Alan D (1989) The benefit of early trabeculectomy versus conventional management in primary open angle glaucoma relative to severity of disease. Eye 3:528-535
5. Sommer A (1989) Intraocular pressure and glaucoma. Am J Ophthalmol 107:186-188
6. Cartwright MJ, Anderson DR (1988) Correlation of asymmetric damage with asymmetric intraocular pressure in normal-tension glaucoma. Arch Ophthalmol 106:898-900
7. Chauhan BC, Drance SM (1990) The influence of intraocular pressure on visual field damage in patients with normal-tension and high-tension glaucoma. Invest Ophthalmol Vis Sci 31:2367-2372
8. Hitchings RA, Wu J, Poinoosawmy D, McNaught A (1995) Surgery for normal tension glaucoma. Br J Ophthalmol 79:402-406
9. Schulzer M, Drance SM, Carter CM, et al. (1990) Biostatistical evidence for two distinct chronic open-angle glaucoma populations. Br J Ophthalmol 74:196-200
10. Caprioli J, Spaeth GL (1985) Comparison of the optic nerve head in high- and low-tension glaucoma. Arch Ophthalmol 103: 1145-1149
11. Drance SM, Douglas GR, Airaksinen PF et al (1987) Diffuse visual field loss in chronic open-angle and low-tension glaucoma. Am J Ophthalmol 104:577-580
12. Caprioli J, Sears M, Miller J (1987) Patterns of early visual field loss in open-angle glaucoma. Am J Ophthalmol 103: 512-517
13. Schumer RA, Podos SM (1994) The nerve of glaucoma! Arch Ophthalmol 112:37-44
14. Flammer J, Guthauser U, Mahler F (1987) Do ocular vasospasms help cause low tension glaucoma? In Greve EL, Heijl A (eds) Seventh International Visual Field Symposium, Amsterdam, September 1986, Martinus Nijhoff/Dr W. Junk, Dordrecht, pp 397-399
15. Rojanapongpun P, Drance SM (1993) The response of blood flow velocity in the ophthalmic artery and blood flow of the finger to warm and cold stimuli in glaucomatous patients. Graefes Arch Clin Exp Ophthalmol 231:375-377
16. Netland PA, Chaturvedi N, et al. (1993) Calcium channel blockers in the management of low-tension and open-angle glaucoma. Am J Ophthalmol 115:608-613
17. Kitazawa Y, Shirai H, et al. (1989) The effect of Ca_2^+-antagonist on visual field in low-tension glaucoma. Graefes Arch Clin Exp Ophthalmol 227:408-412
18. Dugan LL, Choi DW (1994) Excitotoxicity, free radicals, and cell membrane changes. Ann Neurol 35:S17-S21
19. Cummins D, Takahashi N, Caprioli J (1991) Electrophysiology of cultured retinal ganglion cells to investigate basic mechanisms of damage. In Krieglstein GK (ed) Glaucoma update IV, Proceedings of the Glaucoma Society of the International Congress of Ophthalmology, Bali, March 1990, Springer, Berlin, Heidelberg, New York, pp 59-65
20. Olney J (1978) Kainic acid as a tool in neurobiology. In McGreer E, Olney J, McGreer P (eds) Kainic acid as a tool in neurobiology; Raven, New York, pp 95-121
21. Lucas D, Newhouse J (1957) The toxic effects of sodium l-glutamate on the inner layers of the retina. Arch Ophthalmol 58:193-201
22. Choi D (1988) Glutamate neurotoxicity and diseases of the nervous system. Neuron 1:623-634
23. Ehinger B (1989) Glutamate as a retinal neurotransmitter. In: Weiler R, Osbourne N (eds) Neurobiology of the inner retina. Springer, Berlin, Heidelberg, New York, pp 1-14
24. David P, Lusky M, Teichberg V (1988) Involvement of excitatory neurotransmitters in the damage produced in chick embryo retinae by anoxia and extracellular high potassium. Exp Eye Res 46:657-662
25. Zeevalk G, Hyndman A, Nicklas W (1989) Excitatory aminoacid induced toxicity in chick retina: aminoacid release, histology and effects of chloride channel blockers. J Neurochem 53:1610-1619
26. Dreyer EB, Lipton SA (1992) Excitatory amino-acids in glaucoma: A potentially novel etiology of neuronal loss. Invest Ophthalmol Vis Sci 33:1093
27. Schumer RA, Podos SM, Lipton SA, Dreyer EB (1994) Increased glutamate in the vitreous of monkeys with induced glaucoma. Invest Ophthalmol Vis Sci 35:1484
28. Cummins D, Kitano S, Caprioli J (1992) The effects of excitatory amino acids and ischemia on cultured rat retinal ganglion cells. Invest Ophthalmol Vis Sci 33:1031

29. Kittigawa K (1991) Hyperthermia-induced neuronal protection against ischemic injury in gerbils. J Cereb Blood Flow Metab 11:449-452.
30. Barbe M, Tytell M, Gower D, Welch W (1988) Hyperthermia protects against light damage in the rat retina. Science 241:1817-1820
31. Raibowol K, Mizzen L, Welch W (1988) Heat shock is lethal to fibroblasts microinjected with antibodies against hsp70. Science 242:433
32. Kitano S, Caprioli J (1993) Expression of 72k Da HSP in cultured rat retinal ganglion cells: Ischemic tolerance and protective effect of hyperthermia. Invest Ophthalmol Vis Sci 34:1430, 1993
33. Kitano S, Hori S, Koseki Y, Caprioli J (1994) The HSP synthesis inhibitor, quercetin, blocks the protection effect of hyperthermia on anoxic rat retinal ganglion cells in culture. Invest Ophthalmol Vis Sci 35:1868
34. Moncada S, Palmer R et al. (1991) Nitric oxide: physiology, pathophysiology, and pharmacology. Pharmacol Rev 43:109-142
35. Koseki Y, Kitano S, Podos SM, Mittag T, Caprioli J: A nitric oxide synthase inhibitor protects against anoxia in cultured rat retinal ganglion cells. Invest Ophthalmol Vis Sci 35:1968, 1994
36. Pellegrini-Giampietro D, Cherici G et al. (1990) Excitatory amino acid release and free radical formation may cooperate in the genesis of ischemia-induced neuronal damage. J Neurosci 10:1035-1041
37. McNamara J, Fridovich I (1993) Did radicals strike Lou Gehrig? Nature 362: 20-21.
38. Villegas-Perez MP, Vidal-Sanz M, et al. (1988) Influences of peripheral nerve grafts on the survival and regrowth of axotomized retinal ganglion cells in adult rats. J Neurosci 8: 265-280
39. Aguayo AJ, Bray GM, et al. (1990) Synaptic connections made by axons regenerating in the central nervous system of adult mammals. J Exp Biol 153: 199-224

Discussion

Question: Meduri

Do you think that glaucoma is an acute ischemic ganglionar event?

Answer: Caprioli

Certainly glaucoma is a chronic disease, but it may be an acute process that causes death of individual cells. So at a cellular level, the process may be acute and in small regions at a time it could be an acute damage going on. Glaucoma is certainly chronic for the retina, but individual cell death is quite acute.

Question:

How glaucoma filtration affects glutamate levels? Can aqueous humor reflect vitreous concentration?

Answer: Caprioli

I have no idea as for the first question. The highest concentration of glutamate is in the posterior vitreous.

Question:

To Dr. Hoste. What are the possible effects of these drugs on the ocular blood flow?

Answer: Hoste

Prostaglandin 2 can penetrate in the retina during glaucoma treatment; then it may cause vasoconstriction.

Question: Scullica

My question is to Dr. Wilensky. Can brimonidine have an additional effect to timolol if these drugs are combined?

Answer: Wilensky

I cannot give you any answer.

Question: Virno

Does brimocriptine constrict the conjunctival vessels?

Question: Virno

If we use apraclonidine and clonidine we see a vasoconstriction of the conjunctival vessels. I assume that the drugs may cause a vasoconstriction in the ciliary body.

Answer: Wilensky

According to research published in Archives of Ophthalmology in December '95, it seems that brimonidine reduces aqueous production and increases the uveoscleral outflow.

Question: Virno

There is a real antagonism between brimonidine and pilocarpine, but it is a dose related response.

Answer: Wilensky

You get less vasoconstriction with this drug, but I can't say what happens after a long term therapy.